Disorders of Consciousness

Editors

SUNIL KOTHARI
BEI ZHANG

PHYSICAL MEDICINE AND REHABILITATION CLINICS OF NORTH AMERICA

www.pmr.theclinics.com

Consulting Editor
BLESSEN C. EAPEN

February 2024 • Volume 35 • Number 1

ELSEVIER

1600 John F. Kennedy Boulevard • Suite 1800 • Philadelphia, Pennsylvania, 19103-2899

http://www.theclinics.com

**PHYSICAL MEDICINE AND REHABILITATION CLINICS OF NORTH AMERICA Volume 35, Number 1
February 2024 ISSN 1047-9651, 978-0-443-18354-6**

Editor: Megan Ashdown
Developmental Editor: Nitesh Barthwal

Reprints. For copies of 100 or more of articles in this publication, please contact the Commercial Reprints Department, Elsevier Inc., 360 Park Avenue South, New York, NY 10010-1710. Tel.: 212-633-3874; Fax: 212-633-3820; E-mail: reprints@elsevier.com.

Physical Medicine and Rehabilitation Clinics of North America (ISSN 1047-9651) is published quarterly by Elsevier Inc., 360 Park Avenue South, New York, NY 10010-1710. Months of issue are February, May, August, and November. Business and Editorial Offices: 1600 John F. Kennedy Blvd., Suite 1800, Philadelphia, PA 19103-2899. Customer Service Office: 3251 Riverport Lane, Maryland Heights, MO 63043. Periodicals postage paid at New York, NY and additional mailing offices. Subscription price per year is $352.00 (US individuals), $100.00 (US students), $400.00 (Canadian individuals), $100.00 (Canadian students), $506.00 (foreign individuals), and $210.00 (foreign students). For institutional access pricing please contact Customer Service via the contact information below. Foreign air speed delivery is included in all *Clinics* subscription prices. All prices are subject to change without notice. **POSTMASTER:** Send address changes to *Physical Medicine and Rehabilitation Clinics of North America*, Customer Service Office: Elsevier Health Sciences Division, Subscription Customer Service, 3251 Riverport Lane, Maryland Heights, MO 63043. **Customer Service: 1-800-654-2452 (US). From outside of the United States, call 314-447-8871. Fax: 314-447-8029. E-mail: JournalsCustomerService-usa@elsevier.com (for print support); JournalsOnlineSupport-usa@elsevier.com (for online support).**

Physical Medicine and Rehabilitation Clinics of North America is indexed in *Excerpta Medica, MEDLINE/ PubMed (Index Medicus), Cinahl,* and *Cumulative Index to Nursing and Allied Health Literature.*

Contributors

CONSULTING EDITOR

BLESSEN C. EAPEN, MD
Chief, VA Greater Los Angeles Health Care System, Associate Clinical Professor, Division of Physical Medicine and Rehabilitation, Department of Medicine, David Geffen School of Medicine at UCLA, Los Angeles, California, USA

EDITORS

SUNIL KOTHARI, MD
Assistant Professor, H. Ben Taub Department of Physical Medicine and Rehabilitation, Baylor College of Medicine, Attending Physician, TIRR Disorders of Consciousness Program, TIRR Memorial Hermann, Houston, Texas, USA

BEI ZHANG, MD, MSc
Assistant Professor, Division of Physical Medicine and Rehabilitation, Department of Neurology, Texas Tech University Health Sciences Center, Lubbock, Texas, USA

AUTHORS

ELIZABETH ANDERL, PT, DPT
Board-Certified Clinical Specialist in Neurologic Physical Therapy, TIRR Disorders of Consciousness Program, TIRR Memorial Hermann, Houston, Texas, USA

AMANDA APPEL, MD, MPH
Resident Doctor, Departments of Pediatric Rehabilitation Medicine and Pediatrics, Children's Hospital Colorado, Department of Physical Medicine and Rehabilitation, University of Colorado Anschutz Medical Campus, Aurora, Colorado, USA

DAVID B. ARCINIEGAS, MD
Research Director,Marcus Institute for Brain Health, University of Colorado Anschutz Medical Campus, Departments of Neurology and Psychiatry, University of Colorado School of Medicine, Aurora, Colorado, USA; Department of Psychiatry and Behavioral Sciences, University of New Mexico School of Medicine, Albuquerque, New Mexico, USA

ABANA AZARIAH, MD
Clinical Chief, Disorders of Consciousness Program, Attending Physician, Brain Injury and Stroke Program, TIRR Memorial Hermann, Houston, Texas, USA; Assistant Professor, Department of Physical Medicine and Rehabilitation, UT Health, McGovern Medical School

YELENA G. BODIEN, PhD
Site Specific Project Principal Investigator, Department of Physical Medicine and Rehabilitation, Spaulding Rehabilitation Hospital, Charlestown, Massachusetts, USA;

Research Scientist and Associate Director, Department of Neurology, Massachusetts General Hospital, Harvard Medical School, Boston, Massachusetts, USA

BRADLEY CHI, MD
Physical Medicine & Rehabilitation specialist, H. Ben Taub Department of Physical Medicine and Rehabilitation, Baylor College of Medicine, Houston, Texas, USA

SUSAN FAGER, PhD, CCC-SLP
Director of Communication Center of Excellence, Institute for Rehabilitation Science and Engineering, Madonna Rehabilitation Hospitals, Lincoln, Nebraska, USA

DAVID FISCHER, MD
Assistant Professor, Department of Neurology, University of Pennsylvania, Philadelphia, Pennsylvania, USA

JOSEPH T. GIACINO, PhD
Director, Department of Physical Medicine and Rehabilitation, Spaulding Rehabilitation Hospital, Charlestown, Massachusetts, USA; Harvard Medical School, Boston, Massachusetts, USA

KATHERINE GOLDEN, OTD
Occupational Therapist and PhD Student, School of Health and Rehabilitation Sciences, MGH Institute of Health Professions, Boston, Massachusetts, USA

BRIAN D. GREENWALD, MD
Clinical Professor, Medical Director, JFK Johnson Rehabilitation Center for Brain Injuries, JFK Johnson Rehabilitation Institute, Edison, New Jersey, USA

LINDSEY J. GURIN, MD
Neurologist, Departments of Neurology, Psychiatry, and Physical Medicine and Rehabilitation Medicine, NYU Grossman School of Medicine, New York, New York, USA

NICHOLAS GUT, MD
Brain Injury Medicine Fellow, Department of Physical Medicine and Rehabilitation, UT Health, McGovern Medical School, Houston, Texas, USA

STEPHEN HAMPTON, MD
Assistant Professor, Department of Physical Medicine and Rehabilitation, University of Pennsylvania, Philadelphia, Pennsylvania, USA

KRISTEN A. HARRIS, MD
Attending Physician, JFK Johnson Rehabilitation Institute, Edison, New Jersey, USA

CINDY B. IVANHOE, MD
Professor, Physical Medicine and Rehabilitation Department, McGovern Medical School, TIRR Memorial Hermann, Houston, Texas, USA

MICHELLE P. JAFFE, PhD
Clinical Psychologist, Department of Brain Injury Rehabilitation, Park Terrace Care Center, Queens, New York, USA; Co-Owner, BrainMatters Neuropsychological Services, PLLC, Plainview, New York, USA; Senior Psychologist, North Shore University Hospital, Northwell Health, Kings Point, New York, USA

STACEY JOU, MD
Resident Physician, JFK Johnson Rehabilitation Institute, Edison, New Jersey, USA

MARIEL KALKACH APARICIO, MD, MBE
Research Specialist, Department of Neurology, University of Wisconsin-Madison, Madison, Wisconsin, USA; Research Associate at Centro Anahuac de Desarrollo Estrategico en Bioetica (CADEBI), Anahuac University, Mexico City, Mexico; Research Scholar, UNESCO Chair, Rome, Italy

SUNIL KOTHARI, MD
Assistant Professor, H. Ben Taub Department of Physical Medicine and Rehabilitation, Baylor College of Medicine, Attending Physician, TIRR Disorders of Consciousness Program, TIRR Memorial Hermann, Houston, Texas, USA

CHRISTOS LAZARIDIS, MD, EDIC
Professor, Neurosciences Intensive Care Unit, Departments of Neurology and Neurological Surgery, University of Chicago Medicine and Biological Sciences, Chicago, Illinois, USA

GANG LIU, MD, PhD
Department of Rehabilitation Medicine, Huashan Hospital, Fudan University, Shanghai, China

MICHAEL H. MARINO, MD
Director of the Responsiveness Program for Disorders of Consciousness, Moss Rehab, Elkins Park, Pennsylvania, USA; Medical Director of Philadelphia Programming, Remed Residential Brain Injury Center, Paoli, Pennsylvania, USA

BROOKE MURTAUGH, OTD, OTR/L, CBIST
Brain Injury Program Manager, Department of Rehabilitation Programs, Madonna Rehabilitation Hospitals, Lincoln, Nebraska, USA

KATHERINE O'BRIEN, PhD
Clinical Neuropsychologist, TIRR Disorders of Consciousness Program, TIRR Memorial Hermann, Clinical Assistant Professor, Department of Physical Medicine and Rehabilitation, McGovern Medical School, The University of Texas Health Science Center at Houston, Clinical Assistant Professor, H. Ben Taub Department of Physical Medicine and Rehabilitation, Baylor College of Medicine, Houston, Texas, USA

EBONI A. REED, MD
Brain Injury Medicine Fellow, Physical Medicine and Rehabilitation Department, Baylor College of Medicine, Houston, Texas, USA

MARY E. RUSSELL, DO, MS
Assistant Professor, Physical Medicine and Rehabilitation Department, McGovern Medical School, TIRR Memorial Hermann-The Woodlands, Houston, Texas, USA

AMY SHAPIRO-ROSENBAUM, PhD
Program Director, Department of Brain Injury Rehabilitation, Park Terrace Care Center, Queens, New York, USA; Adjunct Faculty and TBI Model System Investigator, TBI Model System, Icahn School of Medicine at Mount Sinai, New York, New York, USA; Co-Owner, BrainMatters Neuropsychological Services, PLLC, Plainview, New York, USA

BETH S. SLOMINE, PhD
Professor, Kennedy Krieger Institute, Departments of Psychiatry, Behavioral Health, and Physical Medicine and Rehabilitation, Johns Hopkins School of Medicine, Baltimore, Maryland, USA

TABATHA SORENSON, OTD, OTR/L, ATP
Occupational Therapist, Department of Occupational Therapy, Madonna Rehabilitation Hospitals, Lincoln, Nebraska, USA

ERIC SPIER, MD
Medical Director, Brain Injury Program, Craig Hospital Englewood, Colorado, USA

STACY J. SUSKAUER, MD
Associate Professor, Departments of Physical Medicine and Rehabilitation, and Pediatrics, Johns Hopkins School of Medicine, Baltimore, Maryland, USA

RUTH TANGONAN, MD
Neurologist, Neurosciences Intensive Care Unit, Department of Neurology, University of Chicago Medicine and Biological Sciences, Chicago, Illinois, USA

JEAN E. WOO, MD
Attending Physician, Disorders of Consciousness Program, Brain Injury and Stroke Program, TIRR Memorial Hermann, Houston, Texas, USA; Assistant Professor, H. Ben Taub Department of Physical Medicine and Rehabilitation, Baylor College of Medicine, Houston, Texas, USA

LINDA B. XU, MD
Neurology Resident, Department of Neurology, University of Pennsylvania, Philadelphia, Pennsylvania, USA

MICHAEL J. YOUNG, MD, MPhil
Neurologist and Brain Injury Specialist, Department of Neurology, Massachusetts General Hospital, Center for Neurotechnology and Neurorecovery, Boston, Massachusetts, USA

BEI ZHANG, MD, MSc
Assistant Professor, Division of Physical Medicine and Rehabilitation, Department of Neurology, Texas Tech University Health Sciences Center, Lubbock, Texas, USA

YI ZHOU, MD
Resident Physician, JFK Johnson Rehabilitation Institute, Edison, New Jersey, USA

Contents

> Providers of patients with disorders of consciousness (DoC) face clinical and ethical challenges that could be lessened by becoming acquainted with the subjective and objective aspects of consciousness. A first step to improving DoC taxonomies, management, and outcomes might be to recognize the shortcomings of the medical concept of consciousness and to improve the terminology used for the clinical parameters assessed. The authors critically review the medical perspective of consciousness represented by three sub-concepts that do not necessarily correlate with one another and discuss how none of them reflects fully the personal subjective nature of consciousness.

> In this article, we discuss the taxonomy associated with the four major disorders of consciousness (DoC): coma, vegetative state or unresponsive wakefulness syndrome, minimally conscious state, and post-traumatic confusional state. We briefly review the history of each disorder and then provide operational definitions and diagnostic criteria for each one. We rely heavily on recently released practice guidelines and, where appropriate, identify knowledge gaps and discuss future directions to advance DoC research and practice.

> Understanding the structural and functional neuroanatomy of core consciousness (ie, wakefulness and awareness) is an asset to clinicians caring for persons with disorders of consciousness. This article provides a primer on the structural and functional neuroanatomy of wakefulness and awareness. The neuroanatomical structures supporting these elements of core consciousness functions are reviewed first, after which brief description of the clinically evaluable relationships between disruption of these structures and disorders of consciousness (ie, brain–behavior relationships) are outlined. Consideration of neuroanatomy at the mesoscale (ie, the mesocircuit hypothesis) as well as in relation to several large-scale neural networks is offered.

There is a clinical need for more accurate diagnosis and prognostication in patients with disorders of consciousness (DoC). There are several neuroimaging modalities that enable detailed, quantitative assessment of structural and functional brain injury, with demonstrated diagnostic and prognostic value. Additionally, longitudinal neuroimaging studies have hinted at quantifiable structural and functional neuroimaging biomarkers of recovery, with potential implications for the management of DoC.

Rehabilitation of patients with disorders of consciousness (DoC) presents unique challenges requiring comprehensive and specialized care. This article reviews the components, organization, and implementation of an inpatient DoC program under the framework of recent evidence-based practice guidelines and minimum competency recommendations. The evidence and clinical applications of these recommendations are elaborated upon with the goal of offering providers a reference to translate guidelines into clinical practice.

Acute disorders of consciousness (DOC) are impairments in arousal and awareness that occur within 28 days of an initial injury and can result from a variety of insults. These states range from coma, unresponsive wakefulness, covert consciousness, minimal consciousness, to confusional state. It is important to perform thorough, serial examinations with particular emphasis on the level of consciousness, brainstem reflexes, and motor responses. Evaluation of acute DOC includes laboratory tests, imaging, and electrophysiology testing. Prognostication in the acute phase of DOC must be done cautiously, using open, frequent communication with families, and by acknowledging significant multidimensional uncertainty.

Behavioral assessment remains the cornerstone of the clinical evaluation of disorders of consciousness (DoC). This article focuses on special considerations in the behavioral assessment of patients with DoC. At the outset, rehabilitation clinicians should be aware of potential biases and their implications in the accuracy of assessments. Assessments should be performed under conditions that maximize the possibility of detecting signs of consciousness and to "set the patient up for success". All therapy disciplines, staff, and family members should be encouraged to share their observations. Assessment with standardized scales should be supplemented by qualitative observations and an Individualized Quantitative Behavioral Assessment.

Over the last 10 years, there have been rapid advances made in technologies that can be utilized in the diagnosis and treatment of patients with a disorder of consciousness (DoC). This article provides a comprehensive review of these modalities including the evidence supporting their potential use in DoC. This review specifically addresses diagnostic, non-invasive therapeutic, and invasive therapeutic technological modalities except for neuroimaging, which is discussed in another article. While technologic advances appear promising for both assessment and treatment of patients with a DoC, high-quality evidence supporting widespread clinical adoption remains limited.

For patients with disorders of consciousness (DoC), treating the medical, neurologic, and neuromuscular complications not only stabilizes their medical disturbances, but minimizes confounding factors that may obscure the ability to accurately identify the level of consciousness and increase the chance of patients' neurologic and functional recovery. Lack of reliable communication and low-level function of patients with DoC make it challenging to diagnose some of the complications. Skilled clinical observation will be imperative to appropriately care for the patients.

Despite the evolving practice of brain injury medicine, consciousness remains enigmatic. Most patients with disorders of consciousness have disordered sleep and return of normal sleep architecture is essential to the emergence of consciousness and the healing brain. In this article we lay a framework for understanding the emergence of consciousness in brain-injured patients. We then explore ways to use that framework to evaluate and tailor treatment of sleep and pain in patients with disorders of consciousness. Although more research is needed to empower better treatment in the future, validated tools now exist for evaluation of emergent consciousness, pain, and sleep.

Pharmacologic treatment of disorders of consciousness remains a critical but challenging task for clinicians. Amantadine has been shown to promote the rate of neurologic recovery for patients with traumatic disorders of consciousness when administered between 4 and 16 weeks, as demonstrated by a well-designed randomized control trial. While there are no large, randomized controlled trials to support the use of other dopaminergic medicines (bromocriptine, levodopa, apomorphine), there is a large body of literature implicating their role in improving alertness and responsiveness in disorders of consciousness. Zolpidem can increase the level of consciousness in a small subset of patients. Zolpidem and intrathecal baclofen likely increase the level of consciousness via the mesocircuit pathway. Psychostimulant medications can be initiated in patients, even without strong evidence to support their use, as long as basic principles of brain injury medicine are followed, and there are systems in place to evaluate therapeutic response.

Historically, there has been a pessimistic view regarding outcomes for patients with disorders of consciousness (DoC). There is a paucity of clinical diagnostic tools and prognostic protocols. Guidelines for the care of patients with DoC require behavioral observation, time, resources, and knowledge of the population. Many nonclinical factors such as patient wishes, family perception, and personal finances can indirectly influence long-term outcomes. Prognostic expectations need to be considered but we health-care professional cannot fully appreciate the decisions and influence of those decisions on the person served or on the care providers involved.

Language and communication deficits are intrinsic to disorders of consciousness. This article will provide an overview of language and communication deficits that can significantly confound the accuracy of diagnostic assessment in these patients. Authors will also discuss interventions to promote early communication using assistive technology and augmentative communication rehabilitation strategies. Finally, this article will discuss the importance of family education as well as ethical considerations connected to the recovery of communication and adaptive strategies to support patient autonomy and enhance self-agency.

Evolving knowledge highlights the deleterious effects of caregiving on the emotional, psychosocial, and financial well-being of caregivers of persons with disorders of consciousness (DoC). Current practice guidelines and minimal competency recommendations emphasize the importance of identifying and addressing DoC caregiver needs. This article serves as a dissemination tool to enhance communication between providers and caregivers. Essential components of education and training are outlined for each level of care. Addressing caregiver needs may mitigate the level of perceived burden, reduce the risk of burnout, and increase care proficiency and likelihood of community discharge, thus potentially reducing long-term costs of care for this population.

Michael J. Young

Patients with disorders of consciousness who survive to discharge following severe acute brain injury may face profoundly complex medical, ethical, and psychosocial challenges during their courses of recovery and rehabilitation. Although issues encountered in caring for such patients during acute hospitalization have received substantial attention, ethical challenges that may arise in subacute and chronic phases have been underexplored. Shedding light on these issues, this article explores the landscape of normative issues in the course of treating and facilitating access to care for persons with disorders of consciousness during rehabilitation and examines potential implications for patients, clinicians, family members, and society.

Beth S. Slomine and Stacy J. Suskauer

Children with acquired brain injury may experience prolonged disorders of consciousness (DoC); research on children with DoC lags behind adult literature. Rigorous evaluation of assessment tools used in children with DoC is lacking, though recent developments may contribute to improvements in care, particularly for assessment of young children and those without overt command following. Literature on prognosis continues to grow, reinforcing that early signs of consciousness suggest better long-term outcome. Although large clinical trials for children with DoC are lacking, single-site and multisite programmatic data inform standards of care and treatment options for children with DoC.

PHYSICAL MEDICINE AND REHABILITATION CLINICS OF NORTH AMERICA

Foreword

Rehabilitation Management of Disorders of Consciousness

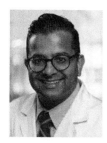

Blessen C. Eapen, MD
Consulting Editor

Disorders of Consciousness (DoC) is a prolonged altered state of consciousness and is typically categorized into three broad categories: coma, vegetative state, or minimally conscious state.

The main goal for the rehabilitation of individuals with DoC is to improve functional and cognitive status of individuals who have experienced a severe brain injury. Individuals with DoC often present unique, complex challenges for health care providers, patients, and families, thus requiring a comprehensive and individualized approach to maximize the chances of recovery.

The assessment, management, and treatment of individuals with DoC are a complex process requiring an interdisciplinary team of providers, typically led by a *physiatrist*. Each rehabilitation plan should be tailored to the individual, taking into account the cause of the diagnosis, functional and cognitive status, and short- and long-term goals. While not all patients will "emerge," from a DoC, the goal of the DoC rehabilitation program is to maximize the functional and cognitive abilities, improve quality of life, and provide the best available support.

In summary, rehabilitation, treatment, and assessment of DoC require a comprehensive team-based approach. The integration of advanced neuroimaging and innovative technology and addressing health care disparities are crucial elements in improving outcomes for individuals with DoC. In addition to the prudent prevention of secondary complications, medication and rehabilitation management and family support contribute to optimizing the quality of care and the potential for recovery in these challenging cases.

I would especially like to thank Dr Kothari and Dr Zhang for their leadership and for providing an in-depth review of current practices in DoC and all of our esteemed

Phys Med Rehabil Clin N Am 35 (2024) xiii–xiv
https://doi.org/10.1016/j.pmr.2023.10.001
1047-9651/24/© 2023 Published by Elsevier Inc.

pmr.theclinics.com

authors for their outstanding work and for sharing their valuable experience and expertise!

Blessen C. Eapen, MD
Division of Physical Medicine and Rehabilation
David Geffen School of Medicine at UCLA
VA Greater Los Angeles Health Care System
11301 Wilshire Boulevard
Los Angeles, CA 90073, USA

E-mail addresses:
beapen@ucla.mednet.edu; blessen.eapen2@va.gov

Preface

Disorders of Consciousness

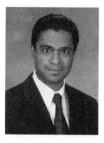   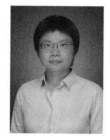

Sunil Kothari, MD   Bei Zhang, MD, MSc

Editors

We are pleased to present this issue of *Physical Medicine and Rehabilitation Clinics of North America* on "Disorders of Consciousness" (DoC). There have been dramatic and exciting changes in the field of DoC in just the last several years. The number of publications on DoC, reflecting research as well as clinical experience, has exploded. There has also been much needed growth in the number of programs and facilities that provide rehabilitation services for these patients. Finally, several national specialty societies have released guidelines addressing the care of these patients, clinically as well as at an institutional level. The aim of this issue is to provide clinicians caring for these patients with a current update on these recent developments.

The issue covers a broad range of topics, encompassing the entire field from the theoretical bases of DoC (eg, models of consciousness, nosology and nomenclature, neuroanatomy, ethics) to bedside care to program development. Notably, it covers the entire trajectory of DoC, addressing assessment and management during the acute, subacute, and chronic phases of recovery. Throughout, the emphasis has been on making the information presented directly relevant to clinicians caring for patients with DoC. The predominant theme of this issue is that we have much to offer these patients, as clinicians and as a health care system. It has become abundantly clear that the nihilism that surrounded the "care" of people with DoC—clinical, ethical, and policy—is completely unjustified and should end.

The authors are well-recognized clinicians and/or renowned scholars in the field of DoC. We are grateful for their expertise and dedication to the content of the issue. Special thanks to Dr Blessen Eapen, who invited us to edit this issue, and Malvika Shah and Nitesh Barthwal from Elsevier, who patiently walked us through every step to its fruition. Finally, we want to acknowledge and thank the patients and families we have been honored to care for. They have both taught and inspired us. It is our

Phys Med Rehabil Clin N Am 35 (2024) xv–xvi
https://doi.org/10.1016/j.pmr.2023.07.008
1047-9651/24/© 2023 Published by Elsevier Inc.

hope that the knowledge contained in this issue will help contribute to improving the care of these vulnerable patients.

Sunil Kothari, MD
H. Ben Taub Department of
Physical Medicine and Rehabilitation
Baylor College of Medicine
TIRR Memorial Hospital
1333 Moursund Street
Houston, TX 77030, USA

Bei Zhang, MD, MSc
Division of Physical Medicine and Rehabilitation
Department of Neurology
Texas Tech University Health Sciences Center
3601 4th Street, STOP 8321
Lubbock, TX 79430, USA

E-mail addresses:
sunil.kothari@memorialhermann.org (S. Kothari)
beizhangmd@gmail.com (B. Zhang)

Conceptualizing Consciousness: a Change in Perspective

The Elephant Still Surprises Those only Touching Its Trunk

Mariel Kalkach Aparicio, MD, MBE[a,b,c,]*,
Christos Lazaridis, MD, EDIC, BPhil[d]

KEYWORDS

- Consciousness • DoC • Neuroethics

KEY POINTS

- There is a high prevalence of misdiagnosis in disorders of consciousness (DoC) syndromes (34–56%).
- Reviewing the different sub-concepts of consciousness underlying this term in the medical field allows to understand what is being measured, and provides a perspective on what cannot be asserted about these patients from behavioral exams.
- Understanding consciousness as subjective experience encompasses states that fall outside of the traditional medical view, such as dreams and mind-wandering—which do not necessarily entail a factual relationship to the external world, can be dissociated from at least one sense of self (narrative or bodily) at a time, and from behavior, but could still be identified with the help of neurotechnology.
- Broadening the concept of consciousness to subjective experience, of which an objective aspect is part, may advance the science of consciousness and help identify the prevalence of DoC patients with a basic form of consciousness (eg, perception), or at the very least promote their more appropriate care and regard.

[a] Department of Neurology, University of Wisconsin, 1685 Highland Avenue, 7th Floor, Madison, WI 53705-2281, USA; [b] Centro Anahuac de Desarrollo Estrategico en Bioetica (CADEBI), Universidad Anahuac Mexico, Edo. Mex. MEX; [c] UNESCO Chair of Bioethics and Human Rights, Rome, ITA; [d] Department of Neurology, The University of Chicago, 5841 South Maryland Avenue, MC 2030, Chicago, IL 60637, USA
* Corresponding author. 1685 Highland Avenue, 7th Floor, Madison, WI 53705-2281
E-mail address: kalkach@neurology.wisc.edu

Phys Med Rehabil Clin N Am 35 (2024) 1–13
https://doi.org/10.1016/j.pmr.2023.06.021

INTRODUCTION

In a multilingual blind kingdom, the ruler asked his blind servants to find out and tell him what an elephant was. The servants went to find an elephant, but because *a priori* knowledge was lacking, each one explored by default the part that was within reach at their arrival. On their return, each one gave a different version of an elephant depending on the part they touched, each using their own different language. Not too dissimilar to this parable, consciousness is studied by different disciplines using different terms. In Medicine, indirect clinical assessments are a frequent form to arrive to diagnoses based on more or less assumptions that relate the measured parameter (eg, blood pressure measured during systole at a specific time) to the phenomenon of interest (eg, blood pressure's most usual state). However, unlike other clinical phenomena measured indirectly, for consciousness, the measurable parameters are not always representative of the phenomenon of interest. This is relevant because providers of patients with disorders of consciousness (DoC) face clinical and ethical challenges that could be eased by becoming acquainted with different concepts or aspects of consciousness. Misdiagnoses (34–56%), prognostic uncertainty, and the potential for mistreatment based on assumptions of reduced agency are salient issues reported in the DoC literature.[1–6] One contributing factor to the misdiagnoses of DoC syndromes is the level of expertise required for the examiner to obtain, observe, and interpret the best behavioral responses possible.[5,7] However, even for a highly trained examiner using the most appropriate scales, there are intrinsic limitations to the physical examination and neurotechnology used for assessment of consciousness.

Consciousness can be understood as a cornerstone faculty or ability which exists and unfolds from an individual's unique point of view, that is, from a "first person perspective" (*I experience it*, 1pp); thus, it is subjective.[8,9] This subjective aspect may seem unfamiliar or irrelevant to the medical approach because providers are requested to assess and measure the patient's state of consciousness. How can a subjective phenomenon that cannot be directly observed, be assessed by clinicians? Or, if not subjective consciousness, then what is being assessed in patients with DoC? The medical approach to consciousness is to *measure its manifestations* through behaviors and neural correlates using indirect clinical parameters and neuroimaging. These interpretations take place from a second- or third-person perspective (*2pp, 3pp*).[8–11] Second-person perspective refers to the observations gathered from one case (hers/his), thus, although one cannot experience someone else's consciousness, one can observe the patient's (*her/his*) behavior (motor, verbal report, brain activity in response to tasks). Third-person perspective refers to the accumulated observations and interpretations of cases (*them*), from which, when gathered through the scientific method, inform clinical scores used in the physical examination (eg, Glasgow Coma Scale, CRS-R, SECONDS, SMART, Rancho) and clinical guidelines.[12] Because the medical approach takes place from a *2pp* or *3pp*, the focus is on what can be tested by the examiner, the "objective" aspect of consciousness. However, despite its objective focus, prognostic difficulties remain.[7,13]

Prognostic difficulties might be linked to misdiagnoses, for which another contributing factor might be the heterogeneity of patients found under the label of each DoC syndrome (ie, coma, Unresponsive Wakefulness Syndrome [UWS] and Minimally Conscious State [MCS]). The predominant syndromic DoC taxonomy informs how patients are grouped in research studies from which prognoses are derived. Under the current classic DoC taxonomy, each syndrome has various possible underlying etiologies for which the prognosis based on a syndromic diagnosis is not straightforward.[14] Proposals have already emerged to try to form new or reform existing DoC taxonomies, for example, based on multimodal cognitive processes[15] or a combination of syndromes and assessment tools.[16] However, to achieve a most successful reform, it is worth considering what is currently, implicitly and explicitly meant by consciousness, and how it is different from what is assessed.

In this article, we critically review the classic medical perspective on consciousness, highlighting three sub-concepts found within it, and present a philosophical perspective of consciousness, and how it could be scientifically identified and made clinically relevant. In other words, the authors lay out the functional perception of the elephant as the trunk and the legs and then briefly present the not-so-widely known tail of the elephant, which may be necessary to have a complete picture of the elephant in the room. Although the approach is conceptual with clinical relevance, we inform our analysis through concepts drawn from Philosophy, which is required to observe the aspects of consciousness left out in the predominant medical perspective. This interdisciplinary analysis informs the medical concept of consciousness using the concepts of "knowledge" by Epistemology and "subjective experience" by Phenomenology. We aim to present the concept of consciousness in a way that fosters providers' awareness of their own assumptions, which could help gauge their interpretation of evidence, management of patients, communication with family members, and thoughts toward reforming the DoC taxonomy.

THE NATURE OF THE PROBLEM

Despite the lack of access to the 1st pp of someone else, the clinical setting requires an assessment of the state or level of consciousness. These measurements are evidence or signs, "correlates" at best, of conscious states but are not an equivalent in nature to consciousness. This means that even if it was known exactly what an electroencephalogram (EEG) or a functional Magnetic Resonance Imaging (fMRI) should look like when someone perceives a red rose, seeing such correlate in the EEG or fMRI would not allow the observer to know or feel exactly what the person is experiencing. In other words, the redness of a red rose a person sees, and the things they recall and feel when seeing it are not guaranteed to be understood or known by someone else merely observing the person's behavior, nor by observing the person's brain activity while perceiving the redness. Furthermore, if an attempt is made to replicate the scene by having someone else observing the same rose's redness from the same physical space and time, although some things might be identified as similar for both individuals, for example, identifying "red" as the rose's color, their experiences will not exactly match. Their experiences are informed by their unique neurologic system, and a life (time and space) of collected information organized in a specific and unique manner.

Providers are required to make judgments about whether a patient "is there" or if they are experiencing pain, or seeing or hearing a loved one, or at least make an educated guess about the potential for recovery of the first-person perspective.[12] Not surprisingly, the solution has been to resort to the only portion of the patient's experience available to the provider for testing: *demonstrable knowledge*. In the previous example, this would mean that the provider focuses on the patient's ability to identify "red" as the rose's color, as supposed to proving their ability to experience "redness". The physical examination requires that the patient *knows* specific elements of their experience, in addition to perceiving redness (environment), and the patient is requested self-related knowledge, for example, "who is that person looking at the rose?" In other words, during the physical examination, the patient is asked to respond verbally or with a corresponding action (eg, squeezing a hand) that indicates they know who, where they are, and why they are there. The provider uses behavioral (verbal, motor, and so forth) and neuroimaging techniques to examine the responses. Thus, it is not only knowing what matters for a patient to be considered conscious but also they must be able to report or demonstrate it.

The concept of consciousness in the clinical setting moves away from being about *any inner subjective experience* to being *an ability to know a specific type of demonstrable (objective knowledge) and demonstrating it.*

APPROACHES
The Objective Aspect of Consciousness

The trunk from the medical perspective
Ideally, one would expect that (1) theoretically defining a clinical parameter will be reflected in two other domains, (2) how that parameter is to be measured, and in (3) how pathologies related to this parameter are to be categorized. Even while focusing on its objective aspect, this conceptual translation does not occur in consciousness. Elsewhere we commented on the fact that the medical perspective is composed of different implicit sub-concepts, which we will refer to as Sub-A, -B and -C. One refers to the *theoretical concept of consciousness* (Sub-A) found in the definitions of classic medical literature, another concept is gathered from what is *implicit in the physical examination* (Sub-B), and yet another is embedded in the *DoC nosology* or taxonomy (Sub-C). In short, *Sub-A* refers to the patient's *ability "to know"* or understand (global state or intransitive consciousness), specifically *themselves, their surroundings, and the relationship* between these two (local state or transitive consciousness), an ability said to be composed of "two elements" *awakeness/arousal* and *awareness/content/object*[11,17–24] **(Fig. 1)**. *Sub-B* refers to the patient's and provider's *ability to demonstrate* that the patient knows what is asked of them. *Sub-C* portrays consciousness as *behavioral incoherence or inconsistencies*, that is, patients who do not respond as expected when asked or given an order (comatose state, unresponsive wakefulness syndrome, and minimally conscious state).

Although the discussion of each sub-concept deserves a separate space, brief acknowledgment of their existence is key to understand the medical perspective. In

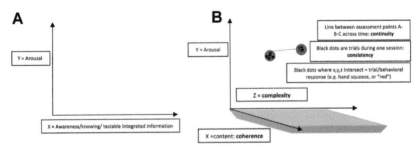

Fig. 1. Clinical parameters considered to be proxies of the consciousness in the physical examination. (*A*) On the left, the classic bidimensional conception of "the elements" of consciousness as "Y" = arousal or awakeness, a background condition for consciousness to exist, and "X" = awareness, the ability of the patient to "know" or content. (*B*) A look at the different behavioral scales reveals that what is called "awareness" is assessed through different clinical parameters as proxies of the content of consciousness. "Y" = arousal, "X" = degree of coherence/matching between the patient's behaviors and the provider's expectations, "Z" = the degree of complexity of the behaviors, consistency is represented by the black dots, where x, y, and z meet at a point in time, and continuity is the trajectory between blue circles or sessions, which gather trials (modified Kalkach 2020).

Sub-A, conceptualizing consciousness as the "ability to know", requires understanding of what is meant by "knowing". Three different forms of "knowing" or types of knowledge can be distinguished: propositional or factual (understanding conceptually what we mean by "the rose is red"), direct or perceptual (seeing red), and procedural or praxis (cutting a flower).[25–27] Drawing these distinctions might be useful while assessing motor or cognitive behaviors, because the cognitive processes, neural signatures, and brain areas underlying each type of "knowing" are different. For example, a patient may perceive their surroundings (direct knowledge), although they may not know what the place is called nor who they are (factual knowledge: semantic and self-related), and some of the brain areas involved in semantic retrieval (factual knowing) are not involved in perception (direct knowing). Understanding Sub-A by outlining the types of "knowing," also allows better observing its difference from Sub-B (requesting a behavioral demonstration), which derives from methodological limitations in the neurological exam: one cannot simply observe consciousness. Recognizing these conceptual distinctions is especially relevant when assessing patients unable to produce verbal responses, in which providers necessarily look for procedural knowledge (eg, "move your arm"). Unfortunately, behavior does not correlate 1:1 to consciousness, a dissociation familiar to anyone who has performed a cognitive task unrelated to a procedural task at the same time (eg, counting while driving); and for which the medical community has evidence in epileptic patients who experience behavioral arrest with preserved awareness (knowledge of their environment) and more recently observed in research utilizing active fMRI paradigms in DoC patients with cognitive-motor dissociation.[4,15,28–30] Last, Sub-C is different from the other two, because although all DoC meet criteria to be an impairment of consciousness within the scope of Sub-A and Sub-B, there are disorders that meet the same criteria per Sub-A and/or Sub-B which are usually excluded from Sub-C such as epilepsy, agnosia, and dementia. Thus, there is a conceptual disconnect between the definition, methods, and taxonomy of the medical perspective of consciousness.

The conceptual disconnect from Sub-A and Sub-B is inherent to the methodological limitations, and despite the lack of 1:1 correlation between consciousness and behavior and the resulting lack of a gold standard, behavioral assessments remain the predominant available tool to "assess consciousness objectively".[7] Therefore, it is worth teasing out what is being valued to assess Sub-B across behavioral scales. Whether in terms of "levels" (eg, Rancho los amigos),[31] numeric values (eg, Glasgow Coma Scale),[32] or syndromic diagnosis (eg, CRS-R),[33] in behavioral scoring, points are granted depending on whether patient behaviors (motor, verbal) meet certain criteria. As a conceptual summary, behaviors may be more highly regarded if they are coherent, that is, match the examiner expectations (eg, "oriented" "attributable to stimuli," "appropriate" or "purposeful"),[32–34] if they show more tacit complexity (eg, less points for reflexes more for "intelligibility"),[31,32] and whether they are consistent or reproducible.[31,33] Although one cannot see a patient's intention to move, the provider can attest to whether the behavior meets her expectation or not, meaning it is *coherent* or not. For example, the patient answering to a name that matches their driver's license, or adequately following an order (eg, "move your finger") would grant them a status of conscious in different ways. If, on the other hand, the verbal or motor responses are out of context from the provider's perspective, she might consider these to be hallucinations, disorientation, automatisms, spontaneous movements, or reflexes, which would not grant them a "fully conscious state" diagnosis. The second aspect the provider implicitly values in the behavior is its *complexity*, a proxy perhaps for the amount or type of integrated information. Complexity here means the number of integrated modalities or processes and networks involved. For example, from two behaviors displayed without coherence, for example, speaking and moving a finger, the first is more likely to gain the patient a status of conscious than the second. However, coherent behaviors even with low complexity, such as eye-blinks,[35] or those not reported in the literature as indicative of consciousness, such as a small finger twitch-like movement, may be considered a consciousness demonstration if these are consistent. *Consistency* refers to the sustained response or reproducibility of the response *when probed* within the same session, as in reproducibility for CRS-R.[33] Finally, *continuity* of the responses across time may be an indicator of stability or improvement of the nervous system's recovery.

The same variables may also be appreciated in the use of neurotechnology to detect covert consciousness. Brain activity assessed through various neuroimaging techniques is considered a more direct surrogate than behavior for different brain processes. For example, the use of active fMRI paradigms where patients are requested to follow commands cognitively as evidence of consciosness, has increased. Cognitive command-following paradigms in consciousness assessments involve many brain processes (eg, sustained attention, response selection, language comprehension) and networks.[29] In fact, a recent literature review revealed the explicit interest in complexity as an indicator of consciousness, using different neuroimaging techniques (EEG, stereo-EEG, TMS-EEG, Magnetoencephalography and fMRI).[36] Consistency in neuroimaging tasks across enough trials is important for statistical accuracy. Coherent behavior in neuroimaging active paradigms refer to finding the same type of brain activity (eg, change in band power in EEG or increased BOLD signal in fMRI), in the same areas as in the controls. Continuity would mean repeating the paradigm in different sessions to observe intersubject changes or persistence.

The Subjective Aspect of Consciousness

Acknowledging the elephant in the room

Consciousness emerges from a unique nervous system, unfolding from a 1pp, and in that sense, it is personal. A bundle of perceptions, ideas, beliefs, and feelings integrate to form a large subjective experience, the whole elephant, so to speak. Within this subjective experience an objective aspect emerges from the overlap in experiences across individuals, from which our shared understanding of the world yields conventions that we call knowledge (Sub-A and Sub-B), a functional and familiar face of consciousness in Medicine, the elephant's trunk. However, parts of the larger subjective experience are independent of objective notions of testable knowledge (ie, facts) or other conventions (eg, language), thus they fall outside of Sub-A's scope. Infants, even those with little cerebral cortex[37], experience states of perceptions and emotions, none of which entail factual knowledge, a sense of autobiographical self, nor verbalization ; yet these subjective states suffice to consider infants conscious in a sense that refers to more than their wake state[38]. Later in life, significant time (~30–50%) is spent in functionally relevant thoughts which are not related to the external environment but instead encompass the internal milieu, such as, mind-wandering or dreaming.[39–41] Because these states do not require a relationship to the environment, their behavioral manifestation (if any) is less specific and meaningful to the external observer. In fact, emotions may or may not show in behavior and could or not naturally be under the control of the subject. Emotional-behavioral dissociation is further supported by evidence from pathological instances such as patients with gelastic and dacrystic crises and in case reports of deep brain stimulation of the subthalamic nucleus.[42,43] The distance between consciousness and behavior seems to be significant in both, physiologic and pathologic states, and it is greater as the content comprises internal states with less relationship with the environment. Therefore, the lack of behavioral expression (Sub-B), does not exclude the possibility of subjective experiences unfolding.

Subjective experience is not separate from what is probed in the clinical exam, it is just a different angle which can remind us of the obvious limitations in the current clinical approach (**Fig. 2**). The value of the personal or autobiographical aspect of consciousness is in fact reflected in the clinical exam because the provider requests patients without verbal impairment to recall their own name. However, the recognition of how clinically valuable this aspect can be, has not gone much further. To exploit the personal aspect of subjective experience, it might be necessary to use novel approaches for patients who cannot demonstrate their subjective experiences. For example, for years, claps and other standardized noises have been used as auditory stimulation in the physical examination, but in the recent years, emotionally-salient songs or sounds have been identified as better stimuli than standardized ones.[44–47] Hence, although behavioral assessments are not reflective of subjective states, personally-focused assesments might be better at triggering measurable behaviors.

In addition to potentially obtaining better behavioral responses, taking the perspective of consciousness as subjective experience, expands the role of neuroimaging for diagnosis. Neuroscientific evidence gathered from dreams and mind-wandering subjective states may be used to create paradigms that identify conscious states in

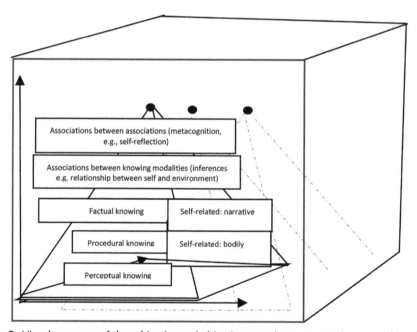

Fig. 2. Visual summary of the subjective and objective experience or consciousness. The cube represents consciousness as subjective experience, which includes all phenomena experienced from 1pp. The pyramid represents the objective aspect of consciousness, "knowing," "access consciousness" the portion which can be measured because it is based on a shared understanding between examiners and patients. The axes x, y, and z, their intersection at one point, and across time represent the measurable clinical aspects of motor and cognitive behavioral observations: arousal, coherency, complexity, and consistency continuity. Inside the pyramid, an example of different content, knowing or experiences.

patients. Some have successfully developed paradigms in which neural correlates for subjective experience (eg, dreaming) can be identified; for example, Siclari and colleagues validated a series of awakenings methods to assess the presence of dream states during sleep using high-density EEG.[48] A study using this paradigm yielded a neural correlate for dreaming, high-frequency activity was increased, and low-frequency activity decreased in parieto-occipital areas during epochs of non-rapid eye movement (REM) sleep dreaming compared with those with no dream reports.[53] Although the study also found increased high-frequency activity in pre-frontal areas during REM sleep dream recall, it can be surprising to those holding a traditional medical view that no prefrontal activity may be required to experience dreams. Evidence from this study and others using dreams as proxies for consciousness could be a foundation to identify the neural correlates of consciousness. The same variables valued in behavioral and active neuroimaging paradigms could be used to assess these states.

DISCUSSION AND CLINICAL RELEVANCE

Recognizing the implicit sub-concepts found within the medical view, allows to see thelimitations and what is excluded from this perspective. The clinical approach to consciousness, which aims to be objective, would seem to be incompatible with a view that endorses the subjective aspect of consciousness, because the latter sounds non-testable. However, specifying what is meant by subjective aspect may be helpful to address this concern. In the same way that procedural knowledge can be tested through fMRI paradigms (eg, "imagine yourself playing tennis"),[30] passive paradigms of subjective experiences unrelated to the environment may be within reach through neurotechnology as demonstrated by Siclari and colleagues.[48,53] The evidence of the brain areas underpinning each concept of "consciousness" keeps growing, including for the notion of subjective experience. In a preliminary study, Gorska and colleagues[54] studied slow wave activity (SWA) in epileptic patients who were classified based on their state of responsiveness and consciousness state during seizures. Consciousness was measured by subjective report and defined as the patients' ability to recall what happened during the seizure and confirmed by the video-EEG (eg, seeing the nurse enter). Delta activity was analyzed for both states, loss of responsiveness (LOR), and loss of consciousness (LOC). SWA activity in the prefrontal area was significantly increased in LOR compared with the responsive states but did not show significant associations for changes in consciousness. On the other hand, SWA was significantly increased in parietal areas in states of LOC compared with those without LOC, but there were no significant changes in this area for responsiveness. These results were further validated through two other data sets. One of these was a sample of intracranial EEG studies in epileptic patients, in which at a group level, significantly higher SWA was observed in the temporal area in sleep without dream recall than in states of dream recall. This evidence supports previous findings in epileptic patients that associate LOC with parieto-occipital areas.[55] Thus, temporo-parietal areas are important for consciousness as subjective experience without involving the patient's ability to express their state, or as narrative self-related content.

Amid all the neuroscientific progress made and the diagnostic and prognostic challenges faced in DoC-care and science of consciousness, the most important task for clinicians is to inform themselves, discuss and decide whether a conceptual renewal of consciousness is pertinent. This will impact clinical and neuroscientific progress because evidence interpretation is influenced by the conceptual framework of consciousness used. Although this may seem obvious, it has been pointed out that the development of scales for DoC is often unaccompanied by an explicit conceptual framework of consciousness.[12] The decision to make is whether it is valid and fair to disregard subjective states or equate them with nonconsciousness because they do not meet criteria for medical definitions focused on one aspect of consciousness and made based on methodological limitations (2pp and 3pp assesments) which themselves have more limitations. The differences between sub-concepts A, B, and C within the medical perspective, should encourage clinicians to reflect and be prudent and specific about what they mean by absence of consciousness and awareness. Deciding on a conceptual framework precedes requesting scientific evidence for consciousness. Evidence pointing at the relevance of theprefrontal and cingulate cortices for metacognition (knowing about knowing) and self awareness, is not evidence that those concepts and their related areas encompass all there is to consciousness. Recent evidence of "mind-body" dissociation through intracranial stimulation of the posterior brain area known as anterior-precuneus, adds to the literature supporting that the precuneus is an essential hub in consciousness-related processes (ie, narrative self, and mind-wandering) as part of the default network[49–51] and outside this network (ie, bodily self)[52]. This and other posterior areas may be key to preserving consciousness in the most essential sense (ie, subjective experience). In addition, paradigms based on dream neuroscience could be performed in DoC patients to recognize subjective experience, but in these populations, there is the limitation of not having a readily available verbal self-report. Thus, an assumption would have to be made based on the extrapolation of scientific studies on the neural correlates of dreams performed on healthy controls, in whom self-report is available; A determined brain activity (eg, decreased SWA in posterior areas) in non-communicative patients could indicate the presence of subjective experience. Correlating these states with outcomes is a separate task, but one that may not be performed if these states or their relevance are not recognized.

Although states such as dreams, mind-wandering, and hallucinations may have little relationship with the external environment, these may not always be devoid of the narrative self (working memory and autobiographical recall) found during wake in healthy people. The literature on lucid dreaming continues to grow, an ability of people to know who they are and to recognize that they are in a fictional environment within a dream state.[53] Through this evidence, it becomes clear that distinguishing content-specific or local states (eg, self-related) is relevant even within unresponsive states. These distinctions are important because the false negatives relevant to this discussion do not refer to a syndromic misdiagnosis but to a global one: to say that a patient is not experiencing anything when they are. The problem with a narrow scope concept of consciousness is that patients who are conscious, even if unresponsive or devoid of narrative self or metacognition, might not be identified as such, and thus not provided a fair clinical management and personal regard by their family and health care personnel.

Hernandez Martin[56] surveyed health care personnel and found that 61% perceived patients in UWS to be devoid of human dignity. Among this sample, the justifications for this perspective were that patients lack intellectual capability, personality or quality of life, they have a poor prognosis, and are dependent or perceived as a burden for others. Providers for whom human dignity is tied to a functional perspective of consciousness may believe they have a responsibility to alleviate the family's burden to make decisions at the end of life and push back against acknowledging that some patients with poor functional prognosis may be conscious in some way. They may argue that recognizing states of subjective experience devoid of objective testable aspects may not be helpful to the patient or the family. However, there is evidence supporting that family members prefer frank communication even in the context of clinical uncertainty.[57,58] In fact, a paternalistic approach that overlooks these states may stall regarding with dignity and providing management, including rehabilitation and palliative care (eg, pain mangement, personalized auditory stimuli or at least control of noises that induce psychosis).

In sum, we suggest that the growth of the science of consciousness and the ethical and clinical challenges faced by various populations of patients (eg, arousal disorders, epilepsies, dementia, agnosia), could be improved if clinical providers become acquainted with the elephant in the room, the subjective aspect of consciousness.

CLINICS CARE POINTS

- There is a high prevalence of misdiagnosis in disorders of consciousness (DoC) syndromes (34–56%) and misclassification of conscious patients (false negatives) related to difficulties in behavioral and neuroscientific evidence interpretation.

- A first step to help decrease misdiagnosis, and reforming DoC taxonomies, might be to improve terminology of a) what is meant by consciousness, and b) what is being/can be clinically examined with the available methods (behavioral or neuroscientific).

- Broadening the composite medical notion of consciousness to include its subjective aspect may help address the current clinical and ethical shortcomings in DoC care.

- Considering the possibility of a patient having subjective experiences without a behavioral responses may lead to increase the utilization of personally-relevant stimuli and the use of neurotechnology in their assessments, rehabilitation, palliative care, and a fair regard in goals of care decision-making.

DISCLOSURE

The authors have nothing to disclose.

ACKNOWLEDGMENTS

The authors thank Dr Melanie Boly and Dr Jose Damian Carrillo Ruiz, for their comments and mentorship in some of the earlier conceptual development of this work; Dr Garrett Mindt, Dr Beril Mat, PhD-candidate Benedetta Cecconi for their comments on this article.

REFERENCES

1. Childs NL, Mercer WN, Childs HW. Accuracy of diagnosis of persistent vegetative state. Neurology 1993;43(8):1465–7.
2. Andrews K, Murphy L, Munday R, et al. Misdiagnosis of the vegetative state: retrospective study in a rehabilitation unit. BMJ 1996;313(7048):13–6.
3. Schnakers C, Vanhaudenhuyse A, Giacino J, et al. Diagnostic accuracy of the vegetative and minimally conscious state: Clinical consensus versus standardized neurobehavioral assessment. BMC Neurol 2009;9(1):35.
4. Peterson A, Cruse D, Naci L, et al. Risk, diagnostic error, and the clinical science of consciousness. NeuroImage Clin 2015;7:588–97.
5. Wade DT. How often is the diagnosis of the permanent vegetative state incorrect? A review of the evidence. Eur J Neurol 2018;25(4):619–25.
6. Wang J, Hu X, Hu Z, et al. The misdiagnosis of prolonged disorders of consciousness by a clinical consensus compared with repeated coma-recovery scale-revised assessment. BMC Neurol 2020;20(1):343.

7. Giacino JT, Katz DI, Schiff ND, et al. Practice guideline update recommendations summary: Disorders of consciousness: Report of the Guideline Development, Dissemination, and Implementation Subcommittee of the American Academy of Neurology; the American Congress of Rehabilitation Medicine; and the National Institute on Disability, Independent Living, and Rehabilitation Research. Neurology 2018;91(10):450–60.
8. Damasio A. The feeling of what happens: body and emotion in the making of consciousness. FL, USA: Harcourt College Publishers; 1999. p. 386.
9. Van Gulick R. Consciousness. Published online June 18, 2004. Available at: https://plato.stanford.edu/archives/spr2018/entries/consciousness/. Accessed January 3, 2023.
10. Searle JR. The mystery of consciousness. London, UK: Granta Books; 1990.
11. Zeman A. Consciousness: a user's guide. CT, USA: Yale University Press; 2004.
12. Seel RT, Sherer M, Whyte J, et al. Assessment scales for disorders of consciousness: evidence-based recommendations for clinical practice and research. Arch Phys Med Rehabil 2010;91(12):1795–813.
13. Schnakers C. Update on diagnosis in disorders of consciousness. Expert Rev Neurother 2020;20(10):997–1004.
14. Edlow BL, Claassen J, Schiff ND, et al. Recovery from disorders of consciousness: mechanisms, prognosis and emerging therapies. Nat Rev Neurol 2021; 17(3):135–56.
15. Bayne T, Hohwy J, Owen AM. Reforming the taxonomy in disorders of consciousness. Ann Neurol 2017;82(6):866–72.
16. Naccache L. Minimally conscious state or cortically mediated state? Brain 2018; 141(4):949–60.
17. Plum F and Posner JB. The Diagnosis of Stupor and Coma. PA, USA: F. A. Davis Co., 1972.
18. Castro P. de. Paciente con alteración de conciencia en urgencias. Anales Sis San Navarra [Internet]. 2008 [Accessed January 3];31(Suppl 1): 87-97. Available at: http://scielo.isciii.es/scielo.php?script=sci_arttext&pid=S1137-662720080002000 08&lng=es.
19. Gosseries O, Vanhaudenhuyse A, Bruno MA, et al. Disorders of consciousness: coma, vegetative and minimally conscious states. In: Cvetkovic D, Cosic I, editors. States of consciousness: experimental insights into meditation, waking, sleep and dreams. The frontiers collection. Berlin, Germany: Springer-Verlag; 2011. p. 29–55. https://doi.org/10.1007/978-3-642-18047-7_2.
20. Salvatore R, Bramanti PC. Chronic disorders of consciousness: from research to clinical practice. Hauppauge, NY, USA: Nova Science Publishers, Inc.; 2013.
21. Snell RS. Clinical neuroanatomy. Philadelphia, PA, USA: Lippincott Williams & Wilkins; 2010.
22. Bayne T, Hohwy J, Owen AM. Are there levels of consciousness? Trends Cogn Sci 2016;20(6):405–13.
23. Manji H, Connolly S, Kitchen N, et al. Oxford handbook of neurology. 2nd edition. Oxford, England, UK: Oxford University Press; 2014.
24. Padilla-Zambrano HS, Ramos-Villegas Y, Manjarreź-Sulbaran J de J, et al. Coma y alteraciones del estado de conciencia: revisión y enfoque para el médico de urgencias. Rev Chil Neurocir 2018;44(1):83–8.
25. Russell BV. —Knowledge by Acquaintance and Knowledge by Description. Proc Aristot Soc 1911;11(1):108–28.
26. Truncellito DA. Epistemology | Internet Encyclopedia of Philosophy. Available at: https://iep.utm.edu/epistemo/. Accessed January 3, 2023.

27. Ichikawa JJ, Steup M. The Analysis of Knowledge. Published online February 6, 2001. Available at: https://plato.stanford.edu/archives/sum2018/entries/knowledge-analysis/. Accessed January 3, 2023.

28. Laureys S, Gosseries O, Tononi G. The neurology of consciousness: cognitive neuroscience and neuropathology. Amsterdam, Netherlands: Academic Press; 2015.

29. Cruse D, Chennu S, Chatelle C, et al. Bedside detection of awareness in the vegetative state: a cohort study. Lancet 2011;378(9809):2088–94.

30. Boly M, Coleman MR, Davis MH, et al. When thoughts become action: an fMRI paradigm to study volitional brain activity in non-communicative brain injured patients. Neuroimage 2007;36(3):979–92.

31. Lin K, Wroten M. Ranchos Los Amigos. In: StatPearls. StatPearls Publishing; 2022. Available at: http://www.ncbi.nlm.nih.gov/books/NBK448151/. Accessed January 3, 2023.

32. Jain S, Iverson LM. Glasgow Coma Scale. In: StatPearls. StatPearls Publishing; 2022. Available at: http://www.ncbi.nlm.nih.gov/books/NBK513298/. Accessed January 3, 2023.

33. Giacino JT, Kalmar K, Whyte J. The JFK coma recovery scale-revised: measurement characteristics and diagnostic utility. Arch Phys Med Rehabil 2004;85(12):2020–9.

34. Gill-Thwaites H, Munday R. The sensory modality assessment and rehabilitation technique (SMART): a comprehensive and integrated assessment and treatment protocol for the vegetative state and minimally responsive patient. Neuropsychol Rehabil 1999;9(3–4):305–20.

35. Mat B, Sanz LRD, Arzi A, et al. New Behavioral Signs of Consciousness in Patients with Severe Brain Injuries. Semin Neurol 2022;42(3):259–72.

36. Sarasso S, Casali AG, Casarotto S, et al. Consciousness and complexity: a consilience of evidence. Neurosci Conscious 2021;niab023. https://doi.org/10.1093/nc/niab023.

37. Merker B. Consciousness without a cerebral cortex: A challenge for neuroscience and medicine. Behav Brain Sci 2007;30(1):63–81.

38. Izard C. Levels of Emotion and Levels of Consciousness. Behav Brain Sci 2007; 30(1):96–8.

39. Smallwood J, Schooler JW. The restless mind. Psychol Bull 2006;132(6):946–58.

40. Kane MJ, Brown LH, McVay JC, et al. For whom the mind wanders, and when: an experience-sampling study of working memory and executive control in daily life. Psychol Sci 2007;18(7):614–21.

41. Baird B, Smallwood J, Schooler JW. Back to the future: autobiographical planning and the functionality of mind-wandering. Conscious Cogn 2011;20(4):1604–11.

42. Okun MS, Raju DV, Walter BL, et al. Pseudobulbar crying induced by stimulation in the region of the subthalamic nucleus. J Neurol Neurosurg Psychiatr 2004; 75(6):921–3.

43. Parvizi J, Coburn KL, Shillcutt SD, et al. Neuroanatomy of pathological laughing and crying: a report of the American neuropsychiatric association committee on research. J Neuropsychiatry Clin Neurosci 2009;21(1):75–87.

44. Heine L, Castro M, Martial C, et al. Exploration of Functional Connectivity During Preferred Music Stimulation in Patients with Disorders of Consciousness. Front Psychol 2015;6. Available at: https://www.frontiersin.org/articles/10.3389/fpsyg.2015.01704. Accessed January 3, 2023.

45. Kempny AM, James L, Yelden K, et al. Patients with a severe prolonged disorder of consciousness can show classical EEG responses to their own name compared with others' names. NeuroImage Clin 2018;19:311–9.
46. Zhu J, Yan Y, Zhou W, et al. Clinical research: auditory stimulation in the disorders of consciousness. Front Hum Neurosci 2019;13:324.
47. Verger J, Ruiz S, Tillmann B, et al. [Beneficial effect of preferred music on cognitive functions in minimally conscious state patients]. Rev Neurol (Paris) 2014; 170(11):693–9.
48. Siclari F, LaRocque J, Postle B, et al. Assessing sleep consciousness within subjects using a serial awakening paradigm. Front Psychol 2013;4. Available at: https://www.frontiersin.org/articles/10.3389/fpsyg.2013.00542. Accessed January 3, 2023.
49. Buckner RL, Carroll DC. Self-projection and the brain. Trends Cogn Sci 2007; 11(2):49–57.
50. Crittenden B.M., Mitchell D.J., Duncan J., Recruitment of the default mode network during a demanding act of executive control. Van Essen D.C., ed. *eLife.* 2015;4:e06481. doi:10.7554/eLife.0648155.
51. Kumral E, Bayam FE, Özdemir HN. Cognitive and Behavioral Disorders in Patients with Precuneal Infarcts. Eur Neurol 2021;84(3):157–67.
52. Lyu D., Stieger J.R., Xin C., et al., Causal evidence for the processing of bodily self in the anterior precuneus. Neuron. 2023:S0896-6273(23)00386-0. https://doi.org/10.1016/j.neuron.2023.05.013.
53. Siclari F, Baird B, Perogamvros L, et al. The neural correlates of dreaming. Nat Neurosci 2017;20(6):872–8.
54. Gorska U, Kozma C, Grobbelaar M, et al. Neural signatures of unresponsiveness vs unconsciousness during epileptic seizures. USA: American Epilepsy Society; 2022. Available at: https://aesnet.org/abstractslisting/neural-signatures-of-unresponsiveness-vs-unconsciousness-during-epileptic-seizures.
55. Juan E, Górska U, Kozma C, et al. Distinct signatures of loss of consciousness during focal impaired awareness versus focal to bilateral tonic clonic seizures. Published online October 14, 2021:2021.10.01.462586. https://doi.org/10.1101/2021.10.01.462586.
56. Hernández Martin I. Consideraciones éticas del personal sanitario sobre el valor dignidad en los pacientes en estado vegetativo. Bioetica 2012;12(2).
57. Blumenthal-Barby JS, Lazaridis C. A woman in her 30s whose family becomes distrustful after an initial prognosis proves inaccurate. Chest 2016;149(4):e115–7.
58. Johnson LSM, Lazaridis C. The sources of uncertainty in disorders of consciousness. AJOB Neurosci 2018;9(2):76–82.

Disorders of Consciousness
Classification and Taxonomy

Katherine Golden, OTD[a], Yelena G. Bodien, PhD[b,c,d],
Joseph T. Giacino, PhD[b,c],*

KEYWORDS

- Disorders of consciousness • Coma • Minimally conscious state • Vegetative state
- Unresponsive wakefulness syndrome • Post-traumatic confusional state
- Cognitive motor dissociation

KEY POINTS

- Recent practice guidelines for the management of patients with disorders of consciousness (DoC) published in the U.S., Europe, and U.K. include evidence-based definitions, diagnostic criteria and assessment methods, improving consistency in terminology and approach to classification.
- While behavioral assessment remains the gold standard for the detection of consciousness and differential diagnosis among DoC, the syndrome of *cognitive motor dissociation* (ie, "covert consciousness") serves as a reminder that behavior is a weak proxy for consciousness.
- A more rational taxonomy that considers behavioral characteristics, as well as underlying pathophysiologic features, is needed to improve DoC classification and treatment precision.

DISORDERS OF CONSCIOUSNESS: AN EVOLVING TAXONOMY
Introduction

Efforts to describe and classify disorders of consciousness date back more than 2 millennia. In 400 B.C., Aristotle offered a simple taxonomy that was centered on self-awareness and distinguished sleep from unconsciousness–"What is (inanimate) is unaware, while what is (animate) is not unaware ... While asleep, the critical

[a] School of Health & Rehabilitation Sciences, MGH Institute of Health Professions, 36 1st Avenue, Boston, MA 02129, USA; [b] Department of Physical Medicine and Rehabilitation, Spaulding Rehabilitation Hospital, 300 1st Avenue, Charlestown, MA, 02129, USA; [c] Center for Neurotechnology and Neurorecovery, Department of Neurology, Massachusetts General Hospital and Harvard Medical School, 55 Fruit Street, Boston, MA 02114, USA; [d] Department of Physical Medicine and Rehabilitation, Harvard Medical School, 25 Shattuck Street, Boston, MA, USA
* Corresponding author. Department of Physical Medicine and Rehabilitation, Spaulding Rehabilitation Hospital, 300 1st Avenue, Charlestown, MA, 02129
E-mail address: jgiacino@mgh.harvard.edu

Phys Med Rehabil Clin N Am 35 (2024) 15–33
https://doi.org/10.1016/j.pmr.2023.06.011

activities, which include thinking, sensing, recalling and remembering, do not function as they do during wakefulness."[1,2] While the construct of consciousness is conceptually grounded in the dichotomy between self-awareness and unawareness, Plum and Posner[3] eloquently posed the central problem, "we can only infer the self-awareness of others by their appearance and their acts." This observation also highlights a critically important limitation of the current diagnostic scheme-all rely almost exclusively on behavioral evidence. Overreliance on behavioral observations and inferential judgement has resulted in confusion and misunderstanding, contributing to alarmingly high rates of diagnostic error.[4–6]

How should we conceptualize a DoC taxonomy that would inform clinical practice and advance the field? Such a taxonomy should aspire to accomplish four aims.[7] Chief among these, it should promote communication between clinicians, and among clinicians, family members, and surrogate decision-makers. This requires the uniform use of diagnostic terms and clinical criteria. Recent multi-organizational guidelines in the U.S., Europe, and U.K. have moved closer to this goal but it has not yet been achieved. Second, a clinically useful taxonomy should demonstrate "goodness of fit." That is, the language used should accurately describe and clearly distinguish the conditions of interest. At present, the existing literature is replete with different terms that refer to the same condition and there is overlap in clinical features that purport to describe distinct conditions. Third, the taxonomy should be feasible to implement. All settings that provide care for this population should have access to the personnel, procedures, and tools that are necessary to identify and classify DoC. This is a second major limitation of present day DoC care. A notable example is the recently defined *cognitive motor dissociation (CMD)* syndrome, which requires the use of specialized functional neuroimaging acquisition and analytic procedures that are generally only available in academic medical centers.[8] The fourth attribute of an effective taxonomy for DoC is that it should facilitate clinical management decisions. The prevailing approach to the treatment of patients with DoC is trial and error. Unique behavioral features and the underlying pathophysiologic substrate are rarely considered in treatment selection, resulting in inconsistency and imprecision in the approach. A rational taxonomy should incorporate knowledge of the neurobiological mechanism underlying the behavioral phenotype as this would inform optimal treatment targets and the likelihood of therapeutic response.

We view the four aims discussed above as aspirational but believe there is a pressing need to move toward a more rational approach to DoC taxonomy. In this article, we provide a brief historical review the major DoCs and then discuss the prevailing operational definitions and diagnostic criteria for each. We rely heavily on current practice guidelines, identify knowledge gaps and, where appropriate, discuss future directions that may have a favorable impact.

Neurobiological Considerations

Existing international practice guidelines recognize four major DoCs: *coma, vegetative state (VS)* (also referred to as *unresponsive wakefulness syndrome (UWS)*), *minimally conscious state (MCS)*, and *post-traumatic confusional state (PTCS)* (also referred to as *emergence from MCS (eMCS)*).[9–11] Disturbance in consciousness is typically caused by either focal injury to the brain stem or diffuse bi-hemispheric injury that results in the widespread disruption of cortical networks responsible for the regulation of arousal and internal and external awareness.[12,13] DoCs may occur following direct insult to specific structures that are integral to sustaining arousal and awareness or indirectly through loss of connectivity between key structures. While the fundamental neurobiological mechanisms required for conscious awareness remain poorly understood, recovery is closely associated with the location and volume of structural damage to the brain.[14]

A major scientific and clinical problem associated with the assessment of DoC is the phenomenon of fluctuation in "state." That is, the level of consciousness may vary moment to moment in patients with DoC. For example, it is not uncommon for a clinician to observe clear and convincing evidence of conscious awareness through command-following on the examination conducted in the morning and then fail to elicit the same behavior on reassessment later in the same day. The pathophysiologic mechanism underlying these fluctuations is unclear but has been linked to instability in the arousal regulation and under-activation of downstream cortical fields brought about by the deafferentation of the central lateral thalamus.[15,16] This instability in the arousal regulation system complicates DoC classification from a diagnostic standpoint as patients may transition in and out of different disorders from examination to examination. While the 40% diagnostic error rate repeatedly reported in DoC literature[4–6] partially reflects insufficient knowledge and misunderstanding among clinicians, it is likely that pathophysiologic oscillations in thalamic gating systems also play a key role.

Challenges to Establishing a Uniform Taxonomy

Over the last three decades, multiple professional organizations[10,17–20] have proposed recommendations for defining and diagnosing DoCs. Earlier efforts were conducted in parallel, sometimes leading to conflicting guidance.[21] More recent initiatives have been decidedly more interdisciplinary, leading to greater consistency across recommendations. There has also been a discernible shift from consensus-based to evidence-based practice recommendations.[9,10] One notable example is the evidence-based recommendations for practice co-sponsored by the American Academy of Neurology (AAN), American Congress of Rehabilitation Medicine (ACRM), and the National Institute on Disability, Independence, and Rehabilitation Research and published concurrently in *Neurology*[9] and *Archives of Physical Medicine and Rehabilitation* in 2018.[22] This partnership between neurology and neurorehabilitation organizations was successful in achieving consensus to discontinue use of the term, *permanent vegetative state*, which had previously been an enduring source of controversy between the 2 disciplines.

Despite increased interdisciplinary collaboration, there is ongoing disagreement on the terminology and diagnostic criteria associated with these conditions, posing considerable clinical and ethical risks to clinicians, patients, and caregivers concerned and living with DoC. Lack of standardization in terminology fosters inappropriate management, inaccurate prognostication, increased caregiver stress, and societal nihilism.[23] Even when there is general consensus among different professional disciplines, widescale adoption and implementation of new recommendations is often slow or incomplete due to delays in knowledge translation, poor dissemination across medical, scientific, and social platforms, and subtle differences in nomenclature.

The remainder of this article provides an historical review of the terminology, definitions, and diagnostic criteria associated with coma, VS, MCS, and PTCS. **Fig. 1** provides a timeline of key developments that have influenced DoC classification. **Fig. 2** shows the distinguishing features of the DoCs covered in this article. Throughout the article, we highlight important knowledge gaps and future directions that may move the field toward a more rational taxonomy for DoC.

Coma

The condition widely referred to as, "coma," is of Greek origin and derives from "koma," meaning deep sleep. Many other terms have been suggested to describe

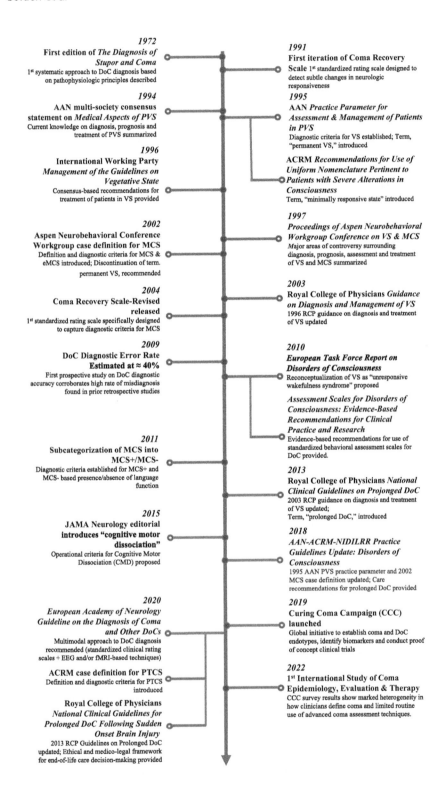

1972
First edition of *The Diagnosis of*
Stupor and Coma
1st systematic approach to DoC diagnosis based
on pathophysiologic principles described

1994
AAN multi-society consensus
statement on *Medical Aspects of PVS*
Current knowledge on diagnosis, prognosis and
treatment of PVS summarized

1996
International Working Party
Management of the Guidelines on
Vegetative State
Consensus-based recommendations for
treatment of patients in VS provided

2002
Aspen Neurobehavioral Conference
Workgroup case definition for MCS
Definition and diagnostic criteria for MCS &
eMCS introduced; Discontinuation of term.
permanent VS, recommended

2004
Coma Recovery Scale-Revised
released
1st standardized rating scale specifically designed
to capture diagnostic criteria for MCS

2009
DoC Diagnostic Error Rate
Estimated at ≈ 40%
First prospective study on DoC diagnostic
accuracy corroborates high rate of misdiagnosis
found in prior retrospective studies

2011
Subcategorization of MCS into
MCS+/MCS-
Diagnostic criteria established for MCS+ and
MCS- based presence/absence of language
function

2015
JAMA Neurology editorial
introduces "cognitive motor
dissociation"
Operational criteria for Cognitive Motor
Dissociation (CMD) proposed

2020
European Academy of Neurology
Guideline on the Diagnosis of Coma
and Other DoCs
Multimodal approach to DoC diagnosis
recommended (standardized clinical rating
scales + EEG and/or fMRI-based techniques)

ACRM case definition for PTCS
Definition and diagnostic criteria for PTCS
introduced

Royal College of Physicians
National Clinical Guidelines for
Prolonged DoC Following Sudden
Onset Brain Injury
2013 RCP Guidelines on Prolonged DoC
updated; Ethical and medico-legal framework
for end-of-life care decision-making provided

1991
First iteration of Coma Recovery
Scale 1st standardized rating scale designed to
detect subtle changes in neurologic
responsiveness

1995
AAN *Practice Parameter for*
Assessment & Management of Patients
in PVS
Diagnostic criteria for VS established; Term,
"permanent VS," introduced

ACRM *Recommendations for Use of*
Uniform Nomenclature Pertinent to
Patients with Severe Alterations in
Consciousness
Term, "minimally responsive state" introduced

1997
Proceedings of Aspen Neurobehavioral
Workgroup Conference on VS & MCS
Major areas of controversy surrounding
diagnosis, prognosis, assessment and treatment
of VS and MCS summarized

2003
Royal College of Physicians *Guidance*
on Diagnosis and Management of VS
1996 RCP guidance on diagnosis and treatment
of VS updated

2010
European Task Force Report on
Disorders of Consciousness
Reconceptualization of VS as "unresponsive
wakefulness syndrome" proposed

Assessment Scales for Disorders of
Consciousness: Evidence-Based
Recommendations for Clinical
Practice and Research
Evidence-based recommendations for use of
standardized behavioral assessment scales for
DoC provided.

2013
Royal College of Physicians *National*
Clinical Guidelines on Prolonged DoC
2003 RCP guidance on diagnosis and treatment
of VS updated;
Term, "prolonged DoC," introduced

2018
AAN-ACRM-NIDILRR Practice
Guidelines Update: Disorders of
Consciousness
1995 AAN PVS practice parameter and 2002
MCS case definition updated; Care
recommendations for prolonged DoC provided

2019
Curing Coma Campaign (CCC)
launched
Global initiative to establish coma and DoC
endotypes, identify biomarkers and conduct proof
of concept clinical trials

2022
1st International Study of Coma
Epidemiology, Evaluation & Therapy
CCC survey results show marked heterogeneity in
how clinicians define coma and limited routine
use of advanced coma assessment techniques.

Dimension			Behavior	Coma	VS/UWS	MCS-	MCS+	PTCS
Awareness	Cognition		Reduced ability to focus or sustain attention					a
			Disorientation to place, time & situation					
			Impaired encoding & recall of new information					
			Symptom fluctuation over course of the day					
			Reliable yes-no responses or functional object use					
	+Language		Consistent command-following				b	
			Reproducible command-following					
			Intelligible speech					
			Object recognition					
			Discernible but unreliable yes-no responses					
	Language		Automatic motor behavior			b		
			Object manipulation &/or localization					
			Visual pursuit &/or fixation					
			Localization to pain					
Arousal			Eyes open spontaneously or to stimulation					
			Continuous eye closure					

Fig. 2. Differential diagnostic criteria for disorders of consciousness. Behaviors associated with DoCs can be conceptualized along two dimensions-arousal (or wakefulness) and awareness (ie, perception of self and environment). The shaded regions of the bars indicate the distinguishing characteristics of each disorder. MCS-, minimally conscious state; MCS+, minimally conscious state plus; PTCS, post traumatic confusional state; VS, vegetative state. [a]All behaviors are required. [b]At least one of these behaviors must be present. (Adapted from Giacino JT, Katz D, Schiff N, Bodien YG. Assessment and Rehabilitative Management of Individuals with Disorders of Consciousness. In: Zasler ND, Katz DI, Zafonte RD, editors. Brain Injury Medicine: Principles and Practice- 3rd edition. New York: Springer Publishing Company, 2022. p. 447-461, with permission.)

this condition, anchoring to either the behavioral or neuropathologic features.[24] For example, the term, cataphora, refers to a hyper-somnolent state while, apallic syndrome, introduced by Kretschmer in 1940, connotes, "without cortex."[25]

In 1972, Plum & Posner published their seminal work, The Diagnosis of Stupor and Coma, offering the first detailed description of the pathophysiologic and clinical characteristics of coma.[3] In subsequent editions, the diagnostic features of coma have largely remained the same. Coma is described as a state of pathological unconsciousness, characterized by complete loss of spontaneous arousal, sustained eye closure despite the introduction of noxious stimulation, and total absence of behaviors associated with "normal" consciousness.[3,13] Neuropathologic studies completed by Plum, Posner, and others have demonstrated that coma can result from severe, diffuse, bi-hemispheric damage to the cortex, underlying white matter, thalamus, or focal lesions of the paramedian tegmentum.[13,26,27] Persons in coma typically remain in this state for approximately 2 to four weeks before transitioning to higher levels of consciousness.

Recently, expert consensus-based criteria for diagnosing coma were established under the auspices of the Curing Coma Campaign (CCC). The CCC is comprised of

Fig. 1. Timeline of events influencing DoC taxonomy over the past five decades. AAN, American Academy of Neurology; ACRM, american congress of rehabilitation medicine; CCC, curing coma campaign; DoC, disorder(s) of consciousness; EEG, electroencephalography; eMCS, emerged from minimally conscious state; fMRI, functional magnetic resonance imaging; MCS-, minimally conscious state-minus; MCS, minimally conscious state; MCS+, minimally conscious state-plus; PTCS, post-traumatic confusional state; PVS, persistent vegetative state; RCP, royal college of physicians; VS, vegetative state.

a multidisciplinary international panel of experts, including scientists, neuro-intensivists, neurorehabilitation specialists, and implementation scientists, who have established a "coma community" with the primary aim of advancing coma science.[28] The expert panel identified the following cardinal features of coma (**Box 1**).

The clinical criteria recommended by both Plum and Posner and the CCC expert panel have an important limitation–they center on the *absence* of specific behaviors. The recently defined condition referred to as *cognitive motor dissociation (CMD)*, in which consciousness is retained in the absence of behavioral evidence (see CMD discussion later in discussion) attests to the inadequacy of these criteria.[8] Moreover, Kondziella and Frontera have argued that some comatose patients may retain spontaneous or stimulus-induced eye-opening, defying traditional diagnostic criteria, which emphasize eye closure as a primary feature, and challenge the longstanding notion that coma is incompatible with arousal.[30] The authors suggest a putative pathophysiologic mechanism for eyes-open coma and call for autopsy and functional imaging studies to further investigate this presentation as a new coma phenotype.

Despite significant advancements in neuroimaging technology, the necessary and sufficient lesion profile underlying coma remains elusive and there is no consensus on the defining clinical characteristics.[27] In 2022, CCC collaborators published the results of an international crowdsourcing survey, the first of its kind, to investigate the point prevalence of coma in the United States and United Kingdom. Findings revealed that the point prevalence rate was approximately four times higher in the U.S. than in the U.K. (31 cases per 100,000 in the U.S. v. 7 cases per 100,000 in the U.K.).[31] Also in 2022, the CCC published the results of the Come Together Survey, which was designed to assess global perspectives on the definition, clinical features, and management strategies associated with coma.[29] Survey results indicated that only 64% of respondents agreed with the cardinal features of coma recommended by the expert panel. There was also substantial variability in assessment methods and treatment strategies routinely used. Findings from this study highlight the pressing need to revisit prevailing diagnostic criteria and management strategies for coma. Current and future efforts to improve longitudinal follow-up with patients who experience coma is also needed to adequately inform policies, protocols, and minimal competency guidelines for equitable management of coma. Furthermore, the CCC is partnering with the National Institute of Health to develop unique common data elements (CDE), or a shared language, for coma.[32] CDEs for coma will streamline standardization and foster international consensus on operational definitions and diagnostic criteria for coma.[33]

Box 1
Diagnostic criteria for coma

All of the following criteria must be met to establish the diagnosis of coma:
- No command-following;
- No intelligible speech or recognizable gesture;
- No volitional movement (reflexive movement such as extensor or flexor posturing, withdrawal from pain, triple flexion may occur);
- No visual pursuit, fixation, saccade to stimuli, or eye opening or closing to command;
- The above criteria are not due to the use of the paralytic agent, active use of sedatives, another neurologic or psychiatric disorder (eg, locked-in syndrome, neuromuscular disorder, catatonia, akinetic mute, abulia, conversion disorder); and
- The patient does not have evidence of cognitive motor dissociation (ie, the covert ability to follow commands) based on electrophysiological or functional imaging, if such testing is available.[29]

Vegetative State

The roots of VS can be tracked back to Aristotle's introduction of the "vegetative faculty" in *De Anima* (*On the Soul*)[2] from the mid-4th century B.C.E.[34] This early conceptualization sparked a French physician, Xavier Bichat (1771–1802),[35] and an American neurologist/endocrinologist, Walter Timme (1874–1956),[36] to extend the concept of a vegetative nervous system. The origin of the concept of vegetative functions emphasized control of autonomic, internal organ systems, such as digestive, cardiovascular, and respiratory processes, which are mediated by the brainstem.[34,37] These functions were classified as foundational, simplistic, automatic internal processes, dichotomized from external processes, which were thought to be responsible for voluntary expression and relation to one's environment.

In 1963, Arnaud and colleagues[38] referred to patients in the early stages of recovery from severe brain injury as, "vie vegetative," denoting "vegetative life." In 1971, in discussing prognostic indicators following severe brain injury, Vapalhati and Troupp modified usage of this term to suggest "vegetative survival."[39] In 1972, Bryan Jennett, a neurosurgeon from Glasgow, and Fred Plum, an American neurologist, published their seminal article entitled, "Persistent Vegetative State After Brain Damage" in *Lancet*, introducing *persistent vegetative state (PVS)* as a diagnostic term.[40] The term, "persistent," was added as a modifier for VS to distinguish patients who were observed to experience prolonged wakefulness without awareness from patients who quickly transitioned to higher states of consciousness following initial injury.[40] Jennett and Plum presciently recognized the potential negative implications of adding "persistent" to VS stating: "Certainly we are concerned to identify an irrecoverable state, although the criteria needed to establish that prediction reliably have still to be confirmed. Until then "persistent" is safer than "permanent" or "irreversible"; but prolonged is not strong enough, and unless it is quantified it is meaningless (p. 735)."[40] In the succeeding years, the definition of PVS was changed to denote an "irreversible state," resulting in clinical confusion and inconsistency in the literature.

In 1994, the American Academy of Neurology (AAN) organized the Multi-Society Task Force on the Vegetative State and published the landmark article, "Medical Aspects of the Persistent Vegetative State," as a 2-part article in the *New England Journal of Medicine*.[17,18] The Task Force report clarified that *persistent VS* was applicable when this condition persisted for at least 1-month post-injury. The authors also introduced the prognostic term, *permanent vegetative state,* to describe patients with an "exceedingly small" chance of regaining consciousness.[17,18,41] It was recommended that this term be applied after 12 months following traumatic brain injury (TBI), and after three months following non-traumatic injury. One year after the publication of the AAN Task Force Report, the American Congress of Rehabilitation Medicine (ACRM) published, "Recommendations for Use of Uniform Nomenclature Pertinent to Patients with Severe Alterations in Consciousness." This position statement advocated for the discontinuation of the term, *persistent VS*, and recommended instead that the diagnosis of VS be accompanied by the length of time post-injury as this would convey prognostic information.[19] Around the same time, the UK-lead "International Working Party on the Management of the Vegetative State: Summary Report" was published by an international group of neurologists, neurosurgeons, neuropsychologists, and neurorehabilitation specialists. The International Working Party proposed three vegetative presentations: hyporesponsive state, reflexic responsive state, and localizing responsive state. The International Working Party recommendations differed from the Multi-Society Task Force guidelines in that the former included localizing responses, including visual tracking, as a feature of the third VS category.[20] Although each group shared the intention of clarity and harmonization of nomenclature, these initiatives were conducted in parallel, resulting in significant differences in nomenclature and defining features. In 2002, the Aspen Neurobehavioral Workgroup published a consensus statement resolving prior discrepancies in some recommendations, including the definition of persistent VS.[42–44] Recent longitudinal studies now clearly indicate that recovery from VS can occur years after injury, substantiating discontinuation of the term, *permanent VS.*[45]

Diagnostic Criteria of the Vegetative State

Vegetative state (VS) is characterized by intermittent periods of wakefulness, evidenced by either spontaneous or stimulus-induced arousal, despite the absence of behavioral signs of conscious awareness (**Box 2**).[17,18] Return of eye opening in patients in VS is the indicative of restoration of reticular system function. Additionally, patients in VS typically do not require mechanical ventilation as the recovery of the reticular system preserves life-sustaining, autonomic functions. Sleep-wake cycles are typically present on EEG.

Is Vegetative State a State or Syndrome ?

There is ongoing disagreement as to whether VS should be characterized as a "state" or a "syndrome." The *Oxford English Dictionary* defines a state as, "the particular condition that someone or something is in at a specific time"[46] whereas a syndrome represents "a group of symptoms which consistently occur together, or a condition characterized by a set of associated symptoms."[47] These subtle differences in language have important clinical implications (see chapter 1 in Jennett B, "The Vegetative State: Medical Facts, Ethical and Legal Dilemmas," for further discussion).[48]

In 2010, the European Task Force on DoC suggested that the term, VS, be replaced with *unresponsive wakefulness syndrome (UWS).*[49] This recommendation was largely motivated by concerns that this term was pejorative and dehumanizing. A similar term, *wakeful unconscious state,* was considered by the Aspen Neurobehavioral Workgroup but was rejected for fear that it would cause confusion given the entrenchment of VS in existing diagnostic coding systems, registries, and databases. The Workgroup also argued that the term, "unresponsive," does not imply unconsciousness–a core feature of VS. The continued use of 2 different terms for this syndrome, mostly along geographic lines, complicates communication between providers and public understanding of an already complex condition.

Box 2
Diagnostic criteria of the vegetative state

All of the following criteria must be met to establish the diagnosis of VS:
- No evidence of awareness of self or environment and an inability to interact with others;
- No evidence of sustained, reproducible, purposeful, or voluntary behavioral responses to visual, auditory, tactile, or noxious stimuli;
- No evidence of language comprehension or expression;
- Intermittent wakefulness manifested by the presence of sleep-wake cycles;
- Sufficiently preserved hypothalamic and brain-stem autonomic functions to permit survival with medical and nursing care;
- Bowel and bladder incontinence; and
- Variably preserved cranial-nerve reflexes (pupillary, oculocephalic, corneal, vestibulo-ocular, gag and spinal reflexes.[17]

Minimally Conscious State

Prior to the introduction of the term MCS, patients with inconsistent or minimal signs of conscious awareness were lumped together with those in VS. The conflation of these 2 groups failed to recognize that early recovery of cognitively mediated behavior, even when minimal, is predictive of further functional recovery.[50,51] The International Working Party on VS considered *transitional vegetative state, inconsistent low awareness state*, and *consistent low awareness state*, but none of these terms achieved broad acceptance.[20] In 1995, the Brain Injury Interdisciplinary Special Interest Group of the ACRM introduced the term, *minimally responsive state,* to reflect evidence of inconsistent interaction with the environment.[19] This term was eventually abandoned as it does not distinguish reflexive from voluntary or cognitively mediated behavior.

In 2002, the Aspen Neurobehavioral Workgroup developed a case definition for the *minimally conscious state.* The Workgroup defined a lower boundary to clearly differentiate MCS from VS, and an upper boundary to mark emergence from MCS. Because the case definition and accompanying diagnostic criteria (**Box 3**) were established by expert consensus, they met with considerable controversy.[52,53] More recently, some experts have advocated for replacing MCS with *cortically mediated state (CMS)*, arguing that CMS simply acknowledges the presence of isolated cortical connectivity, whereas consciousness requires sustained and complex integration of cortical networks.[54] Others argue that MCS should not be replaced by CMS because it negates border between MCS and eMCS.[55]

The hallmark feature of MCS is behavioral fluctuation, which complicates diagnostic assessment and contributes to the 40% rate of misdiagnosis.[4–6] It is also essential to be alert to common confounding factors such as sedating medications, occult illness, subclinical seizure, and unrecognized hydrocephalus.[56] These problems can be mitigated to some extent by conducting serial assessments.[57] Confounding conditions will be discussed in greater detail in articles six and seven on DoC assessment measures. Early detection of MCS is essential in view of its favorable prognostic implications and the potential harmful effects of misdiagnosis on family members.[58]

Box 3
Diagnostic criteria of MCS

To establish the diagnosis of MCS, at least one of the following behaviors must be demonstrated on a reproducible or sustained basis:
- Following simple commands;
- Gestural or verbal yes/no responses regardless of accuracy;
- Intelligible verbalization;
- Purposeful behavior including movements or affective behaviors that occur in contingent relation to relevant environmental stimuli and are not due to reflexive activity, including:
  - Vocalizations or gestures that occur in direct response to the linguistic content of questions
  - Reaching for objects that demonstrates a clear relationship between object location and direction of reach
  - Touching or holding objects in a manner that accommodates the size and shape of the object
  - Pursuit eye movement or sustained fixation that occurs in direct response to moving or salient stimuli
  - Appropriate smiling or crying in response to the linguistic or visual content of emotional but not to neutral topics or stimuli.[42]

Minimally Conscious State Subtypes: Minimally Conscious State +/−

In 2011, in the Coma Science Group in Belgium proposed that MCS be subcategorized into MCS plus (MCS+) and MCS minus (MCS-) based on behavioral signs of preserved language function.[59] Functional connectivity studies have shown that patients in MCS + have higher cerebral metabolism in left hemisphere cortical areas encompassing the language network, compared to patients with MCS-, who have demonstrably less connectivity between Broca's region and language cortices.[60] The MCS plus/minus distinction appears to be clinically relevant as patients in MCS + demonstrate less functional disability on standardized outcome measures.[51,61] The 11th revision of the International Statistical Classification of Diseases and Related Health Problems (ICD-11) now includes MCS- and MCS + as diagnostic categories (**Box 4**), which may support population-based mechanistic studies of DoC.[62]

Minimally Conscious State Subtypes: Akinetic Mutism, Hyperkinetic Mutism

Akinetic mutism (AM) is characterized by spontaneous visual pursuit with minimal to no behavioral evidence of command following, vocalization, emotional expression, and other forms of goal-directed behavior.[63–65] Increased behavioral activity may be prompted by exposure to high intensity stimuli or neurostimulants.[66] The basis for the severely reduced level of behavioral activity in AM is the downregulation of frontal-subcortical circuits that regulate drive functions responsible for behavioral initiation and persistence.[26] The "telephone effect" described by Fisher in 1983 illustrates the mechanism underlying AM.[67] The patient initially presents as mute and motionless but when exposed to a ringing telephone, picks up the receiver and begins speaking fluently. The ringing phone represents a salient sensory cue that initiates a temporary reversal in depressed drive triggering the release of overlearned behaviors.[67]

AM is usually caused by the bilateral or orbito-basal cortex. Patients with AM appear attentive but exhibit little to no speech or movement[14] despite maintaining intrinsic capability to move and speak.[19,26,68] The lesion profile usually includes the involvement of the anterior cingulate bilaterally, medial frontal cortex, paramedian mesodiencephalon, globus pallidus, caudate nucleus and/or medial forebrain bundle.[14,69] *Hyperkinetic mutism* is a related condition characterized by heightened vigilance and non-goal-directed motor activity.[14] Bilateral temporal, parietal, and occipital junction lesions are presumed responsible for the ballistic, continuous and unrestrained movements.[67,70,71]

Box 4
Diagnostic criteria of MCS plus/minus

The diagnosis of MCS plus requires at least one clearly discernible language sign, including:
• Response to command;
• Intelligible verbalization; or
• Intentional communication (at least 2 instances of a verbal or gestural yes or no signal, regardless of accuracy).

The diagnosis of MCS minus requires at least one clearly discernible behavioral sign of awareness, including:
• Visual pursuit or fixation;
• Object localization;
• Localization to noxious stimulation;
• Object manipulation;
• Automatic motor behavior.[61]

Differentiating Vegetative State and Minimally Conscious State from Locked-in Syndrome

The *locked-in syndrome (LIS)* is not a DoC, but may be misdiagnosed as VS or MCS due to the severely limited or total loss of speech and movement.[72,73] LIS may arise from mass lesions, infection, trauma, or demyelinating disorders that affect the ventral pons or caudal ventral midbrain,[73] resulting in quadriplegia, apnea, bulbar palsy (ie, anarthria and dysphagia), and sensory dysfunction.[73,74] The distinguishing feature of LIS is the preservation of vertical eye movements and voluntary blinking as these behaviors allow affected patients to communicate.[64,75,76] In rare cases, ocular mobility is also impaired, making it virtually impossible to distinguish from VS on bedside examination.

Emergence from Minimally Conscious State and the Posttraumatic Confusional State

The Aspen Neurobehavioral Workgroup proposed that functional communication and/ or functional object should demarcate the upper boundary of MCS, signaling emergence from MCS (eMCS).[42] Functional communication was defined as accurate verbal or gestural yes-no responses to six consecutive situational orientation questions (eg, "Am I touching my nose?") on 2 consecutive examinations. Functional object use is demonstrated through generally appropriate use of at least 2 different objects on 2 consecutive evaluations. (eg, hairbrush, cup, pen). Both behaviors require the integration of multiple cortical networks to support the cognitive processes (eg, language comprehension, attention, motor control) that underlie them. Some have argued that functional communication should not be a criterion for eMCS as some patients who never experienced DoC also have difficulty meeting the threshold for functional communication.[77,78] Recent evidence suggests that consistent command-following recovers at nearly the same time[79] and is as difficulty to achieve[80] as functional communication and functional object and, for these reasons, should also mark the transition to eMCS.

Work by neurologists C.P Symonds and W.R. Russell in the early-mid 1900's observed that the period after sustaining a blow to the head is marked by a "clouded consciousness" and a constellation of symptoms, including profound disorientation in space and time, restlessness, perceptual disturbances, labile emotions, and so forth. The term they used to describe their observations was *post-traumatic amnesia (PTA)*, which "is taken to end at the time from which the patient can give a clear and consecutive account of what was happening around him."[81]

In the 1990's, Stuss and colleagues[82] proposed that *post traumatic confusional state (PTCS)* replace PTA based on observations that PTA was typically accompanied by distractibility, impaired judgement, perceptual disturbance, restlessness, sleep disorder, confabulation, and emotional or behavioral dysregulation, among other symptoms. In 2020, the American Congress of Rehabilitation Medicine Disorders of Consciousness Special Interest Group published a case definition for PTCS.[83] This evidence-informed case definition characterizes patients meeting criteria for eMCS but with ongoing symptoms of confusion that impede functional independence, limit cooperation in rehabilitation, interfere with personal safety, and limit appropriate engagement with others and the environment. Nearly all patients emerging from MCS meet the criteria for PTCS based on the presence of ongoing cognitive impairment, disorientation, agitation, and symptom fluctuation (**Box 5**).[50]

To meet the criteria for recovery from PTCS, patients must demonstrate significant improvement in all core features and 5 associated features of PTCS such that deficits

---

Box 5
Core features to establish the diagnosis of PTCS

All four of the following core features must be present to establish the diagnosis of PTCS:[83]
- Disturbances of attention: Reduced ability to focus or sustain attention
- Disorientation: Impaired orientation to place, time, and situation
- Disturbances of memory: Impaired ability to encode and recall new information
- Fluctuation: The character and severity of the disturbance waxes and wanes during the course of the day

In addition to the four core features, PTCS can include any of the following:
- Emotional and/or behavioral disturbances: Including but not limited to agitation/restlessness and/or hypoactivity; irritability, impulsivity, disinhibition, aggression and/or decreased responsiveness; affective lability and/or flattening
- Sleep-wake cycle disturbance: Excessive sleep, insufficient sleep, alteration of normal sleep pattern, or decreased level of arousal
- Delusions: Fixed false beliefs
- Perceptual disturbance: Illusions, hallucinations
- Confabulation: False memory

---

in attention, orientation, memory, and behavioral consistency no longer have a major impact on the patient's functional independence for basic self-care and safety awareness. Most patients eventually recover from PTCS, though ongoing assistance is typically still required to meet basic needs.[50] No single measure assesses all symptoms of confusion, but the Confusion Assessment Protocol,[84] a multidimensional tool derived from previously validated measures, addresses most aspects of PTCS.

Although similarities in the symptom profiles associated with PTCS and delirium have been noted,[85–88] for patients with DoC PTCS is considered a positive prognostic indicator and an expected milestone of ongoing recovery. Conversely, delirium is associated with a decline in function and a worse prognosis.[89–91] Moreover, the pathophysiological mechanisms resulting in PTCS are likely to differ significantly compared to those underlying other causes of delirium such as infection and anesthesia.[92] Consistent use of the term PTCS to characterize patients who demonstrate the symptoms described above is necessary to support research and clinical practice specific to the effects of brain injury. For example, given that PTCS has been studied primary in TBI, whether the results of prior studies can be applied to non-traumatic etiologies (eg, cardiac arrest) is an area requiring further study.

Cognitive Motor Dissociation

The diagnostic accuracy of DoC has improved a significant with the development and dissemination of standardized assessments. However, the behavioral output required to clearly demonstrate awareness on these assessments may be masked by the disconnection of efferent pathways, peripheral injury, contracture, or hypotonicity, and other factors. Advanced neuroimaging and electrophysiological techniques, such as task-based functional magnetic resonance imaging (fMRI) and EEG assess consciousness by instructing patients to covertly follow a command (eg, imagine opening and closing your hand) while recording signals from the brain. Volitional brain activity is measured during the task and compared to resting brain activity levels.

Cognitive motor dissociation (CMD), or covert consciousness, describes patients who lack behavioral signs of awareness (ie, diagnosis of coma, VS, MCS-) yet exhibit evidence of command-following on fMRI or EEG assessment.[93] This phenomenon was first demonstrated using task-based fMRI to show the preservation of volitional brain activity and neural networks in patients who lack motoric output, self-expression, or appear unresponsive on bedside examination.[94] Various terms have been used, such as *functional locked-in syndrome*,[59] *covert cognition*,[95] *non-behavioral MCS*,[96] and *CMD*,[8] to describe this distinct, subgroup of patients with DoC. CMD may be present in up to 15-20% of patients with subacute-to chronic DoC.[97,98]

There is also evidence suggesting that CMD may be present in as many 15% of patients during the acute period (ie, first 7 days post-onset), early detection of CMD is associated with recovery of at least partial functional independence at 1-year post injury[99] and favorable recovery occurs earlier in patients with CMD as compared to those without CMD.[100]

The term, *covert cortical processing (CCP),* has recently been proposed to describe a patients with DoC who do not show evidence of language comprehension on behavioral examination (eg, MCS-), but exhibit fMRI or EEG responses to spoken words or phrases.[93,101–106] Although CCP cannot provide definitive evidence of volitional cognitive processing, it may be a useful predictor of ongoing recovery.[107]

The 2018 AAN-ACRM-NIDILRR and the 2020 European Academy of Neurology DoC guidelines both recommend the use of advanced neuroimaging and EEG methods to assess for CMD in some circumstances.[9,10] These approaches are currently only available in select academic centers and their utility across healthcare systems is still being debated.[11,108,109] Nevertheless, when complemented by standardized behavioral evaluation, the direct assessment of consciousness via fMRI and EEG, has the potential to fundamentally change diagnosis, prognosis, and treatment for patients with DoC.[101]

SUMMARY

DoC taxonomy has progressed over the last 50 years as multidisciplinary practice guidelines have improved the consistency of nomenclature and diagnostic criteria. Recent work by the Neurocritical Care Society's Curing Coma Campaign provides an excellent example of international and interprofessional collaboration making strides toward clarity of diagnostic criteria and operational definitions within coma research. However, global consensus has not yet been achieved, compromising communication between clinicians and consumers, hindering epidemiologic studies, and complicating outcomes research. Future efforts should aim to establish a more rational DoC taxonomy that integrates behavioral and pathophysiologic characteristics.

CLINICS CARE POINTS

- Clinicians should adhere to evidence-based practice guidelines, such as those published by AAN-ACRM-NIDILLR in 2018, when conducting diagnostic assessment in patients with DoC.

- Despite advancements in DoC taxonomy, areas of ambiguity and disagreement persist, compromising diagnostic accuracy, prognostication, and family/caregiver counseling.

- Global interdisciplinary initiatives such as the Curing Coma Campaign provide an unprecedented opportunity for clinicians and investigators to establish uniform guidelines for a rational DoC taxonomy.

DISCLOSURE

No disclosures.

ACKNOWLEDGEMENTS

The contents of this manuscript were developed with support from the National Institute on Disability, Independent Living, and Rehabilitation Research (NIDILRR grant numbers: 90DPTB0011, 90DPTB0027). NIDILRR is a Center within the United States Administration for Community Living (ACL), Department of Health and Human Services (HHS) and the VA TBI Model System. The contents of this publication do not necessarily represent the policy of NIDILRR, ACL, HHS, and you should not assume endorsement by the United States Federal Government.

REFERENCES

1. Young MJ, Bodien YG, Giacino JT, et al. The neuroethics of disorders of consciousness: a brief history of evolving ideas. Brain 2021;144(11):3291–310.
2. Polansky R., Arstotle's de Anima: A Critical Commentary. Cambridge University Press, 2007. Book 1 of *Aristotle's de Anima*.
3. Plum F, Posner JB. The diagnosis of stupor and coma. Contemp Neurol Ser 1972;10:1–286.
4. Andrews K, Murphy L, Munday R, et al. Misdiagnosis of the vegetative state: retrospective study in a rehabilitation unit. BMJ 1996;313(7048):13–6.
5. Schnakers C, Vanhaudenhuyse A, Giacino J, et al. Diagnostic accuracy of the vegetative and minimally conscious state: clinical consensus versus standardized neurobehavioral assessment. BMC Neurol 2009;9(1):35.
6. Childs NL, Mercer WN, Childs HW. Accuracy of diagnosis of persistent vegetative state. Neurology 1993;43(8):1465.
7. Reed GM. Toward ICD-11: Improving the clinical utility of WHO's international classification of mental disorders. Prof Psychol Res Pr 2010;41(6):457–64.
8. Schiff ND. Cognitive motor dissociation following severe brain injuries. JAMA Neurol 2015;72(12):1413.
9. Giacino JT, Katz DI, Schiff ND, et al. Practice guideline update recommendations summary: disorders of consciousness: report of the guideline development, dissemination, and implementation subcommittee of the American academy of neurology; the American congress of rehabilitation medicine; and the national institute on disability, independent living, and rehabilitation research. Neurology 2018;91(10):450–60.
10. Kondziella D, Bender A, Diserens K, et al. European academy of neurology guideline on the diagnosis of coma and other disorders of consciousness. Eur J Neurol 2020;27(5):741–56.
11. Royal College of Physicians. Prolonged disorders of consciousness following sudden onset brain injury: National clinical guidelines. London: RCP; 2020.
12. Laureys S, Schiff ND. Coma and consciousness: paradigms (re)framed by neuroimaging. Neuroimage 2012;61(2):478–91.
13. Posner JB, Saper CB, Schiff ND, Plum F. Pathophysiology of signs and symptoms of coma. In: Posner JB, Saper CB, Schiff ND, Plum F, editors. Plum and Posner's diagnosis of stupor and coma. 4th ed. New York, NY: Oxford University Press; 2007. p. 3–37.
14. Schiff ND, Plum F. The role of arousal and "gating" systems in the neurology of impaired consciousness. J Clin Neurophysiol 2000;17(5):438–52.
15. Kinomura S, Larsson J, Gulyás B, et al. Activation by attention of the human reticular formation and thalamic intralaminar nuclei. Science 1996;271(5248):512–5.

16. Schiff ND. Central thalamic deep-brain stimulation in the severely injured brain: rationale and proposed mechanisms of action. Ann N Y Acad Sci 2009;1157(1): 101–16.
17. Medical aspects of the persistent vegetative state. N Engl J Med 1994;330(21): 1499–508.
18. Medical aspects of the persistent vegetative state. N Engl J Med 1994;330(22): 1572–9.
19. American Congress of Rehabilitation Medicine. Recommendations for use of uniform nomenclature pertinent to patients with severe alterations in consciousness. Arch Phys Med Rehabil 1995;76(2):205–9.
20. Andrews K. International working party on the management of the vegetative state: summary report. Brain Inj 1996;10(11):797–806.
21. Giacino J, Whyte J. The vegetative and minimally conscious states: current knowledge and remaining questions. J Head Trauma Rehabil 2005;20(1):30–50.
22. Giacino JT, Katz DI, Schiff ND, et al. Practice guideline update recommendations summary: disorders of consciousness. Arch Phys Med Rehabil 2018; 99(9):1699–709.
23. Giacino JT, Bodien YG, Zuckerman D, et al. Empiricism and rights justify the allocation of health care resources to persons with disorders of consciousness. AJOB Neuroscience 2021;12(2–3):169–71.
24. Koehler PJ, Wijdicks EFM. Historical study of coma: looking back through medical and neurological texts. Brain 2008;131(3):877–89.
25. Kretschmer E. Das apallische Syndrom. Z f d g Neur u Psych 1940;169(1): 576–9.
26. Giacino JT, Fins JJ, Laureys S, et al. Disorders of consciousness after acquired brain injury: the state of the science. Nat Rev Neurol 2014;10(2):99–114.
27. Fischer DB, Boes AD, Demertzi A, et al. A human brain network derived from coma-causing brainstem lesions. Neurology 2016;87(23):2427–34.
28. Provencio JJ, Hemphill JC, Claassen J, et al. The curing coma campaign: framing initial scientific challenges—proceedings of the first curing coma campaign scientific advisory council meeting. Neurocritical Care 2020; 33(1):1–12.
29. Helbok R, Rass V, Beghi E, et al. The curing coma campaign international survey on coma epidemiology, evaluation, and therapy (COME TOGETHER). Neurocritical Care 2022;37(1):47–59.
30. Kondziella D, Frontera JA. Pearls & Oy-sters: eyes-open coma. Neurology 2021; 96(18):864–7.
31. Kondziella D, Amiri M, Othman MH, et al. Incidence and prevalence of coma in the UK and the USA. Brain Communications 2022;4(5):fcac188.
32. Olson DM, Hemphill JC, The Curing Coma Campaign and its Executive Committe. The curing coma campaign: challenging the paradigm for disorders of consciousness. Neurocritical Care 2021;35(Suppl 1):1–3.
33. Claassen J, Akbari Y, Alexander S, et al. Proceedings of the first curing coma campaign NIH symposium: challenging the future of research for coma and disorders of consciousness. Neurocritical Care 2021;35(S1):4–23.
34. Adams ZM, Fins JJ. The historical origins of the vegetative state: received wisdom and the utility of the text. J Hist Neurosci 2017;26(2):140–53.
35. Bichat X. Recherches physiologiques sur la vie et la mort. Translated by Tobias Watkins. Philadelphia: Smith and Maxwell; 1809.

36. Timme W, Davis TK and Riley HA, The vegetative nervous system: an investigation of the most recent answers, In: Proceedings of the association of nervous and mental diseases, 1928, 3-11, Williams & Wilkins; Baltimore, MD.

37. Plum F, Schiff N, Ribary U, et al. The American Association for Research into Nervous and Mental Diseases, Coordinated expression in chronically unconscious persons. Phil Trans Roy Soc Lond B 1998;353(1377):1929–33.

38. Arnould M, Vigouroux R, Vigouroux M. Etats frontiers entre la vie et la mort en neuron-tramatologie. Neurochirurgica (Stuttg) 1963;(6):1–21.

39. Vapalahti M, Troupp H. Prognosis for patients with severe brain injuries. BMJ 1971;3(5771):404–7.

40. Jennett B, Plum F. Persistent vegetative state after brain damage. Lancet 1972; 299(7753):734–7.

41. Practice parameters [RETIRED]: assessment and management of patients in the persistent vegetative state (Summary statement). Neurology 1995;45(5): 1015–8.

42. Giacino JT, Ashwal S, Childs N, et al. The minimally conscious state: definition and diagnostic criteria. Neurology 2002;58(3):349–53.

43. Giacino JT, Zasler ND, Katz DI, et al. Development of practice guidelines for assessment and management of the vegetative and minimally conscious states. J Head Trauma Rehabil 1997;12(4):79–89.

44. Giacino J, Kalmar K. Diagnostic and prognostic guidelines for the vegwive and minimally conscious states. Neuropsychol Rehabil 2005;15(3–4):166–74.

45. Estraneo A, Moretta P, Loreto V, et al. Late recovery after traumatic, anoxic, or hemorrhagic long-lasting vegetative state. Neurology 2010;75(3):239–45.

46. Definition of state noun from the Oxford Advanced American Dictionary. Published online 2023. Available at: https://www.oxfordlearnersdictionaries.com/us/definition/american_english/state_1. Accessed May 1, 2023.

47. "Syndrome." Oxford Advanced American Dictionary. Published online 2023. Available at: https://www.oxfordlearnersdictionaries.com/us/definition/american_english/syndrome#:~:text=syndrome-,noun,is%20associated%20with%20frequent%20coughing. Accessed May 1, 2023.

48. Howard RS. The Vegetative state: Medical Facts, Ethical and Legal Dilemmas. Brain 2002;125(12):2782.

49. Laureys S., Celesia G.G., Cohadon F., et al., the European Task Force on Disorders of Consciousness, Unresponsive wakefulness syndrome: a new name for the vegetative state or apallic syndrome, BMC Med, 8(1), 2010, 68.

50. Bodien YG, Martens G, Ostrow J, et al. Cognitive impairment, clinical symptoms and functional disability in patients emerging from the minimally conscious state. NRE 2020;46(1):65–74.

51. Giacino JT, Sherer M, Christoforou A, et al. Behavioral recovery and early decision making in patients with prolonged disturbance in consciousness after traumatic brain injury. J Neurotrauma 2020;37(2):357–65.

52. Shewmon DA. The minimally conscious state: definition and diagnostic criteria. Neurology 2002;58(3):506 [author reply: 506-507].

53. Coleman D. The minimally conscious state: definition and diagnostic criteria. Neurology 2002;58(3):506 [author reply: 506-507].

54. Naccache L. Minimally conscious state or cortically mediated state? Brain 2018; 141(4):949–60.

55. Bayne T, Hohwy J, Owen AM. Reforming the taxonomy in disorders of consciousness. Ann Neurol 2017;82(6):866–72.

56. Whyte J, Nordenbo AM, Kalmar K, et al. Medical complications during inpatient rehabilitation among patients with traumatic disorders of consciousness. Arch Phys Med Rehabil 2013;94(10):1877–83.

57. Wannez S, Heine L, Thonnard M, et al, Coma Science Group collaborators. The repetition of behavioral assessments in diagnosis of disorders of consciousness. Ann Neurol 2017;81(6):883–9.

58. Demertzi A, Antonopoulos G, Heine L, et al. Intrinsic functional connectivity differentiates minimally conscious from unresponsive patients. Brain 2015;138(9):2619–31.

59. Bruno MA, Vanhaudenhuyse A, Thibaut A, et al. From unresponsive wakefulness to minimally conscious PLUS and functional locked-in syndromes: recent advances in our understanding of disorders of consciousness. J Neurol 2011;258(7):1373–84.

60. Bruno MA, Majerus S, Boly M, et al. Functional neuroanatomy underlying the clinical subcategorization of minimally conscious state patients. J Neurol 2012;259(6):1087–98.

61. Thibaut A, Bodien YG, Laureys S, et al. Minimally conscious state "plus": diagnostic criteria and relation to functional recovery. J Neurol 2020;267(5):1245–54.

62. World Health Organization (WHO). International Classification of Diseases, Eleventh Revision (ICD-11). Published online 2021 2019 Licensed under Creative Commons Attribution-NoDerivatives 3.0 IGO license (CC BY-ND 3.0 IGO). Available at: https://icd.who.int/browse. Accessed May 1, 2023.

63. Cairns H, Oldfield RC, Pennybacker JB, et al. Akinetic mutism with an epidermoid cyst of the 3rd ventricle. Brain 1941;64(4):273–90.

64. Giacino J. Disorders of consciousness: differential diagnosis and neuropathologic features. Semin Neurol 1997;17(02):105–11.

65. Formisano R, D'Ippolito M, Risetti M, et al. Vegetative state, minimally conscious state, akinetic mutism and Parkinsonism as a continuum of recovery from disorders of consciousness: an exploratory and preliminary study. Funct Neurol 2011;26(1):15–24.

66. Nagaratnam N, Nagaratnam K, Ng K, et al. Akinetic mutism following stroke. J Clin Neurosci 2004;11(1):25–30.

67. Fisher MC. Honored guest presentation: abulia minor vs. Agitated behavior. Neurosurgery 1984;31(Supplement 1):9–31.

68. Tibbetts PE. The anterior cingulate cortex, akinetic mutism, and human volition. Brain Mind 2001;2(3):323–41.

69. Royal College of Physicians. *Prolonged disorders of consciousness: national clinical guidelines.* London: RCP; 2020.

70. Inbody S, Jankovic J. Hyperkinetic mutism. Neurology 1987;37(9):1566.

71. Hesselink JMK, van Gijn J, Verwey JC. Hyperkinetic mutism. Neurology 1987;37(9):1566.

72. Laureys S, Pellas F, Van Eeckhout P, et al. The locked-in syndrome : what is it like to be conscious but paralyzed and voiceless? Prog Brain Res 2005;150:495–611. Elsevier.

73. M Das J, Anosike K, Asuncion RMD. Locked-in Syndrome. In: StatPearls. StatPearls Publishing; 2022. Available at: http://www.ncbi.nlm.nih.gov/books/NBK559026/. Accessed December 13, 2022.

74. Patterson JR, Grabois M. Locked-in syndrome: a review of 139 cases. Stroke 1986;17(4):758–64.

75. Giacino JT, Schnakers C, Rodriguez-Moreno D, et al. Behavioral assessment in patients with disorders of consciousness: gold standard or fool's gold? Prog Brain Res 2009;177:33–48. Elsevier.

76. Rodriguez Moreno D, Schiff ND, Giacino J, et al. A network approach to assessing cognition in disorders of consciousness. Neurology 2010;75(21):1871–8.

77. Nakase-Richardson R, Yablon SA, Sherer M, et al. Serial yes/no reliability after traumatic brain injury: implications regarding the operational criteria for emergence from the minimally conscious state. J Neurol Neurosurg Psychiatr 2008;79(2):216–8.

78. Nakase-Richardson R, Yablon SA, Sherer M, et al. Emergence from minimally conscious state: Insights from evaluation of posttraumatic confusion. Neurology 2009;73(14):1120–6.

79. Golden K, Erler KS, Wong J, et al. Should consistent command-following be added to the criteria for emergence from the minimally conscious state? Arch Phys Med Rehabil 2022;103(9):1870–3.

80. Weaver JA, Cogan AM, O'Brien KA, et al. Determining the hierarchy of coma recovery scale-revised rating scale categories and alignment with aspen consensus criteria for patients with brain injury: a rasch analysis. J Neurotrauma 2022;39(19–20):1417–28.

81. Symonds CP, Ritchie Russell W. Accidental head injuries. Lancet 1943;241(6227):7–10.

82. Stuss DT, Binns MA, Carruth FG, et al. The acute period of recovery from traumatic brain injury: posttraumatic amnesia or posttraumatic confusional state? J Neurosurg 1999;90(4):635–43.

83. Sherer M, Katz DI, Bodien YG, et al. Post-traumatic confusional state: a case definition and diagnostic criteria. Arch Phys Med Rehabil 2020;101(11):2041–50.

84. Sherer M, Nakase-Thompson R, Yablon SA, et al. Multidimensional assessment of acute confusion after traumatic brain injury. Arch Phys Med Rehabil 2005;86(5):896–904.

85. Slooter AJC, Otte WM, Devlin JW, et al. Updated nomenclature of delirium and acute encephalopathy: statement of ten Societies. Intensive Care Med 2020;46(5):1020–2.

86. Ropper AH, Samuels MA, Klein JP. Chapter 20. Delirium and other acute confusional states. In: Adams and victor's principles of neurology, 10e. The McGraw-Hill Companies; 2014. Available at: accessmedicine.mhmedical.com/content.aspx?aid=57615881. Accessed December 13, 2022.

87. Morandi A, Pandharipande P, Trabucchi M, et al. Understanding international differences in terminology for delirium and other types of acute brain dysfunction in critically ill patients. Intensive Care Med 2008;34(10):1907–15.

88. Disorders of attention: a frontier in neuropsychology. Phil Trans Roy Soc Lond B 1982;298(1089):173–85.

89. Pompei P, Foreman M, Rudberg MA, et al. Delirium in hospitalized older persons: outcomes and predictors. J Am Geriatr Soc 1994;42(8):809–15.

90. Brooks PB. Postoperative delirium in elderly patients. AJN, American Journal of Nursing 2012;112(9):38–49.

91. Pandharipande PP, Girard TD, Jackson JC, et al. Long-term cognitive impairment after critical illness. N Engl J Med 2013;369(14):1306–16.

92. Sherer M, Katz DI, Bodien YG. Seeking clarity about confusion. Arch Phys Med Rehabil 2021;102(2):339–40.

93. Edlow BL, Claassen J, Schiff ND, et al. Recovery from disorders of consciousness: mechanisms, prognosis and emerging therapies. Nat Rev Neurol 2021; 17(3):135–56.
94. Owen AM, Coleman MR, Boly M, et al. Detecting awareness in the vegetative state. Science 2006;313(5792):1402.
95. Schnakers C, Giacino JT, Løvstad M, et al. Preserved covert cognition in noncommunicative patients with severe brain injury? Neurorehabil Neural Repair 2015;29(4):308–17.
96. Gosseries O, Zasler ND, Laureys S. Recent advances in disorders of consciousness: focus on the diagnosis. Brain Inj 2014;28(9):1141–50.
97. Kondziella D, Friberg CK, Frokjaer VG, et al. Preserved consciousness in vegetative and minimal conscious states: systematic review and meta-analysis. J Neurol Neurosurg Psychiatr 2016;87(5):485–92.
98. Schnakers C, Hirsch M, Noé E, et al. Covert cognition in disorders of consciousness: a meta-analysis. Brain Sci 2020;10(12):930.
99. Claassen J, Doyle K, Matory A, et al. Detection of brain activation in unresponsive patients with acute brain injury. N Engl J Med 2019;380(26):2497–505.
100. Egbebike J, Shen Q, Doyle K, et al. Cognitive-motor dissociation and time to functional recovery in patients with acute brain injury in the USA: a prospective observational cohort study. Lancet Neurol 2022;21(8):704–13.
101. Edlow BL, Chatelle C, Spencer CA, et al. Early detection of consciousness in patients with acute severe traumatic brain injury. Brain 2017;140(9):2399–414.
102. Menon D, Owen A, Williams E, et al. Cortical processing in persistent vegetative state. Lancet 1998;352(9123):200.
103. Schiff ND, Plum F. Cortical function in the persistent vegetative state. Trends Cogn Sci 1999;3(2):43–4.
104. Coleman MR, Davis MH, Rodd JM, et al. Towards the routine use of brain imaging to aid the clinical diagnosis of disorders of consciousness. Brain 2009; 132(9):2541–52.
105. Fernández-Espejo D, Junqué C, Vendrell P, et al. Cerebral response to speech in vegetative and minimally conscious states after traumatic brain injury. Brain Inj 2008;22(11):882–90.
106. Di HB, Yu SM, Weng XC, et al. Cerebral response to patient's own name in the vegetative and minimally conscious states. Neurology 2007;68(12):895–9.
107. Sokoliuk R, Degano G, Banellis L, et al. Covert speech comprehension predicts recovery from acute unresponsive states. Ann Neurol 2021;89(4):646–56.
108. Wade DT, Turner-Stokes L, Playford ED, et al. Prolonged disorders of consciousness: a response to a "critical evaluation of the new UK guidelines". Clin Rehabil 2022;36(9):1267–75.
109. Scolding N, Owen AM, Keown J. Prolonged disorders of consciousness: a critical evaluation of the new UK guidelines. Brain 2021;144(6):1655–60.

Structural and Functional Neuroanatomy of Core Consciousness

A Primer for Disorders of Consciousness Clinicians

David B. Arciniegas, MD[a,b,c,d,*], Lindsey J. Gurin, MD[e,f,g],
Bei Zhang, MD, MSc[h]

KEYWORDS

- Consciousness • Coma • Unresponsive wakefulness state • Vegetative state
- Minimally conscious state • Neuroanatomy

KEY POINTS

- Core consciousness comprises wakefulness (arousal) and awareness.
- Wakefulness reflects the integrated and coordinated activation within and between brainstem neuronal groups (the ascending reticular activating system), the thalamus, and widespread excitatory efferents to the neocortex, with corresponding desynchronized cortical activity (a hallmark of wakefulness).
- Awareness reflects the integrated and coordinated activity within and between systems serving wakefulness with cortical areas within which ascending sensory, interoceptive, and motor information is presented and associatively processed.
- Emerging perspectives suggest that an account of phenomenal consciousness is usefully informed by consideration of alteration in anterior forebrain dynamics at the "mesocircuit" scale (ie, the mesocircuit hypothesis) as well as consequent and co-occurring alterations the large-scale default mode, salience, and central executive networks.

[a] Marcus Institute for Brain Health, University of Colorado Anschutz Medical Campus, Aurora, CO 80045, USA; [b] Department of Neurology, University of Colorado School of Medicine, Aurora, CO 80045, USA; [c] Department of Psychiatry, University of Colorado School of Medicine, Aurora, CO 80045, USA; [d] Department of Psychiatry and Behavioral Sciences, University of New Mexico School of Medicine, Albuquerque, NM 87131, USA; [e] Department of Neurology, NYU Grossman School of Medicine, New York, NY 10017, USA; [f] Department of Psychiatry, NYU Grossman School of Medicine, New York, NY 10016, USA; [g] Department of Physical Medicine & Rehabilitation, NYU Grossman School of Medicine, New York, NY 10016, USA; [h] Division of Physical Medicine and Rehabilitation, Department of Neurology, Texas Tech University Health Sciences Center, Lubbock, TX 79430, USA
* Corresponding author. 12348 E Montview Boulevard, Aurora, CO 80045.
E-mail address: david.arciniegas@cuanschutz.edu

Phys Med Rehabil Clin N Am 35 (2024) 35–50
https://doi.org/10.1016/j.pmr.2023.09.002

INTRODUCTION

The "hard problem" of explaining phenomenal consciousness and its relationship to brain-based physical processes has long occupied thinkers in fields ranging from neuroscience to philosophy to quantum physics.[1–3] The subjective (ie, individual experiential) nature of consciousness presents challenges to its objective study. As such, the assessment and scientific study of consciousness and its disorders in clinical contexts has relied first and foremost on observable behaviors as bases for drawing inferential conclusions about an individual patient's state of consciousness. Such observations and inferences define the disorders of consciousness, a set of syndromes in which the most basic elements of consciousness are demonstrably impaired; these include coma (defined by unresponsiveness without wakefulness or awareness), the unresponsive wakefulness syndrome (UWS, also known as vegetative state [VS]), and the minimally conscious state (MCS).

At the most basic levels, two fundamental functions establish core consciousness, or *sentience*: wakefulness (or arousal) and awareness. *Wakefulness*, the clinical manifestation of spontaneous or stimulus-induced activation of a brainstem-diencephalic set of structures and their modulatory projections to other subcortical and cortical systems, is a prerequisite for awareness. Awareness reflects the ability of the brain to engage in information processing at a level of complexity beyond the merely reflexive or automatic; it manifests clinically by cognitively mediated behavioral evidence of self-awareness and/or environmental awareness, even if such is rudimentary and present only inconsistently.[4,5] Both wakefulness and awareness are required for higher, more complex aspects of consciousness to develop, including sapience—that is, a state of (self-awareness and/or other) awareness that provides consciousness with a capacity for thought and rationality.[6] Impairments of wakefulness and/or awareness manifest clinically as disorders of consciousness. These include *coma*, in which both arousal and awareness are absent[7]; the UWS, in which arousal is preserved but there is no demonstrable evidence of awareness[8]; and the MCS, in which arousal is preserved and there is definite, although inconsistent, demonstrable evidence of at least rudimentary awareness of the self and/or environment.[4,9] *Cognitive-motor dissociation* (CMD),[10] a recent addition to the disorders of consciousness spectrum, in which there is functional neuroimaging-based (eg, functional magnetic resonance imaging-based [fMRI]) and/or clinical neurophysiologic (eg, electroencephalographic [EEG])—but not behavioral—evidence of at least minimal awareness, marks the first major departure from reliance on clinical (or "bedside") behavioral evidence for the diagnosis of disorders of consciousness and highlights the potential of advanced neurodiagnostic techniques to facilitate future discovery and expand clinical care in this area.

Indeed, modern neuroscientific technologies have made possible the visualization of neural activity (both preserved and impaired) in response to specific stimuli among persons with these disorders.[10–13] Although interpretation of such activity in relation to its experiential correlates does not fully obviate inferential reasoning regarding states of consciousness, its use in clinical practice reduces reliance on clinically observable motor behavior as a basis for inferentially drawing conclusions about an individual's state of consciousness—a distinct improvement in the fidelity of clinical assessment, particularly in patients whose clinical presentations are consistent with a disorder of consciousness (especially UWS) but in whom there is concern for CMD. These technologies have also facilitated a broader and more nuanced understanding and study of the clinical manifestations of consciousness and its impairments in these syndromes as well as an evidence-informed approach to clinical assessment and treatment.

In the service of supporting the evidence-informed work of disorders of consciousness clinicians, this article provides a primer on the structural and functional neuroanatomy of wakefulness and awareness. The neuroanatomical structures supporting these elements of core consciousness functions are reviewed first, after which brief description of the clinically evaluable relationships between disruption of these structures and disorders of consciousness (ie, brain–behavior relationships) are outlined. Consideration of neuroanatomy at the mesoscale (ie, the "mesocircuit hypothesis") as well as in relation to several large-scale neural networks is offered. Additionally, the distinction between the absence of wakefulness and the active process of sleep, as well as disruptions of the latter in the context of disorders of consciousness, is made. Implications for evaluation and treatment in relation to these neuroanatomic considerations also are noted, as are issues in need of further investigation.

NEUROANATOMY OF WAKEFULNESS AND AWARENESS

Arousal, the physiologic state of wakefulness and alertness, is a prerequisite for awareness and higher levels of consciousness, cognition, emotion, social behavior, and volitional and goal-directed motor behavior.[14] The level of arousal and the neural systems that support this most basic function establish both the context and capacity for other cognitive, emotional, and behavioral functions and, hence, the content of consciousness. In other words, wakefulness establishes readiness for and precipitates awareness.[15] Arousal occurs along a continuum and may be diminished, as in drowsiness, somnolence, or sleep; absent, as in coma; or heightened, as in the hyperarousal of hypomania, mania, posttraumatic stress disorders, or severe anxiety.

Wakefulness reflects the integrated and coordinated activation within and between brainstem neuronal groups (including noradrenergic, dopaminergic, histaminergic, orexin, serotonergic, and cholinergic neuronal groups/nuclei; collectively, the ascending reticular activating system [ARAS]) and basal forebrain cholinergic neurons projections to the thalamus (the reticulothalamic core) and other neocortical regions (ie, the reticulocortical projections), which provides widespread excitatory input to the neocortex and desynchronizes cortical activity (a hallmark of wakefulness).[16–19] Key features of the distributed neural networks supporting wakefulness are their multiplicity and redundancy, which together permit fine-tuning of an individual's response to the environment; these features also provide for the preservation of function in the face of failure of (eg, injury or insult to) many, although not all, single components within these networks.[20–22] These distributed reticulocortical, reticulothalamic, and thalamocortical networks establish this core component of consciousness and adjust the level of arousal to the requirements of the individual and environment (**Fig. 1**).

Wakefulness is both phenomenologically and neurobiologically in tension with sleep, with both circadian and shorter period cycles driving toward either wakefulness or sleep.[20,23] Proper functioning of both the arousal and sleep systems facilitates normal sleep–wake cycles.

Impaired arousal due to brain injury must be distinguished from the normal variations in arousal that occur in healthy individuals and also from alterations in arousal that follow administration of sedating medications (including at doses that may not be sedating among persons without brain injuries) or occur with toxic-metabolic disturbances.[24] Importantly, among patients with severe acquired brain injury, the capacity for arousal must be determined before evaluating motor and cognitive functions, and impairments of arousal must be considered when interpreting findings from such examinations.

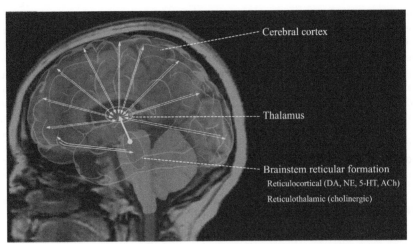

Fig. 1. The components of core consciousness: wakefulness and awareness. The brainstem reticular formation includes reticulothalamic and reticulocortical components. The reticulo-thalamic component is comprised principally by the cholinergic pedunculopontine and LDT nuclei (designated Ch5 and 6, respectively) and their efferents to the thalamus (ie, the dorsal tegmental pathway of Shute and Lewis). The reticulocortical component includes cell groups providing acetylcholine (Ch1 and 2 to the hippocampus; Ch4 to neocortical areas), dopamine (ventral tegmental area to limbic and neocortical areas; substantia nigra to basal ganglia), norepinephrine (locus ceruleus to limbic and neocortical areas), serotonin (dorsal and median raphe nuclei to widespread cerebral areas), orexin (lateral and posterior hypo-thalamic neurons to brainstem, diencephalic, and basal forebrain nuclei involved in the modulation of wakefulness), and histamine (tuberomammillary nuclear cells to widespread cerebral areas), schematically represented here by modulatory efferents to cortex and their top–down cortical afferents to these brainstem nuclei (*curved arrows*). Thalamocortical and corticothalamic projections (*straight arrows*) support the integration of systems supporting wakefulness with the areas necessary for awareness. The most relevant thalamic targets of the brainstem reticular nuclei to the disorders of consciousness include the intralaminar and reticular nuclei, which support activation and sampling, gating, and focusing of thalamo-cortical outputs, respectively. Together, these thalamic nuclei are part of the higher order (ie, nonsensory) thalamus and form extensive cortico-thalamo-cortical pathways, repre-sented here with pairs of thalamic efferent and afferent pathways.

As noted earlier, awareness—in clinical contexts—refers to cognitively mediated (ie, conscious) and behaviorally observable evidence of self-perception and action and/or environmental perception and action, even if such is rudimentary and present only inconsistently.[4] In this context, Lemaire and colleagues (2022) describe metag-nostic and metapractic aspects of consciousness, the former referring to the seman-tic (ie, meaningful) recognition of information received by sensory cortices, including somesthetic and interoceptive areas, whereas the latter refers to volitional (ie, willful) goal-directed sequencing of motor acts.[25] Both are higher level (ie, conscious or cognitive) aspects of the more fundamental information processing functions to which they are connected (ie, recognition and action, respectively) and yield observ-able behaviors related to an individual's internal drives and/or environmental de-mands.[25] Accordingly, awareness reflects the integrated and coordinated activity within and between systems serving wakefulness with cortical areas to and within which ascending sensory, interoceptive, and motor information is presented and associatively processed.

Ascending Reticular Activating System

The notion of an arousal system originating in the brainstem with ascending projections to cortex dates back to the mid-twentieth century. With the advent of EEG in 1925, a means of visualizing cortical activity associated with sleep and wakefulness became available; using it, early investigators sought to map the anatomy of arousal using animal brain lesion and stimulation paradigms. Bremer famously showed that transection at the level of the midbrain—but not the medulla—in cats caused the EEG to take on an appearance resembling sleep,[26,27] and subsequent investigators using lesional paradigms provided additional support for the existence of an upper brainstem system necessary for arousal. Other researchers used electrical stimulation to characterize the ascending projections originating from this crucial area. Demonstrating that stimulation to select brainstem and subcortical brain regions in anesthetized cats could produce an EEG appearance of arousal, Moruzzi and Magoun (1949) proposed the existence of a diffuse arousal-promoting network extending from the upper medulla to the thalamus that they called the ARAS.[28]

Initially believed to be a largely homogenous network, the ARAS is now understood to comprise a collection of distinct nuclei located in the midbrain and upper pons that provide stimulating input to the cortex directly and indirectly via thalamic and other subcortical relays. These nuclei and their associated projections, operating in parallel and in communication with each other, together give rise to a resilient subcortical arousal system in which substantial anatomic redundancy limits the ability of any single focal injury to abolish consciousness irreversibly.[29] The subcortical arousal systems are conceptually and structurally organized according to the dominant neurotransmitter produced by their respective nuclei of origin.

Ascending arousal system nuclei send projections to the cortex via one of two main routes: a dorsal, primarily cholinergic pathway that reaches the thalamus and a ventral, serotoninergic-noradrenergic pathway that reaches the hypothalamus and basal forebrain.[29] The cholinergic pedunculopontine tegmental (PPT, or Ch5) and laterodorsal tegmental (LDT, or Ch6) nuclei—collectively the Ch5–6 complex—project to the reticular nuclei of the thalamus,[21] which modulates excitatory (ie, glutamatergic) and inhibitory (ie, gamma-aminobutyric acid [GABA]) neurotransmission therein and permits the thalamus to provide tonic stimulation to the cortex.

Several other nuclei contribute stimulating inputs to the ascending arousal system. These include the basal forebrain cholinergic nuclei, which compromise the medial septal nucleus (Ch1) and vertical limb of the diagonal band of Broca (Ch2), both of which project via the fornix to the hippocampus, and the nucleus basalis of Meynert (Ch4), which projects broadly to limbic, paralimbic, and neocortical areas; the dopaminergic substantia nigra and ventral tegmental area in the midbrain; the noradrenergic locus coeruleus in the pons; the serotonergic raphe nuclei in the midbrain, pons, and upper medulla, and particularly the ascending projections of the median and dorsal raphe nuclei; the histaminergic cell group in the tuberomammillary nucleus; and orexin-producing neurons of the lateral and posterior hypothalamus and perifornical area.[30,31] The ascending arousal system receives modulatory (inhibitory) GABAergic projections from the ventrolateral preoptic nucleus (VLPO).[32]

These parallel systems work in an integrated and coordinated fashion to support the necessary level of arousal given prevailing (ie, in-the-moment) internal and environmental demands.[14] Although anatomic redundancy confers resilience to the effects of lesions to the systems subserving wakefulness, the high concentration of neuronal cell groups/nuclei in the upper brainstem (midbrain and pons) supporting this aspect of core consciousness creates vulnerability to compromise via destructive lesions.[26]

Indeed, relatively small lesions of key brainstem and diencephalic structures can cause profound suppression of arousal; examples of this can be seen in brainstem stroke and traumatic diffuse axonal injury and/or hemorrhage within the brainstem (ie, Duret hemorrhage).[33] In contrast, thalamic lesions without extension to the upper brainstem[34,35] and unilateral cortical injuries (even when large) have minimal direct influence on arousal, although such lesions may indirectly compromise wakefulness when large enough to exert mass effect (ie, compression) of the brainstem structures responsible for arousal. Otherwise, widespread regions of cortex bilaterally must be disrupted before arousal is impaired; examples of this include systemic toxic-metabolic disturbances, deep sedation, or generalized seizures.[14,36]

Coma due to brain injury is a state of "unarousable unawareness."[14] Although the phenomena characterizing coma are of variable duration, those occurring for seconds to minutes are more typically referred to by the term "loss of consciousness" (LOC) rather than as coma *per se*. Those that last beyond the durations in which LOC is the term more typically used (eg, mild traumatic brain injury, in which LOC is less than 30 minutes) are often described using the term coma. In general, coma progresses to higher states of consciousness (eg, UWS/VS, MCS, and posttraumatic confusional state) or to a prolonged condition, the latter of which often concludes either by the occurrence of brain death or by the withdrawal of life-sustaining care.[37–39] The emergence of spontaneous eye opening marks the transition from coma to UWS and indicates functional recovery of basic brainstem arousal mechanisms, although normal sleep–wake cycles may still be absent.[40,41]

Thalamus

The thalamus is a critical information processing hub and relay station for ascending arousal pathways. Bilateral thalamic injury—especially to the central thalamus—can cause disorders of consciousness.[41–44] The thalamic targets of the brainstem reticular nuclei include, among others, the intralaminar and reticular nuclei, which support activation, sampling, gating, and focusing of thalamocortical outputs.[45] Together, these thalamic nuclei are part of the higher order (ie, nonsensory) thalamus and form extensive cortico-thalamo-cortical pathways that are essential for the development of wakefulness and awareness.[18]

The location of thalamic damage seems to influence disability associated with traumatic brain injury, with neuronal loss in the mediodorsal parvocellularis, rostral center medial, central lateral, and paracentral nuclei observed in moderately disabled patients; in the mediodorsal magnocellularis, caudal center medial, rhomboid, and parafascicular nuclei in severely disabled patients; and in all of the above as well as the centromedian nucleus in patients with UWS/VS.[43] Because the central thalamus is particularly important to selective attention, sustained attention (vigilance), and working memory,[41] bilateral focal injuries to, deafferentation of, or destruction of efferents from the central thalamic subnuclei seem to produce disorders of consciousness. Damage in these areas may impair wakefulness and disturb basic attentional functions; the latter may be predicated on impaired arousal but may also be impaired themselves as a function of thalamic injury. Because these basic cognitive functions are required for awareness of and responsiveness to self and environment, thalamic (and, in particular, central thalamic) injury or dysfunction may contribute substantially to disruptions of core consciousness.[36,46] That said, the role of the thalamus in disorders of consciousness remains incompletely defined, a subject of at least occasional debate, and in need of further investigation, reflecting the complexity of the anatomy, connectivity, and function of this brain structure.[34,47–49]

Neural Circuitry of Core Consciousness at a Mesoscopic Scale

Schiff (2009),[41] extending the proposal by Bohland and colleagues (2009)[50] for a mesoscopic anatomic analysis for understanding neuroanatomical connectivity and corresponding brain–behavior relationships, suggests that large-scale forebrain dysfunction of the sort that is foundational to the disorders of consciousness develops via three general mechanisms: widespread death of forebrain neurons; widespread deafferentation and neuronal disconnection; and circuit-level functional disturbances resulting from deafferentation and neuronal disconnection. Although neuronal death is not reversible, recovery after severe brain injury may include at least partial restoration of afferentation across networks serving wakefulness and awareness (as well as higher cortical functions), both adaptive and potentially maladaptive.[51]

Schiff (2009)[52] posits that the negative consequences of alteration in anterior forebrain dynamics and corresponding alterations are best understood at the "mesocircuit" scale as reflecting global decreases of excitatory neurotransmission and consequent changes in background cerebral activity levels. Anchored to a frontal-subcortical model of information processing (eg, motor, and, by extension, cognitive, emotional, and social-behavioral) as described, among others, by Mega and Cummings (1994),[53] and as outlined in **Fig. 2**, a broad decrease in background synaptic activity and

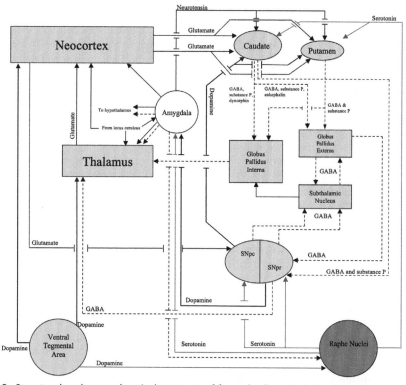

Fig. 2. Structural and neurochemical anatomy of frontal-subcortical circuitry relevant to disorders of consciousness. Solid lines indicate excitatory connections and dashed lines indicate inhibitory connections. Abbreviations: GABA, gamma-aminobutyric acid; SNpc, substantia nigra pars compacta; SNpr, substantia nigra pars reticulata. *Adapted from* Arciniegas DB. Diminished Motivation and Apathy. In Arciniegas DB, Beresford TP (eds). Neuropsychiatry: An Introductory Approach. Cambridge, Cambridge University Press, 2001, p.471.

excitatory neurotransmission will predictably result in diminished activation of the medium spiny neurons (MSNs) of the striatum (caudate and putamen). The MSNs maintain activity in the anterior forebrain via inhibitory projections to the globus pallidus interna (GPi), which, in turn, inhibits the central thalamus; MSN activation thereby reciprocally disinhibits central thalamic neurons, which increases thalamocortical transmission. Frontal cortex is innervated by thalamocortical projections from the central thalamus that, in a closed-loop circuit manner, project back to MSNs in the striatum.

Thalamocortical projections drive cortical excitation more robustly than do cortico-cortical projections. Accordingly, diminished thalamic output due to severe brain injury would be expected, under this hypothesis, to broadly diminish cortical activity.[41] As MSNs require relatively high levels of both dopamine and also background thalamostriatal and corticostriatal input in order to activate, broadly diminished cortical activity due to severe brain injuries sharply reduces MSN output. This hypothesis further holds that the anterior cingulate cortex features importantly among the prefrontal cortical areas to which this general circuit architecture and dynamics apply[53] because it is innervated by the anterior intralaminar nuclei (central lateral nucleus) and provides diffuse regulatory input on the rostral striatum.[41]

Reduced activity of the striatal MSNs to the GPi releases the latter structure from inhibition; this, in turn, results in the GPi tonically inhibiting the central thalamus. Following the circuit architecture noted above, inhibition of the central thalamus further and broadly reduces cortical and anterior forebrain activity. Conversely, interventions that augment function within these circuits—for example, agents that directly or indirectly augment dopaminergic function, stabilize glutamatergic function, inhibit GABA function at the alpha-1 subunit (which is densely expressed in the GPi), or otherwise enhance background cortical activity (as neurostimulation therapies may do)—may restore activity within these circuits and improve awareness and other cognitive functions.

Consistent with this hypothesis and this mesocircuit (mesoscale) perspective, the disorders of consciousness are associated with EEG evidence of diminished cortical activity, *vis-a-vis* diffuse slow wave (delta) activity, reflecting decreased firing rate of subcortical activating systems, excessive inhibition of the thalamus by the GPi, and/or large-scale cortical deafferentation.[47] Activity in these states is characterized by fMRI and/or EEG evidence of decreased cortical integration and, instead, increased modularity—that is, anatomic circuits and networks operating relatively separately from one another and, thereby, less adaptively. Cerebral EEG demonstrates the progression from diffuse slow wave activity (ie, delta, then to theta—the baseline frequencies associated with cortex freed from thalamic input and thalamocortical circuits without other inputs, respectively)[47,54,55] to faster frequencies (ie, alpha—the frequency of activated cortex ready to engage in information processing)[55] in association with the clinical progression from coma or UWS/VS to MCS and to behavioral evidence of consciousness.[52] These changes are interpreted as reflecting improved cortical activation and integration as systems subserving wakefulness and awareness, including anterior forebrain dynamics, recovery structurally and functionally after brain injury. The elements of the wakefulness-supporting and awareness-supporting systems considered in this mesocircuit perspective also constitute potential targets of intervention, particularly deep brain stimulation of the central lateral thalamus, given its essential role in promoting cortical activation and integration[56]; or vagal nerve stimulation, given the activity-promoting effects in the reticular formation, forebrain, and thalamus.[57]

Large-Scale Networks

The interactions between the neuroanatomical substrates of core consciousness (ie, wakefulness and awareness) and cortical areas, including large-scale cortical networks, in the development of consciousness has been and remains a subject of neuroscientific study and neurophilosophical inquiry.[3,25,58–60] Emerging perspectives suggest that an account of phenomenal consciousness is usefully informed by the anatomy and function of three key large-scale networks: the default mode, salience, and central executive networks.[3,25,61,62]

The *default mode network* refers to a set of structures that are functionally connected when a person is awake and at rest cognitively (ie, wakeful rest)[63,64]—for example, while daydreaming, thinking about others or themselves, thinking about past or future, or allowing their mind to wander nonspecifically from topic to topic.[65] In such states, a network of functionally connected structures activates; this network is principally composed of discrete, bilateral, and symmetric cortical areas in the medial prefrontal, medial and lateral parietal, and medial and lateral temporal cortices, with three major subdivisions: ventral medial prefrontal cortex, dorsal medial prefrontal cortex, and the posterior cingulate cortex and adjacent precuneus plus the lateral parietal cortex (approximately Brodmann area 39).[64,66] Subcortical structures, including the basal forebrain nuclei as well as the anterior and mediodorsal thalamic nuclei, are also involved in this network.[67] Given the function of this network, it stands to reason and has been observed in practice that activity of the default mode network is reduced among persons with UWS/VS (ie, in which awareness of self and environment is absent) and more typical in its activation among those with MCS (in which both the capacity for awareness is restored, even if such awareness is intermittent and/or inconsistently demonstrated).[68,69] Such observations suggest that the default mode network is an important element of the structural and functional neuroanatomy of core consciousness; these observation also raise the prospect, as has been suggested by clinical study, that this network (or key elements of it) may be useful diagnostic markers, and potentially prognostic markers, in the clinical assessment of persons with disorders of consciousness.[69,70]

The *salience network* (also known as the midcingulate-anterior insular network or the ventral attentional network)[71]—which has as key elements the dorsal anterior cingulate cortex and anterior insula—detects and filters salient stimuli and activates (ie, recruits) task-relevant functional networks. This network also facilitates detection, integration of sensory and emotional stimuli,[72] as well as switching between the default mode network (ie, internally directed cognition) and the central executive network (ie, externally directed cognition, described below).[73] As with the default mode network, compromised function of the salience network, along with the default mode network and the information processing domain-specific networks needed for auditory and visual function, distinguishes UWS/VS from MCS.[74,75]

The *central executive network* (also known as the frontoparietal network or lateral frontoparietal network) is principally composed of the dorsolateral prefrontal cortex (particularly the middle frontal gyrus) and the posterior parietal cortex (approximately the intraparietal sulcus).[72] As its name implies, this network supports executive function as well as sustained attention and working memory.[72] Given the higher level cognitive functions subserved by this network, disrupted functional connectivity of this network among persons with disorders of consciousness is not unexpected—and such disruptions distinguish between UWS/VS and MCS,[74,76] with lesser disruptions correlating with higher levels of consciousness[77] as measured by the Coma Recovery Scale-Revised.[78]

These large-scale networks, and particularly structures in the central executive network, constitute potential targets for noninvasive neurostimulation treatments (eg, transcranial direct cortical stimulation, repetitive transcranial magnetic stimulation [rTMS]) aimed at adaptively altering cortical activity and, through such activation, improving integration and function of the networks subserving wakefulness and awareness.[79,80]

SLEEP

As noted above, wakefulness is phenomenologically and neurobiologically in tension with sleep, with both circadian and shorter-period cycles driving toward either wakefulness or sleep.[20,23,81] Accordingly, a brief commentary on sleep and its neural mechanisms is needed in order to understand that tension and to distinguish the absence of wakefulness from the active process that is sleep.

Sleep–wake states are influenced by both circadian rhythms (the "circadian clock") and a hypothalamic switching circuitry (the so-called sleep/wake switch).[82,83] The circadian clock has its neurobiological bases in genetic feedback loops, the timing of the expression of which is relatively fixed; that is, clock genes code for clock proteins that are enzymatically transformed into transcription factors that suppress or activate the expression the genes of other clock proteins.[84] This clock is synchronized to day/night cycles predominantly by light, via the reticulothalamic tract projections from photosensitive retinal ganglion cells to the suprachiasmatic nucleus (SCN) as well as by other cues (including exercise, temperature, meals and their timing, and social interactions) that provide nonphotic entrainment via inputs from the thalamus and midbrain raphe nuclei to the SCN.[85] The SCN projects to other hypothalamic nuclei and the pineal gland, the secretion of melatonin from which regulates sleep, temperature, hormone fluctuations, and other bodily functions.[82]

The sleep switch reflects the reciprocal influences of the VLPO on the ARASs subserving wakefulness.[82,83] During sleep, VLPO inhibitory projections to the monoaminergic nuclei—especially the histaminergic tuberomammillary nucleus and the orexin-releasing lateral hypothalamus—decrease activity in the wakefulness-promoting ARAS, which in turn disinhibits (ie, releases) VLPO neurons to continue doing so, thereby maintaining sleep. During wakefulness, these same wakefulness-promoting systems project to the VLPO and inhibit its function, thereby disinhibiting (ie, releasing) them and further promoting wakefulness. This reciprocal relationship is analogous to a "flip-flop" switch in which the two halves of that switch each strongly inhibit each other and create a bistable feedback loop—one in which there are two possible stable firing patterns and no intermediate state. In humans, this sleep switch adaptively maintains either wakefulness or sleep, with only brief periods of transition between these states.[83]

Although the neuroanatomy and neurophysiology of sleep is more complex than the circadian and sleep-switch processes described briefly here, the structural and functional anatomy of these systems renders them vulnerable to damage and/or dysfunction that not only disturbs wakefulness and awareness but also impairs the regulation of sleep–wake cycles and the bistable sleep-switch for wakefulness and sleep. Consistent with this suggestion are the disturbances of sleep–wake cycles and abnormalities of sleep neurophysiology commonly observed among persons with disorders of consciousness, the delayed recovery of which are negative prognostic indicators in persons with UWS/VS.[86] Conversely, the recovery of sleep–wake cycles and normalization of sleep physiology may be a useful marker of neural recovery of the systems required not only for sleep but also, given their reciprocal influences, for those required for wakefulness and awareness—and, as such, are possible positive prognostic indicators for recovery and potential targets of treatment in person with disorders of consciousness.

SUMMARY

Understanding the structural and functional neuroanatomy of core consciousness (ie, wakefulness and awareness) is an asset to clinicians caring for persons with disorders of consciousness. Although the neuroscience of wakefulness and awareness remain active areas of investigation, consistent evidence regarding several brain–behavior relationships informs this area of study. Wakefulness (arousal) is supported by brainstem-forebrain-diencephalic systems; its development reflects the integrated and coordinated activation within and between brainstem neuronal groups (eg, the ARAS) and basal forebrain cholinergic neurons innervating the thalamus and other neocortical regions; and widespread excitatory efferents to the neocortex, with corresponding desynchronized cortical activity (a hallmark of wakefulness). Awareness reflects the integrated and coordinated activity within and between systems serving wakefulness with cortical areas to and within which ascending sensory, interoceptive, and motor information is presented and associatively processed. Its development reflects anterior forebrain dynamics and corresponding activity within frontal-subcortical circuits in which the central thalamus is a key node for global cortical activation.

Predictable and clinically evaluable relationships follow on disruption of the structure and function of the neural systems subserving wakefulness and awareness, and the nature of those disruptions informs not only the clinical presentation of disorders of consciousness but also the interventions (especially pharmacologic agents and/or neurostimulation methods) that may be offered to modify or remediate them. Additionally, distinguishing between the absence of wakefulness and the active process of sleep permits consideration of the interaction between the neural systems supporting consciousness and those producing sleep in relation to clinical presentation and treatment.

The current state of the science provides clinicians with deeper insights into the nature of these conditions and their clinical, ethical, and neurophilosophical implications than at any prior time. Although increasing access to practical, reliable, advanced neurodiagnostic methods will no doubt continue to further the scientific study and clinical assessment of the neural systems supporting core consciousness, it is hoped that the present primer on the structural and functional neuroanatomy of wakefulness and awareness will provide clinicians with information that enhances their medical knowledge about the disorders of consciousness and provides a context into which extant and emerging findings from the assessment and treatment literature can be placed.

CLINICS CARE POINTS

- Relatively small lesions of key brainstem and diencephalic structures can cause profound suppression of wakefulness. By contrast, thalamic lesions and unilateral cortical injuries usually have minimal direct influence on arousal; widespread regions of cortex must be disrupted bilaterally before wakefulness is impaired.

- The structural and functional (including neurochemical) anatomy of the frontal-subcortical circuits reveals multiple potential targets of pharmacotherapies for disorders of consciousness aimed at restoring activity within these circuits and improving awareness and other cognitive functions; these include agents that inhibit GABA function at the alpha-1 subunit in the GPi, directly or indirectly augment dopaminergic function, stabilize glutamatergic function, and/or augment cholinergic function.

- The elements of the wakefulness-supporting and awareness-supporting networks, especially at the mesocircuit scale and large-network scale, are potential targets of anatomically targeted treatments for disorders of consciousness, including deep brain stimulation, rTMS, transcranial direct current stimulation, or vagal nerve stimulation.

- The delayed recovery of sleep–wake cycle and abnormalities of sleep neurophysiology are negative prognostic indicators in persons with UWS/VS.

DECLARATIONS OF INTERESTS

The authors have no declarations of interests or disclosures to provide in relation to this work.

DISCLOSURES

None.

ACKNOWLEDGMENT

The authors gratefully acknowledge the support from the Marcus Institute for Brain Health at the University of Colorado Anschutz Medical Campus for the development of this work.

REFERENCES

1. Chalmers D. The Conscious Mind: in Search of a Fundamental Theory. New York, NY: Oxford University Press; 1997.
2. Dennett DC. Facing up to the hard question of consciousness. Philos Trans R Soc Lond B Biol Sci 2018;373(1755):20170342.
3. Churchland PS. A neurophilosophical slant on consciousness research. Prog Brain Res 2005;149:285–93.
4. Giacino JT, Ashwal S, Childs N, et al. The minimally conscious state: definition and diagnostic criteria. Neurology 2002;58(3):349–53.
5. Blumenfeld H. Chapter 1 - Neuroanatomical Basis of Consciousness. In: Laureys S, Gosseries O, Tononi G, editors. The Neurology of Conciousness. Second Edition. San Diego, CA: Academic Press; 2016. p. 3–29.
6. Yolles M. Consciousness, sapience and sentience—a metacybernetic view. Systems 2022;10(6):254.
7. Plum F, Posner JB. The diagnosis of stupor and coma. Contemp Neurol Ser 1972; 10:1–286.
8. Laureys S, Celesia GG, Cohadon F, et al. Unresponsive wakefulness syndrome: a new name for the vegetative state or apallic syndrome. BMC Med 2010;8:68.
9. Giacino JT, Katz DI, Schiff ND, et al. Comprehensive systematic review update summary: Disorders of consciousness: Report of the Guideline Development, Dissemination, and Implementation Subcommittee of the American Academy of Neurology; the American Congress of Rehabilitation Medicine; and the National Institute on Disability, Independent Living, and Rehabilitation Research. Neurology 2018;91(10):461–70.
10. Schiff ND. Cognitive motor dissociation following severe brain injuries. JAMA Neurol 2015;72(12):1413–5.
11. Cruse D, Chennu S, Chatelle C, et al. Bedside detection of awareness in the vegetative state: a cohort study. Lancet Lond Engl 2011;378(9809):2088–94.
12. Owen AM. Detecting consciousness: a unique role for neuroimaging. Annu Rev Psychol 2013;64:109–33.
13. Cruse D, Chennu S, Fernández-Espejo D, et al. Detecting awareness in the vegetative state: electroencephalographic evidence for attempted movements to command. PLoS One 2012;7(11):e49933.
14. Anderson CA, Filley CM, Arciniegas DB, et al. Arousal. In: Arciniegas DB, Anderson AC, Filley CM, editors. Behavioral Neurology & Neuropsychiatry. Cambridge, UK: Cambridge University Press; 2013. p. 88–97.

15. Di Perri C, Stender J, Laureys S, et al. Functional neuroanatomy of disorders of consciousness. Epilepsy Behav EB 2014;30:28–32.
16. Parvizi J, Damasio A. Consciousness and the brainstem. Cognition 2001;79(1–2):135–60.
17. Pfaff D, Ribeiro A, Matthews J, et al. Concepts and mechanisms of generalized central nervous system arousal. Ann N Y Acad Sci 2008;1129:11–25.
18. Saalmann YB. Intralaminar and medial thalamic influence on cortical synchrony, information transmission and cognition. Front Syst Neurosci 2014;8:83.
19. Mesulam MM. Attentional networks, confusional states, and neglect syndromes. In: Mesulam MM, editor. Principles of Behavioral and Cognitive Neurology. Second Edition. Oxford, UK: Oxford University Press; 2000. p. 174–256.
20. Rosenwasser AM. Functional neuroanatomy of sleep and circadian rhythms. Brain Res Rev 2009;61(2):281–306.
21. Arciniegas DB. Cholinergic dysfunction and cognitive impairment after traumatic brain injury. Part 1: the structure and function of cerebral cholinergic systems. J Head Trauma Rehabil 2011;26(1):98–101.
22. Pfaff D. Brain arousal and information theory: neural and genetic mechanisms. Cambridge, MA: Harvard University Press; 2005.
23. Herzog ED. Neurons and networks in daily rhythms. Nat Rev Neurosci 2007;8(10):790–802.
24. Arciniegas DB, Quinn DK, Silver JM. Pharmacotherapy of Cognitive Impairment. In: Zasler N, Katz DI, Zafonte R, editors. Brain Injury Medicine. Third edition. NY: Springer Publishing Company; 2023. p. 1137–49.
25. Lemaire JJ, Pontier B, Chaix R, et al. Neural correlates of consciousness and related disorders: From phenotypic descriptors of behavioral and relative consciousness to cortico-subcortical circuitry. Neurochirurgie 2022;68(2):212–22.
26. Grady FS, Boes AD, Geerling JC. A century searching for the neurons necessary for wakefulness. Front Neurosci 2022;16:930514.
27. Bremer F. Cerveau "isolé" et physiologie du sommeil. Paris): CR Soc Biol; 1935.
28. Moruzzi G, Magoun HW. Brain stem reticular formation and activation of the EEG. Electroencephalogr Clin Neurophysiol 1949;1(4):455–73.
29. Goldfine AM, Schiff ND. Consciousness: its neurobiology and the major classes of impairment. Neurol Clin 2011;29(4):723–37.
30. Burt J, Alberto CO, Parsons MP, et al. Local network regulation of orexin neurons in the lateral hypothalamus. Am J Physiol Regul Integr Comp Physiol 2011;301(3):R572–80.
31. Arciniegas DB. Executive function. In: Arciniegas DB, Anderson AC, Filley CM, editors. Behavioral Neurology & Neuropsychiatry. Cambridge, MA: Cambridge University Press; 2013. p. 225–49.
32. Brudzynski SM. The ascending mesolimbic cholinergic system–a specific division of the reticular activating system involved in the initiation of negative emotional states. J Mol Neurosci MN 2014;53(3):436–45.
33. Izzy S, Mazwi NL, Martinez S, et al. Revisiting grade 3 diffuse axonal injury: not all brainstem microbleeds are prognostically equal. Neurocrit Care 2017;27(2):199–207.
34. Lutkenhoff ES, Chiang J, Tshibanda L, et al. Thalamic and extrathalamic mechanisms of consciousness after severe brain injury. Ann Neurol 2015;78(1):68–76.
35. Hindman J, Bowren MD, Bruss J, et al. Thalamic strokes that severely impair arousal extend into the brainstem. Ann Neurol 2018;84(6):926–30.

36. Schiff ND, Plum F. The role of arousal and "gating" systems in the neurology of impaired consciousness. J Clin Neurophysiol Off Publ Am Electroencephalogr Soc 2000;17(5):438–52.

37. Giacino JT, Whyte J, Nakase-Richardson R, et al. Minimum competency recommendations for programs that provide rehabilitation services for persons with disorders of consciousness: A Position Statement of the American Congress of Rehabilitation Medicine and the National Institute on Disability, independent living and rehabilitation research traumatic brain injury model systems. Arch Phys Med Rehabil 2020;101(6):1072–89.

38. Turgeon AF, Lauzier F, Simard JF, et al. Mortality associated with withdrawal of life-sustaining therapy for patients with severe traumatic brain injury: a Canadian multicentre cohort study. CMAJ Can Med Assoc J J Assoc Medicale Can 2011; 183(14):1581–8.

39. Taran S, Gros P, Gofton T, et al. The reticular activating system: a narrative review of discovery, evolving understanding, and relevance to current formulations of brain death. Can J Anaesth J Can Anesth 2023;70(4):788–95.

40. Kobylarz EJ, Schiff ND. Neurophysiological correlates of persistent vegetative and minimally conscious states. Neuropsychol Rehabil 2005;15(3–4):323–32.

41. Schiff ND. Recovery of consciousness after brain injury: a mesocircuit hypothesis. Trends Neurosci 2010;33(1):1–9.

42. Adams JH, Graham DI, Jennett B. The neuropathology of the vegetative state after an acute brain insult. Brain J Neurol 2000;123(Pt 7):1327–38.

43. Maxwell WL, MacKinnon MA, Smith DH, et al. Thalamic nuclei after human blunt head injury. J Neuropathol Exp Neurol 2006;65(5):478–88.

44. Maxwell WL, Pennington K, MacKinnon MA, et al. Differential responses in three thalamic nuclei in moderately disabled, severely disabled and vegetative patients after blunt head injury. Brain J Neurol 2004;127(Pt 11):2470–8.

45. Anderson AC, Arciniegas DB, Hall DA, et al. Behavioral Neuroanatomy. In: Arciniegas DB, Anderson AC, Filley CM, editors. Behavioral Neurology & Neuropsychiatry. Cambridge, MA: Cambridge University Press; 2013. p. 12–31.

46. Castaigne P, Lhermitte F, Buge A, et al. Paramedian thalamic and midbrain infarct: clinical and neuropathological study. Ann Neurol 1981;10(2):127–48.

47. Koch C, Massimini M, Boly M, et al. Neural correlates of consciousness: progress and problems. Nat Rev Neurosci 2016;17(5):307–21.

48. Wilke M, Mueller KM, Leopold DA. Neural activity in the visual thalamus reflects perceptual suppression. Proc Natl Acad Sci U S A 2009;106(23):9465–70.

49. Panagiotaropoulos TI, Kapoor V, Logothetis NK. Subjective visual perception: from local processing to emergent phenomena of brain activity. Philos Trans R Soc Lond B Biol Sci 2014;369(1641). 20130534.

50. Bohland JW, Wu C, Barbas H, et al. A proposal for a coordinated effort for the determination of brainwide neuroanatomical connectivity in model organisms at a mesoscopic scale. PLoS Comput Biol 2009;5(3). e1000334.

51. McGinn MJ, Povlishock JT. Cellular and molecular mechanisms of injury and spontaneous recovery. Handb Clin Neurol 2015;127:67–87.

52. Schiff ND, Nauvel T, Victor JD. Large-scale brain dynamics in disorders of consciousness. Curr Opin Neurobiol 2014;25:7–14.

53. Mega MS, Cummings JL. Frontal-subcortical circuits and neuropsychiatric disorders. J Neuropsychiatry Clin Neurosci 1994;6(4):358–70.

54. Chennu S, Finoia P, Kamau E, et al. Spectral signatures of reorganised brain networks in disorders of consciousness. PLoS Comput Biol 2014;10(10). e1003887.

55. Arciniegas DB, Anderson A, Rojas DC. Electrophysiological Assessment. In: Silver JM, McAllister TW, Arciniegas DB, editors. Textbook of Traumatic Brain Injury. Third Edition. Cambridge, UK: American Psychiatric Association Publishing; 2019. p. 151–62.

56. Schiff ND. Mesocircuit mechanisms in the diagnosis and treatment of disorders of consciousness. Presse Medicale Paris Fr 1983 2022;52(2):104161.

57. Corazzol M, Lio G, Lefevre A, et al. Restoring consciousness with vagus nerve stimulation. Curr Biol CB 2017;27(18):R994–6.

58. Baars BJ, Geld N, Kozma R. Global Workspace Theory (GWT) and Prefrontal Cortex: Recent Developments. Front Psychol 2021;12:749868.

59. Fox MD, Snyder AZ, Vincent JL, et al. The human brain is intrinsically organized into dynamic, anticorrelated functional networks. Proc Natl Acad Sci U S A 2005; 102(27):9673–8.

60. Owen AM, Schiff ND, Laureys S. A new era of coma and consciousness science. Prog Brain Res 2009;177:399–411.

61. Chand GB, Dhamala M. Interactions Among the Brain Default-Mode, Salience, and Central-Executive Networks During Perceptual Decision-Making of Moving Dots. Brain Connect 2016;6(3):249–54.

62. Trambaiolli LR, Peng X, Lehman JF, et al. Anatomical and functional connectivity support the existence of a salience network node within the caudal ventrolateral prefrontal cortex. Elife 2022;11:e76334.

63. Raichle ME, MacLeod AM, Snyder AZ, et al. A default mode of brain function. Proc Natl Acad Sci U S A 2001;98(2):676–82.

64. Raichle ME. The brain's default mode network. Annu Rev Neurosci 2015;38: 433–47.

65. Gusnard DA, Raichle ME, Raichle ME. Searching for a baseline: functional imaging and the resting human brain. Nat Rev Neurosci 2001;2(10):685–94.

66. Greicius MD, Krasnow B, Reiss AL, et al. Functional connectivity in the resting brain: a network analysis of the default mode hypothesis. Proc Natl Acad Sci U S A 2003;100(1):253–8.

67. Alves PN, Foulon C, Karolis V, et al. An improved neuroanatomical model of the default-mode network reconciles previous neuroimaging and neuropathological findings. Commun Biol 2019;2:370.

68. Hannawi Y, Lindquist MA, Caffo BS, et al. Resting brain activity in disorders of consciousness: a systematic review and meta-analysis. Neurology 2015;84(12): 1272–80.

69. Bodien YG, Chatelle C, Edlow BL. Functional Networks in Disorders of Consciousness. Semin Neurol 2017;37(5):485–502.

70. Silva S, de Pasquale F, Vuillaume C, et al. Disruption of posteromedial large-scale neural communication predicts recovery from coma. Neurology 2015;85(23): 2036–44.

71. Uddin LQ, Yeo BTT, Spreng RN. Towards a Universal Taxonomy of Macro-scale Functional Human Brain Networks. Brain Topogr 2019;32(6):926–42.

72. Seeley WW, Menon V, Schatzberg AF, et al. Dissociable intrinsic connectivity networks for salience processing and executive control. J Neurosci Off J Soc Neurosci 2007;27(9):2349–56.

73. Sridharan D, Levitin DJ, Menon V. A critical role for the right fronto-insular cortex in switching between central-executive and default-mode networks. Proc Natl Acad Sci U S A 2008;105(34):12569–74.

74. Demertzi A, Antonopoulos G, Heine L, et al. Intrinsic functional connectivity differentiates minimally conscious from unresponsive patients. Brain J Neurol 2015; 138(Pt 9):2619–31.

75. Qin P, Wu X, Huang Z, et al. How are different neural networks related to consciousness? Ann Neurol 2015;78(4):594–605.

76. Demertzi A, Gómez F, Crone JS, et al. Multiple fMRI system-level baseline connectivity is disrupted in patients with consciousness alterations. Cortex J Devoted Study Nerv Syst Behav 2014;52:35–46.

77. Bruno MA, Majerus S, Boly M, et al. Functional neuroanatomy underlying the clinical subcategorization of minimally conscious state patients. J Neurol 2012; 259(6):1087–98.

78. Giacino JT, Kalmar K, Whyte J. The JFK Coma Recovery Scale-Revised: measurement characteristics and diagnostic utility. Arch Phys Med Rehabil 2004; 85(12):2020–9.

79. Liu S, Gao Q, Guan M, et al. Effectiveness of transcranial direct current stimulation over dorsolateral prefrontal cortex in patients with prolonged disorders of consciousness: A systematic review and meta-analysis. Front Neurol 2022;13: 998953.

80. O'Neal CM, Schroeder LN, Wells AA, et al. Patient Outcomes in Disorders of Consciousness Following Transcranial Magnetic Stimulation: A Systematic Review and Meta-Analysis of Individual Patient Data. Front Neurol 2021;12:694970.

81. Andrillon T. How we sleep: From brain states to processes. Rev Neurol (Paris) 2023. S0035-S3787(23)00997-00999.

82. Tallavahjula S, Rodgers J, Slater J. Sleep and Sleep-Wake Disorders. In: Silver JM, McAllister TW, Arciniegas DB, editors. Textbook of Traumatic Brain Injury. Third Edition. Washington, DC: American Psychiatric Association Publishing; 2019. p. 373–93.

83. Saper CB, Chou TC, Scammell TE. The sleep switch: hypothalamic control of sleep and wakefulness. Trends Neurosci 2001;24(12):726–31.

84. Lück S, Thurley K, Thaben PF, et al. Rhythmic degradation explains and unifies circadian transcriptome and proteome data. Cell Rep 2014;9(2):741–51.

85. Toh KL. Basic science review on circadian rhythm biology and circadian sleep disorders. Ann Acad Med Singapore 2008;37(8):662–8.

86. Raciti L, Raciti G, Militi D, et al. Sleep in Disorders of Consciousness: A Brief Overview on a Still under Investigated Issue. Brain Sci 2023;13(2):275.

Neuroimaging in Disorders of Consciousness and Recovery

Linda B. Xu, MD[a],*, Stephen Hampton, MD[b], David Fischer, MD[a],*

KEYWORDS

- Disorders of consciousness • Neuroimaging • Longitudinal
- Magnetic resonance imaging

KEY POINTS

- Neuroimaging biomarkers address a clinical need for more accurate diagnosis and prognostication in patients with disorders of consciousness (DoC).
- Various neuroimaging modalities evaluate structural and functional brain changes in DoC, with demonstrated diagnostic and prognostic value.
- Longitudinal studies have developed potential structural and functional neuroimaging biomarkers of recovery, with clinical implications for the management of DoC.

INTRODUCTION

Disorders of consciousness (DoC) encompass a range of conditions of disrupted arousal and/or awareness secondary to acquired brain injury.[1] Despite a significant socioeconomic burden of disease,[2] management of these patients remains challenging due to limitations in diagnostic and prognostic accuracy.[3,4] Consequently, outcomes are highly variable; some patients die or have life-sustaining treatment withdrawn, others recover consciousness, while still others may remain in a persistent unresponsive state for years without evidence of recovery.[5,6] Understanding the natural history of DoC is a topic of ongoing research, with important implications for decisions to maintain or withdraw life-sustaining treatment, as well as for the development of rehabilitation strategies and therapeutic targets.[7]

Existing diagnostic and prognostic tools include bedside clinical assessments, serum and cerebrospinal fluid biomarkers, neurophysiologic studies, and neuroimaging studies.[8-10] The JFK Coma Recovery Scale—Revised (CRS-R) is a widely used

ᵃ Department of Neurology, University of Pennsylvania, 3400 Spruce Street, Philadelphia, PA 19104, USA; ᵇ Department of Physical Medicine and Rehabilitation, University of Pennsylvania, 1800 Lombard Street, Philadelphia, PA 19146, USA
* Corresponding authors.
E-mail addresses: linda.xu@pennmedicine.upenn.edu (L.B.X.); david.fischer@pennmedicine.upenn.edu (D.F.)

Phys Med Rehabil Clin N Am 35 (2024) 51–64
https://doi.org/10.1016/j.pmr.2023.06.017
1047-9651/24/© 2023 Elsevier Inc. All rights reserved.

bedside assessment that categorizes DoC based on level of arousal and awareness,[11] including (1) the unresponsive wakeful state (UWS), or vegetative state (VS), defined as arousal without awareness, and (2) the minimally conscious state (MCS), defined as arousal with minimal and/or fluctuating awareness, which is further subdivided based on the absence (MCS-) or presence (MCS+) of language function.[12] Bedside assessments are relatively inexpensive and noninvasive, but their sensitivity is limited by examiner error, fluctuating patient exams, and sensorimotor impairment.[13–15] Neuroimaging assessments are less susceptible to these limitations and allow for objective and detailed characterization of brain structure and function in DoC.

While initial neuroimaging studies focused on structural changes seen on conventional magnetic resonance imaging (MRI), advances in neuroimaging technology now enable quantification of white matter tract structural integrity, cerebral metabolism and blood flow, and functional connectivity across brain networks.[16] These studies have attempted to differentiate patients with DoC from healthy controls, as well as UWS from MCS, particularly when neuroimaging findings may be discordant from clinical assessments. Prognostication efforts have also used various neuroimaging modalities to predict clinical outcome and likelihood of recovery of consciousness.

Here, we review neuroimaging studies in disorders of consciousness, with an additional focus on longitudinal neuroimaging assessments–that is, repeated neuroimaging assessments over time. Recovery after acquired brain injury may occur over years,[5,6] and evaluation in the acute phase may not accurately reflect the potential for long-term recovery.[17] Studies using longitudinal neuroimaging assessments may provide insight into the structural and functional correlates of recovery in DoC and offer strategies for more accurate prognostication.

STRUCTURAL IMAGING
Conventional Neuroimaging

Conventional structural neuroimaging, such as computed tomography (CT) and magnetic resonance imaging (MRI), is frequently acquired clinically and is relatively accessible to obtain and interpret. Studies using conventional CT and MRI have identified common regions of brain injury in DoC, which may shed light on brain regions critical to maintaining consciousness.

Studies using conventional neuroimaging have identified the corpus callosum and rostral dorsolateral brainstem as commonly injured regions in DoC.[18,19] Within the brainstem, injury to the pontine/midbrain tegmentum is associated with coma,[20,21] and nuclei in this region, including the parabrachial nucleus and locus coeruleus, are known to be critical for arousal.[21] Cortical lesions associated with loss of consciousness also exhibit functional connectivity to the brainstem tegmentum.[22] When separated by etiology, patients with traumatic brain injury (TBI) are more likely to have brainstem, hypothalamus, and cerebellar lesions,[23] which may be more susceptible to acceleration/deceleration forces against the skull base, while patients with anoxic injury have disproportionate involvement of the occipital lobes, potentially related to the failure of cerebral autoregulation.[24]

Patterns of injury observed acutely may have prognostic implications for recovery. Patients who remain in a vegetative state for greater than 12 months after TBI, compared to those who recover consciousness within 12 months, have more lesions in the corpus callosum, corona radiata, and dorsolateral brainstem, as well as more brain areas affected overall.[19] In patients with intracranial hemorrhage, presence of structural lesions in the midbrain peduncle and pontine tegmentum predicted impaired consciousness at the time of ICU discharge.[25] In patients with anoxic brain injury, injury to the occipital lobes may be associated with more severe and persistent impairments in consciousness.[24] A quantitative assessment of anoxic injury also has prognostic value; a small percentage of brain volume (<10–15%) with severe diffusion restriction (apparent diffusion coefficient <650–700 × 10^{-6} mm^2/s) predicts a favorable outcome with high sensitivity.[26,27]

Longitudinal Conventional Imaging

Studies have used conventional neuroimaging to evaluate structural brain changes over time in DoC (**Fig. 1**). Patients with chronic DoC demonstrate widespread cortical and subcortical atrophy.[23,28,29] The precise changes observed over time differ between patients who do and do not recover consciousness. One study combined seven

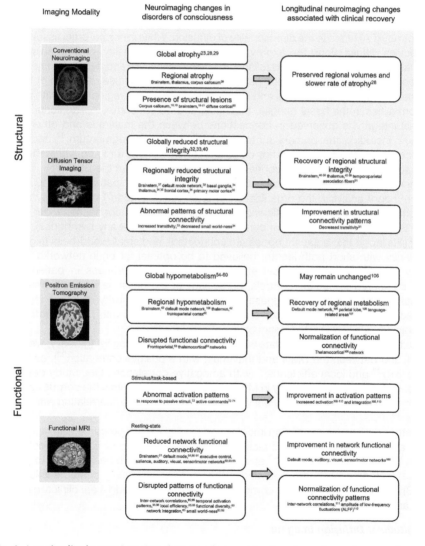

Fig. 1. Longitudinal neuroimaging changes observed in disorders of consciousness in association with clinical recovery.

measures of structural injury, including diffuse cortical atrophy, brainstem and/or thalamus degeneration, and corpus callosum lesions, to distinguish UWS from MCS with a sensitivity of 82.4%.[30] Structural features that discriminate between UWS and MCS include the degree of regional atrophy of the subcortical gray matter, long-ranging white matter tracts, and default mode network[28] (DMN; a functional brain network linked to consciousness and performance of internally directed tasks[31,32]). Rates of gray matter atrophy are also faster in UWS compared to MCS.[28] Patients with MCS+ , distinguished by retained language ability, demonstrate preserved left hemisphere volume compared to patients with MCS-.[23]

Diffusion Imaging

Diffusion tensor imaging (DTI) is a form of MRI that characterizes white matter tract structural integrity and connectivity based on properties of water molecule diffusion across tissues. Mean diffusivity (MD) refers to the overall degree of diffusion, while fractional anisotropy (FA) refers to the directionality of diffusion. While in normal brain tissue, water molecules diffuse along the axon with a coherent directionality, or high anisotropy, axonal injury would be expected to increase overall diffusivity and decrease anisotropy.

Compared to healthy controls, patients with DoC have diffuse reduction of FA and elevation of MD across cortical and subcortical white matter regions,[32,33] with greater abnormalities in the basal ganglia, thalamus, and frontal cortex.[34] Additional loss of axonal integrity is observed in connections between the thalamus and other structures,[35] including the primary motor cortex,[36] brainstem tegmentum,[37] and DMN, particularly involving the posterior cingulate cortex[32] (PCC, a region within the DMN that acts as a primary hub of connectivity between regions of the DMN[38]).

There is also evidence of altered structural connectivity patterns in DoC. Using graph theory analysis, the organization of brain region ("node") connectivity can be described based on local efficiency (average number of connections per node), path length (average number of connections required to link any two nodes), transitivity (likelihood that adjacent nodes are connected), and small world-ness (high local efficiency with short path length, believed to be optimal for brain networks[39]). One study reported decreased local efficiency and small world-ness in patients with DoC compared to healthy controls, particularly at the basal ganglia, thalamus, and frontal cortex,[34] generally suggestive of disrupted connectivity. Another study reported increased local efficiency and transitivity in patients with DoC, hypothesized to indicate locally restricted connectivity after injury.[33]

Multiple DTI measures correlate with CRS-R score, including FA (globally, within the DMN, and between the DMN and thalamus, with a positive correlation[32]), as well as transitivity[33] and local efficiency[34] (with a negative correlation). One study describes regions of increased anisotropy in MCS compared to UWS within the corpus callosum and multiple right-sided structures, with right-sided anisotropy correlating with CRS-R score.[40]

Metrics derived from diffusion imaging can predict clinical outcome with high sensitivity and specificity, in some cases outperforming standard clinical prognostication tools.[41,42] Both whole-brain[42,43] and ROI-based[44,45] FA have been shown to predict clinical outcome, with an area under the receiver operating characteristic curve (AUC) as high as 0.95,[42] while a composite DTI score predicted 1-year clinical outcome with an AUC of 0.84.[41]

Longitudinal Diffusion Imaging

Longitudinal DTI studies demonstrate potential for improvement, and even normalization, of white matter structural integrity after injury, with associated clinical recovery (see **Fig. 1**). In patients with recovery of consciousness, regional increases in structural connectivity have been observed within the ascending activating system of the brainstem,[46–49] particularly between the tegmentum and thalamus,[50] as well as at the temporoparietal associative fibers.[51]

One case report of repeated 7T DTI assessments in a patient with TBI found an initial decrease in left hemisphere connectivity at 1.5 months post-injury, followed by increased right hemisphere connectivity at 7.5 months, and finally increased left hemisphere connectivity again at 17.5 months.[52] These changes may reflect right-sided compensation for left hemisphere injury in the early chronic phase and were associated with clinical recovery from UWS to MCS. Regional recovery of structural connectivity may continue into the chronic phase of injury; in a patient with MCS for 19 years, initial imaging showed diffusely decreased FA, with focally increased FA above the level of healthy controls within the parieto-occipital white matter. On follow-up imaging 18 months later, this focally increased region had normalized, but a new area of increased FA was noted at the cerebellum, with associated clinical improvement in motor function and dysarthria.[53]

FUNCTIONAL IMAGING
Positron Emission Tomography

Positron emission tomography (PET) quantifies cerebral glucose metabolism (via fluorodeoxyglucose PET, or FDG-PET) or cerebral blood flow (via ^{15}O-radiolabeled water PET), both of which are linked to neuronal functional activity. PET can be used to map functional connectivity between brain regions by identifying temporal correlations in metabolic demand.

Patients with DoC demonstrate marked global hypometabolism, often below 50% of healthy controls.[54–60] A global metabolism of at least 42% of normal cortical activity may be required for the emergence of consciousness.[59] Hypometabolism can diffusely affect the cortical and subcortical gray matter, although some studies suggest relative preservation of metabolism in infratentorial structures.[54,57] Some patients demonstrate isolated regions of preserved metabolism, with intact behaviors reflective of those regions[58,61]; for instance, a patient with relatively preserved metabolism in language-related areas maintained the ability to produce isolated words.[58,62] Functional connectivity has also been found to be altered in DoC, including both thalamocortical connectivity[63] and connectivity between the premotor/prefrontal cortices and PCC.[64]

Patients with UWS demonstrate greater hypometabolism compared to those with MCS.[59,62] Patients with MCS demonstrate at least partially preserved activation within cortical networks and the frontoparietal association cortices,[65,66] and the absence of complete hypometabolism in the frontoparietal cortex can distinguish MCS from UWS with high sensitivity, potentially outperforming standardized clinical assessment.[67] Notably, the European Academy of Neurology currently recommends the use of PET, in addition to clinical and EEG-based measures, in the classification of patients with DoC.[68] Using PET paired with visual stimuli, patients without behavioral signs of consciousness on clinical assessment have demonstrated cerebral metabolism patterns comparable to those with MCS[69] and have been categorized as "non-behavioral MCS" or "MCS*."[70]

Patients with MCS+ demonstrate relatively preserved metabolism in language-related areas, while patients with MCS- demonstrate functional disconnection (poor temporal correlation of metabolic demand) between language-related areas.[12,71] Patients with MCS+ also demonstrate higher overall cerebral metabolism compared to those with MCS-.[71]

In terms of prognostication, global hypometabolism was not found to correlate with clinical outcome in two initial studies.[57,60] However, complete hypometabolism of the frontoparietal region was found to predict poor outcome (lack of recovery of consciousness by 12 months) with 92% accuracy.[67]

Functional Magnetic Resonance Imaging

Functional MRI (fMRI) assesses neuronal activity based on cerebral blood flow, using blood oxygen level dependent (BOLD) signal. fMRI studies include stimulus-based fMRI, task-based fMRI, and resting-state fMRI (rsfMRI).

Stimulus-based functional magnetic resonance imaging

In stimulus-based fMRI, patients are passively presented with stimuli of various sensory modalities, including tactile[72] and auditory[72–74] stimuli. In general, while patients with UWS are restricted to low-level activation of primary sensory cortices, patients with MCS demonstrate additional activation of higher-order association cortices similar to healthy controls.[72,73]

Task-based functional magnetic resonance imaging

In task-based fMRI, functional activation patterns are assessed as patients are given active commands, including language-based[75–77] and motor imagery tasks.[67,74,77–79] Notably, a subset of patients with no evidence of consciousness on clinical assessment can willfully modulate their brain activity in response to commands, similar to healthy controls.[67,73,74,76–80] This mismatch between the level of consciousness evident clinically and through technological assessment is termed cognitive motor dissociation (CMD), or "covert consciousness."[81] In some cases, these activation patterns can be used to facilitate communication,[78–80] for instance, instructing patients to complete a specific motor imagery task to respond "yes" versus "no" to a question.[78,79]

Resting-state functional magnetic resonance imaging

rsfMRI measures temporal correlations in BOLD signal between brain regions (ie, functional connectivity) while a patient is at rest. Studies using rsfMRI demonstrate widespread reduction of connectivity in DoC,[82–84] with disproportionate disruption of connectivity at functional "hubs," or areas of high interconnectedness.[85–87] Dysfunction is observed in several brain networks, most notably including the DMN,[84,86–91] thalamus,[86] and a functional brain network associated with the dorsolateral brainstem.[21] Connectivity in functional networks involved in extrinsic awareness may also correlate with level of consciousness, including in the executive control (ECN, involved in externally directed task performance[92]), salience (SN, diverts attention and resources between internal and external stimuli[92]), auditory, sensorimotor, and visual networks.[82,83,93]

Networks involved in intrinsic representation (eg, the DMN) are normally anticorrelated (ie, have a negative temporal correlation) with networks involved in external processing (eg, the SN and ECN),[94] and the strength and temporal pattern of this relationship is disrupted in patients with DoC.[95,96] Functional diversity, network integration, network complexity, and small world-ness are also reduced across multiple cortical networks and the DMN in patients with DoC.[83,89,95]

Compared to UWS, patients with MCS have increased functional connectivity overall,[82,93] as well as increased connectivity and local efficiency of the DMN/PCC[38,84,91] and SN.[91] Functional connectivity of the auditory network has demonstrated particularly high discriminatory power between UWS and MCS.[82] While patients with UWS favor low-complexity, low-efficiency states, patients with MCS spend more time in high-complexity, high-efficiency states and transition between states more often.[95,97]

Poor connectivity within and between the DMN/PCC,[88,90,98–104] SN,[101,104] and ECN[101,103] predicts poor clinical outcome. The degree of anticorrelation between the DMN and SN,[101] as well as whole brain cortico-cortical connectivity,[105] is also predictive of outcome. Notably, measures of functional connectivity may outperform both conventional clinical biomarkers[103] and diffusion-based prognostic biomarkers.[101,105]

Longitudinal Functional Studies

Studies have used PET to evaluate longitudinal changes in cerebral metabolism in DoC, showing evidence of metabolic recovery over time (see **Fig. 1**). A patient with hypoxic brain injury was imaged at 15 days (in UWS) and 37 days (after recovery of consciousness) post-injury. Initially, the patient had a 38% decrease in global metabolism compared to healthy controls, with regional hypometabolism in the primary sensorimotor cortices, parietal association cortices, and precuneus (PCu) of the DMN. After recovery of consciousness, global hypometabolism remained unchanged, but regional metabolism improved in the parietal lobes and PCu.[106] Patients who recovered from MCS- to MCS+ were also imaged before and after recovery, demonstrating improvement of regional hypometabolism, particularly within the PCu, thalamus, and language-related areas.[107]

Longitudinal studies using fMRI demonstrate increased activation and functional integration of multiple brain networks after recovery of consciousness (see **Fig. 1**).[108–110] Using stimulus-based fMRI paradigms, patients before recovery lacked differential activation between speech and non-speech stimuli[110] or demonstrated isolated left temporal activation in response to speech.[108] After recovery of consciousness, patients demonstrated robust activation in language areas[109,110] and integrated activation across multiple brain regions.[108,110] Similar improvements were demonstrated using visuospatial tasks, with the degree of activation reaching the range of healthy controls.[109]

In a patient with severe TBI, functional connectivity patterns across ten resting-state networks were found to improve in association with the clinical recovery of consciousness, including the DMN, sensorimotor, visual, and auditory networks.[109] Features of inter-network connectivity were also shown to recover over time, as initially absent inter-network anticorrelations and intra-network correlations within the DMN normalized after recovery of consciousness.[111] Amplitude of low-frequency fluctuations (ALFF), a measure of spontaneous neuronal activity at rest, normalized within the PCu in patients who demonstrated some degree of clinical improvement, while remaining unchanged in those without improvement.[112]

SUMMARY

Neuroimaging in DoC has provided a wealth of information in the last decades. With the advancement of neuroimaging technologies, the initial identification of brain regions injured in DoC has evolved to the characterization of complex structural and functional brain networks. Multimodal neuroimaging combining structural and functional techniques will likely be integral in the ongoing optimization of diagnosis and prognostication in DoC.

Findings in longitudinal neuroimaging studies suggest the potential for quantifiable structural and functional recovery. Updated research has demonstrated that the natural history of DoC is less pessimistic than once believed, and recovery in the chronic phase does occur.[113] Neuroimaging biomarkers provide a complement to clinical bedside assessments and may be valuable to track longitudinally, particularly in patients with prolonged unconsciousness. Elucidating the structural and functional changes that occur over time after acquired brain injury will likely have significant implications both in deepening our understanding of the natural history of DoC and in optimizing the long-term management of this patient population.

CLINICS CARE POINTS

- Bedside clinical assessments provide valuable diagnostic and prognostic information but may be limited by both examiner and patient factors.
- Quantifiable global and regional changes in brain volume, structural integrity, cerebral metabolism, and functional connectivity are observed in patients with DoC and show promise as diagnostic and prognostic biomarkers.
- Longitudinal neuroimaging may offer quantifiable structural and functional biomarkers of recovery, with potential implications in the long-term management of patients with DoC.

DISCLOSURE

The authors have no disclosures to report.

REFERENCES

1. Giacino JT, Fins JJ, Laureys S, et al. Disorders of consciousness after acquired brain injury: the state of the science. Nat Rev Neurol 2014;10(2):99–114.
2. Peterson A, Aas S, Wasserman D. What Justifies the Allocation of Health Care Resources to Patients with Disorders of Consciousness? AJOB Neurosci 2021;12(2–3):127–39.
3. Elmer J, Torres C, Aufderheide TP, et al. Association of early withdrawal of life-sustaining therapy for perceived neurological prognosis with mortality after cardiac arrest. Resuscitation 2016;102:127–35.
4. Pratt AK, Chang JJ, Sederstrom NO. A Fate Worse Than Death: Prognostication of Devastating Brain Injury. Crit Care Med 2019;47(4):591–8.
5. Katz DI, Polyak M, Coughlan D, et al. Natural history of recovery from brain injury after prolonged disorders of consciousness: outcome of patients admitted to inpatient rehabilitation with 1-4 year follow-up. Prog Brain Res 2009;177:73–88.
6. Nakase-Richardson R, Whyte J, Giacino JT, et al. Longitudinal outcome of patients with disordered consciousness in the NIDRR TBI Model Systems Programs. J Neurotrauma 2012;29(1):59–65.
7. Hammond FM, Katta-Charles S, Russell MB, et al. Research Needs for Prognostic Modeling and Trajectory Analysis in Patients with Disorders of Consciousness. Neurocrit Care 2021;35(Suppl 1):55–67.
8. Edlow BL, Claassen J, Schiff ND, et al. Recovery from disorders of consciousness: mechanisms, prognosis and emerging therapies. Nat Rev Neurol 2021;17(3):135–56.
9. Fischer D, Edlow BL, Giacino JT, et al. Neuroprognostication: a conceptual framework. Nat Rev Neurol 2022;18(7):419–27.
10. Sandroni C, D'Arrigo S, Cacciola S, et al. Prediction of good neurological outcome in comatose survivors of cardiac arrest: a systematic review. Intensive Care Med 2022;48(4):389–413.
11. Giacino JT, Kalmar K, Whyte J. The JFK Coma Recovery Scale-Revised: measurement characteristics and diagnostic utility. Arch Phys Med Rehabil 2004;85(12):2020–9.

12. Bruno MA, Majerus S, Boly M, et al. Functional neuroanatomy underlying the clinical subcategorization of minimally conscious state patients. J Neurol 2012;259(6):1087–98.
13. Andrews K, Murphy L, Munday R, et al. Misdiagnosis of the vegetative state: retrospective study in a rehabilitation unit. BMJ 1996;313(7048):13–6.
14. Schnakers C, Vanhaudenhuyse A, Giacino J, et al. Diagnostic accuracy of the vegetative and minimally conscious state: clinical consensus versus standardized neurobehavioral assessment. BMC Neurol 2009;9:35.
15. van Erp WS, Lavrijsen JC, Vos PE, et al. The vegetative state: prevalence, misdiagnosis, and treatment limitations. J Am Med Dir Assoc 2015;16(1):85.
16. Fischer D, Newcombe V, Fernandez-Espejo D, et al. Applications of Advanced MRI to Disorders of Consciousness. Semin Neurol 2022;42(3):325–34.
17. Giacino JT, Katz DI, Schiff ND, et al. Practice guideline update recommendations summary: Disorders of consciousness: Report of the Guideline Development, Dissemination, and Implementation Subcommittee of the American Academy of Neurology; the American Congress of Rehabilitation Medicine; and the National Institute on Disability, Independent Living, and Rehabilitation Research. Neurology 2018;91(10):450–60.
18. Kampfl A, Franz G, Aichner F, et al. The persistent vegetative state after closed head injury: clinical and magnetic resonance imaging findings in 42 patients. J Neurosurg 1998;88(5):809–16.
19. Kampfl A, Schmutzhard E, Franz G, et al. Prediction of recovery from post-traumatic vegetative state with cerebral magnetic-resonance imaging. Lancet 1998;351(9118):1763–7.
20. Parvizi J, Damasio AR. Neuroanatomical correlates of brainstem coma. Brain 2003;126(Pt 7):1524–36.
21. Fischer DB, Boes AD, Demertzi A, et al. A human brain network derived from coma-causing brainstem lesions. Neurology 2016;87(23):2427–34.
22. Snider SB, Hsu J, Darby RR, et al. Cortical lesions causing loss of consciousness are anticorrelated with the dorsal brainstem. Hum Brain Mapp 2020;41(6):1520–31.
23. Guldenmund P, Soddu A, Baquero K, et al. Structural brain injury in patients with disorders of consciousness: A voxel-based morphometry study. Brain Inj 2016;30(3):343–52.
24. Snider SB, Fischer D, McKeown ME, et al. Regional Distribution of Brain Injury After Cardiac Arrest: Clinical and Electrographic Correlates. Neurology 2022;98(12):e1238–47.
25. Rohaut B, Doyle KW, Reynolds AS, et al. Deep structural brain lesions associated with consciousness impairment early after hemorrhagic stroke. Sci Rep 2019;9(1):4174.
26. Bevers MB, Scirica BM, Avery KR, et al. Combination of Clinical Exam, MRI and EEG to Predict Outcome Following Cardiac Arrest and Targeted Temperature Management. Neurocrit Care 2018;29(3):396–403.
27. Hirsch KG, Fischbein N, Mlynash M, et al. Prognostic value of diffusion-weighted MRI for post-cardiac arrest coma. Neurology 2020;94(16):e1684–92.
28. Annen J, Frasso G, Crone JS, et al. Regional brain volumetry and brain function in severely brain-injured patients. Ann Neurol 2018;83(4):842–53.
29. Lutkenhoff ES, Chiang J, Tshibanda L, et al. Thalamic and extrathalamic mechanisms of consciousness after severe brain injury. Ann Neurol 2015;78(1):68–76.

30. Morozova S, Kremneva E, Sergeev D, et al. Conventional Structural Magnetic Resonance Imaging in Differentiating Chronic Disorders of Consciousness. Brain Sci 2018;8(8). https://doi.org/10.3390/brainsci8080144.

31. Buckner RL, Andrews-Hanna JR, Schacter DL. The brain's default network: anatomy, function, and relevance to disease. Ann N Y Acad Sci 2008;1124:1–38.

32. Fernandez-Espejo D, Soddu A, Cruse D, et al. A role for the default mode network in the bases of disorders of consciousness. Ann Neurol. Sep 2012; 72(3):335–43.

33. Tan X, Zhou Z, Gao J, et al. Structural connectome alterations in patients with disorders of consciousness revealed by 7-tesla magnetic resonance imaging. Neuroimage Clin 2019;22:101702.

34. Weng L, Xie Q, Zhao L, et al. Abnormal structural connectivity between the basal ganglia, thalamus, and frontal cortex in patients with disorders of consciousness. Cortex 2017;90:71–87.

35. Zheng ZS, Reggente N, Lutkenhoff E, et al. Disentangling disorders of consciousness: Insights from diffusion tensor imaging and machine learning. Hum Brain Mapp 2017;38(1):431–43.

36. Stafford CA, Owen AM, Fernandez-Espejo D. The neural basis of external responsiveness in prolonged disorders of consciousness. Neuroimage Clin 2019;22:101791.

37. Snider SB, Bodien YG, Bianciardi M, et al. Disruption of the ascending arousal network in acute traumatic disorders of consciousness. Neurology 2019;93(13): e1281–7.

38. Crone JS, Schurz M, Holler Y, et al. Impaired consciousness is linked to changes in effective connectivity of the posterior cingulate cortex within the default mode network. Neuroimage 2015;110:101–9.

39. Watts DJ, Strogatz SH. Collective dynamics of 'small-world' networks. Nature 1998;393(6684):440–2.

40. Tan X, Zhou Z, Gao J, et al. White matter connectometry in patients with disorders of consciousness revealed by 7-Tesla magnetic resonance imaging. Brain Imaging Behav 2022;16(5):1983–91.

41. Galanaud D, Perlbarg V, Gupta R, et al. Assessment of white matter injury and outcome in severe brain trauma: a prospective multicenter cohort. Anesthesiology 2012;117(6):1300–10.

42. Velly L, Perlbarg V, Boulier T, et al. Use of brain diffusion tensor imaging for the prediction of long-term neurological outcomes in patients after cardiac arrest: a multicentre, international, prospective, observational, cohort study. Lancet Neurol 2018;17(4):317–26.

43. Betz J, Zhuo J, Roy A, et al. Prognostic value of diffusion tensor imaging parameters in severe traumatic brain injury. J Neurotrauma 2012;29(7):1292–305.

44. Luyt CE, Galanaud D, Perlbarg V, et al. Diffusion tensor imaging to predict long-term outcome after cardiac arrest: a bicentric pilot study. Anesthesiology 2012; 117(6):1311–21.

45. Tollard E, Galanaud D, Perlbarg V, et al. Experience of diffusion tensor imaging and 1H spectroscopy for outcome prediction in severe traumatic brain injury: Preliminary results. Crit Care Med 2009;37(4):1448–55.

46. Jang SH, Chang CH, Jung YJ, et al. Change of ascending reticular activating system with recovery from vegetative state to minimally conscious state in a stroke patient. Medicine (Baltim) 2016;95(49):e5234.

47. Jang SH, Hyun YJ, Lee HD. Recovery of consciousness and an injured ascending reticular activating system in a patient who survived cardiac arrest: A case report. Medicine (Baltim) 2016;95(26):e4041.

48. Jang SH, Kim SH, Lim HW, et al. Recovery of injured lower portion of the ascending reticular activating system in a patient with traumatic brain injury. Am J Phys Med Rehabil 2015;94(3):250–3.

49. Jang SH, Lee HD. Recovery of multiply injured ascending reticular activating systems in a stroke patient. Neural Regen Res 2017;12(4):671–2.

50. Snider SB, Bodien YG, Frau-Pascual A, et al. Ascending arousal network connectivity during recovery from traumatic coma. Neuroimage Clin 2020;28: 102503.

51. Tan X, Gao J, Zhou Z, et al. Spontaneous Recovery from Unresponsive Wakefulness Syndrome to a Minimally Conscious State: Early Structural Changes Revealed by 7-T Magnetic Resonance Imaging. Front Neurol 2017;8:741.

52. Li X, Tan X, Wang P, et al. Chronic disorders of consciousness: a case report with longitudinal evaluation of disease progression using 7 T magnetic resonance imaging. BMC Neurol 2020;20(1):396.

53. Voss HU, Ulug AM, Dyke JP, et al. Possible axonal regrowth in late recovery from the minimally conscious state. J Clin Invest. Jul 2006;116(7):2005–11.

54. Beuthien-Baumann B, Handrick W, Schmidt T, et al. Persistent vegetative state: evaluation of brain metabolism and brain perfusion with PET and SPECT. Nucl Med Commun 2003;24(6):643–9.

55. DeVolder AG, Goffinet AM, Bol A, et al. Brain glucose metabolism in postanoxic syndrome. Positron emission tomographic study. Arch Neurol 1990;47(2): 197–204.

56. Levy DE, Sidtis JJ, Rottenberg DA, et al. Differences in cerebral blood flow and glucose utilization in vegetative versus locked-in patients. Ann Neurol 1987; 22(6):673–82.

57. Rudolf J, Ghaemi M, Ghaemi M, et al. Cerebral glucose metabolism in acute and persistent vegetative state. J Neurosurg Anesthesiol 1999;11(1):17–24.

58. Schiff N, Ribary U, Plum F, et al. Words without mind. J Cogn Neurosci 1999; 11(6):650–6.

59. Stender J, Mortensen KN, Thibaut A, et al. The Minimal Energetic Requirement of Sustained Awareness after Brain Injury. Curr Biol 2016;26(11):1494–9.

60. Tommasino C, Grana C, Lucignani G, et al. Regional cerebral metabolism of glucose in comatose and vegetative state patients. J Neurosurg Anesthesiol 1995;7(2):109–16.

61. Schiff ND, Ribary U, Moreno DR, et al. Residual cerebral activity and behavioural fragments can remain in the persistently vegetative brain. Brain 2002;125(Pt 6):1210–34.

62. Stender J, Kupers R, Rodell A, et al. Quantitative rates of brain glucose metabolism distinguish minimally conscious from vegetative state patients. J Cereb Blood Flow Metab 2015;35(1):58–65.

63. Laureys S, Faymonville ME, Luxen A, et al. Restoration of thalamocortical connectivity after recovery from persistent vegetative state. Lancet 2000; 355(9217):1790–1.

64. Laureys S, Goldman S, Phillips C, et al. Impaired effective cortical connectivity in vegetative state: preliminary investigation using PET. Neuroimage 1999;9(4): 377–82.

65. Boly M, Faymonville ME, Peigneux P, et al. Auditory processing in severely brain injured patients: differences between the minimally conscious state and the persistent vegetative state. Arch Neurol 2004;61(2):233–8.

66. Boly M, Faymonville ME, Schnakers C, et al. Perception of pain in the minimally conscious state with PET activation: an observational study. Lancet Neurol 2008; 7(11):1013–20.

67. Stender J, Gosseries O, Bruno MA, et al. Diagnostic precision of PET imaging and functional MRI in disorders of consciousness: a clinical validation study. Lancet 2014;384(9942):514–22.

68. Kondziella D, Bender A, Diserens K, et al. European Academy of Neurology guideline on the diagnosis of coma and other disorders of consciousness. Eur J Neurol 2020;27(5):741–56.

69. Menon DK, Owen AM, Williams EJ, et al. Cortical processing in persistent vegetative state. Wolfson Brain Imaging Centre Team. Lancet 1998;352(9123):200.

70. Thibaut A, Panda R, Annen J, et al. Preservation of Brain Activity in Unresponsive Patients Identifies MCS Star. Ann Neurol 2021;90(1):89–100.

71. Aubinet C, Cassol H, Gosseries O, et al. Brain Metabolism but Not Gray Matter Volume Underlies the Presence of Language Function in the Minimally Conscious State (MCS): MCS+ Versus MCS- Neuroimaging Differences. Neurorehabil Neural Repair 2020;34(2):172–84.

72. Schiff ND, Rodriguez-Moreno D, Kamal A, et al. fMRI reveals large-scale network activation in minimally conscious patents. Neurology 2005;64(3):514–23.

73. Di HB, Yu SM, Weng XC, et al. Cerebral response to patient's own name in the vegetative and minimally conscious states. Neurology 2007;68(12):895–9.

74. Edlow BL, Chatelle C, Spencer CA, et al. Early detection of consciousness in patients with acute severe traumatic brain injury. Brain 2017;140(9):2399–414.

75. Rodriguez Moreno D, Schiff ND, Giacino J, et al. A network approach to assessing cognition in disorders of consciousness. Neurology 2010;75(21):1871–8.

76. Monti MM, Rosenberg M, Finoia P, et al. Thalamo-frontal connectivity mediates top-down cognitive functions in disorders of consciousness. Neurology 2015; 84(2):167–73.

77. Owen AM, Coleman MR, Boly M, et al. Detecting awareness in the vegetative state. Science 2006;313(5792):1402.

78. Bardin JC, Fins JJ, Katz DI, et al. Dissociations between behavioural and functional magnetic resonance imaging-based evaluations of cognitive function after brain injury. Brain 2011;134(Pt 3):769–82.

79. Monti MM, Vanhaudenhuyse A, Coleman MR, et al. Willful modulation of brain activity in disorders of consciousness. N Engl J Med 2010;362(7):579–89.

80. Naci L, Owen AM. Making every word count for nonresponsive patients. JAMA Neurol 2013;70(10):1235–41.

81. Schiff ND. Cognitive Motor Dissociation Following Severe Brain Injuries. JAMA Neurol 2015;72(12):1413–5.

82. Demertzi A, Antonopoulos G, Heine L, et al. Intrinsic functional connectivity differentiates minimally conscious from unresponsive patients. Brain 2015;138(Pt 9):2619–31.

83. Martinez DE, Rudas J, Demertzi A, et al. Reconfiguration of large-scale functional connectivity in patients with disorders of consciousness. Brain Behav 2020;10(1):e1476.

84. Vanhaudenhuyse A, Noirhomme Q, Tshibanda LJ, et al. Default network connectivity reflects the level of consciousness in non-communicative brain-damaged patients. Brain 2010;133(Pt 1):161–71.

85. Achard S, Delon-Martin C, Vertes PE, et al. Hubs of brain functional networks are radically reorganized in comatose patients. Proc Natl Acad Sci U S A 2012; 109(50):20608–13.

86. Crone JS, Soddu A, Holler Y, et al. Altered network properties of the fronto-parietal network and the thalamus in impaired consciousness. Neuroimage Clin 2014;4:240–8.

87. Wu X, Zou Q, Hu J, et al. Intrinsic Functional Connectivity Patterns Predict Consciousness Level and Recovery Outcome in Acquired Brain Injury. J Neurosci 2015;35(37):12932–46.

88. Koenig MA, Holt JL, Ernst T, et al. MRI default mode network connectivity is associated with functional outcome after cardiopulmonary arrest. Neurocrit Care 2014;20(3):348–57.

89. Luppi AI, Craig MM, Pappas I, et al. Consciousness-specific dynamic interactions of brain integration and functional diversity. Nat Commun 2019;10(1):4616.

90. Norton L, Hutchison RM, Young GB, et al. Disruptions of functional connectivity in the default mode network of comatose patients. Neurology 2012;78(3):175–81.

91. Qin P, Wu X, Huang Z, et al. How are different neural networks related to consciousness? Ann Neurol 2015;78(4):594–605.

92. Liang X, Zou Q, He Y, et al. Topologically Reorganized Connectivity Architecture of Default-Mode, Executive-Control, and Salience Networks across Working Memory Task Loads. Cereb Cortex 2016;26(4):1501–11.

93. Medina JP, Nigri A, Stanziano M, et al. Resting-State fMRI in Chronic Patients with Disorders of Consciousness: The Role of Lower-Order Networks for Clinical Assessment. Brain Sci 2022;12(3). https://doi.org/10.3390/brainsci12030355.

94. Fox MD, Snyder AZ, Vincent JL, et al. The human brain is intrinsically organized into dynamic, anticorrelated functional networks. Proc Natl Acad Sci U S A 2005; 102(27):9673–8.

95. Demertzi A, Tagliazucchi E, Dehaene S, et al. Human consciousness is supported by dynamic complex patterns of brain signal coordination. Sci Adv 2019;5(2):eaat7603.

96. Di Perri C, Amico E, Heine L, et al. Multifaceted brain networks reconfiguration in disorders of consciousness uncovered by co-activation patterns. Hum Brain Mapp 2018;39(1):89–103.

97. Cao B, Chen Y, Yu R, et al. Abnormal dynamic properties of functional connectivity in disorders of consciousness. Neuroimage Clin 2019;24:102071.

98. Guo H, Liu R, Sun Z, et al. Evaluation of Prognosis in Patients with Severe Traumatic Brain Injury Using Resting-State Functional Magnetic Resonance Imaging. World Neurosurg 2019;121:e630–9.

99. Kondziella D, Fisher PM, Larsen VA, et al. Functional MRI for Assessment of the Default Mode Network in Acute Brain Injury. Neurocrit Care 2017;27(3):401–6.

100. Peran P, Malagurski B, Nemmi F, et al. Functional and Structural Integrity of Frontoparietal Connectivity in Traumatic and Anoxic Coma. Crit Care Med. Aug 2020; 48(8):e639–47.

101. Sair HI, Hannawi Y, Li S, et al. Early Functional Connectome Integrity and 1-Year Recovery in Comatose Survivors of Cardiac Arrest. Radiology 2018;287(1): 247–55.

102. Silva S, de Pasquale F, Vuillaume C, et al. Disruption of posteromedial large-scale neural communication predicts recovery from coma. Neurology 2015; 85(23):2036–44.

103. Song M, Yang Y, He J, et al. Prognostication of chronic disorders of consciousness using brain functional networks and clinical characteristics. Elife 2018;7doi. https://doi.org/10.7554/eLife.36173.

104. Wu GR, Di Perri C, Charland-Verville V, et al. Modulation of the spontaneous hemodynamic response function across levels of consciousness. Neuroimage 2019;200:450–9.

105. Pugin D, Hofmeister J, Gasche Y, et al. Resting-State Brain Activity for Early Prediction Outcome in Postanoxic Patients in a Coma with Indeterminate Clinical Prognosis. AJNR Am J Neuroradiol 2020;41(6):1022–30.

106. Laureys S, Lemaire C, Maquet P, et al. Cerebral metabolism during vegetative state and after recovery to consciousness. J Neurol Neurosurg Psychiatry 1999;67(1):121.

107. Aubinet C, Panda R, Larroque SK, et al. Reappearance of Command-Following Is Associated With the Recovery of Language and Internal-Awareness Networks: A Longitudinal Multiple-Case Report. Front Syst Neurosci 2019;13:8.

108. Bekinschtein T, Tiberti C, Niklison J, et al. Assessing level of consciousness and cognitive changes from vegetative state to full recovery. Neuropsychol Rehabil 2005;15(3–4):307–22.

109. Kazazian K, Norton L, Gofton TE, et al. Cortical Function in Acute Severe Traumatic Brain Injury and at Recovery: A Longitudinal fMRI Case Study. Brain Sci 2020;10(9). https://doi.org/10.3390/brainsci10090604.

110. Tomaiuolo F, Cecchetti L, Gibson RM, et al. Progression from Vegetative to Minimally Conscious State Is Associated with Changes in Brain Neural Response to Passive Tasks: A Longitudinal Single-Case Functional MRI Study. J Int Neuropsychol Soc 2016;22(6):620–30.

111. Threlkeld ZD, Bodien YG, Rosenthal ES, et al. Functional networks reemerge during recovery of consciousness after acute severe traumatic brain injury. Cortex 2018;106:299–308.

112. Zou Q, Wu X, Hu J, et al. Longitudinal recovery of local neuronal activity and consciousness level in acquired brain injury. Hum Brain Mapp 2017;38(7): 3579–91.

113. Giacino JT, Katz DI, Whyte J. Neurorehabilitation in disorders of consciousness. Semin Neurol 2013;33(2):142–56.

Disorders of Consciousness Programs
Components, Organization, and Implementation

Kristen A. Harris, MD*, Yi Zhou, MD, Stacey Jou, MD,
Brian D. Greenwald, MD

KEYWORDS

- Disorders of consciousness • Inpatient rehabilitation • Acquired brain injury

KEY POINTS

- Inpatient rehabilitation is recommended to maximize functional recovery and family training for patients with disorders of consciousness.
- Recommendations published by the American Academy of Neurology/American Congress of Rehabilitation Medicine and American Congress of Rehabilitation Medicine/National Institute on Disability, Independent Living and Rehabilitation Research Traumatic Brain Injury Model Systems provide a useful framework for the components of an effective rehabilitation program for patients with disorders of consciousness.
- Implementation of published guidelines into clinical practice requires familiarity with supporting evidence and available resources.

INTRODUCTION

Disorders of consciousness (DoC) exist on a continuum of pathologic altered consciousness resulting from severe acquired brain injury, with etiologies varying from traumatic brain injury to ischemic and hemorrhagic stroke, anoxic injury, malignancy, infection, and metabolic disorders. Patients with DoC have unique rehabilitation needs. Following acute hospitalization and medical stabilization, patients with DoC require multidisciplinary rehabilitation care from providers with specialized training in brain injury medicine. Recent guidelines have outlined best practices in caring for patients with DoC. In this study, we review practice guidelines including the 2018 update by the American Academy of Neurology/American Congress of Rehabilitation Medicine (AAN/ACRM) and subsequent minimum competency recommendations

JFK Johnson Rehabilitation Institute/Hackensack Meridian School of Medicine, Rutgers Robert Wood Johnson Medical School, 65 James Street, Edison, NJ 08820, USA
* Corresponding author.
E-mail address: Kristen.harris@hmhn.org

Phys Med Rehabil Clin N Am 35 (2024) 65–77
https://doi.org/10.1016/j.pmr.2023.06.014
pmr.theclinics.com

published by the American Congress of Rehabilitation Medicine and the National Institute on Disability, Independent Living and Rehabilitation Research (NIDILRR) Traumatic Brain Injury Model Systems in 2020.[1,2] Evidence supporting current guidelines is elaborated upon, and we include suggestions on how to operationalize recommendations into clinical practice.

The states of impaired consciousness in DoC consist of coma, vegetative state/unresponsive wakefulness (VS/UWS), and minimally conscious state (MCS), distinguished fundamentally by characteristic levels of arousal and awareness. The states of impaired consciousness in DoC have implications on evaluation, prognostication, therapy approach, and medical management. During recovery, patients do not necessarily progress sequentially through each state of disordered consciousness, which impacts medical rehabilitation management, rehabilitation therapies, and family counseling.

DISCUSSION
Acute Care Evaluation of Patients with Disorders of Consciousness

The first recommendation of the AAN/ACRM indicates that patients with DoC should be referred to an inpatient rehabilitation program with the goals of assessment and intervention for impaired consciousness, minimizing medical complications, maintaining overall health, promoting mobilization, and establishing means of communication. Typical qualifiers for inpatient neurorehabilitation, including anticipated tolerance of 3 hours of therapy per day, may not pertain to patients with DoC when advocating for acceptance to a dedicated DoC rehabilitation program. An acute care brain injury consult service can facilitate early diagnosis, family counseling, and post-acute placement for patients with DoC. Early support for specialized medical management of patients with DoC can positively impact recovery. One study supports that patients followed by a dedicated brain injury medicine consult service during their acute hospital stay had a higher likelihood of emergence from MCS during inpatient rehabilitation than those followed by a general physical medicine and rehabilitation consult service.[3] Admission to inpatient rehabilitation is critical for patients with DoC, with a large retrospective review demonstrating that patients discharged to home or inpatient rehabilitation had a significantly lower 3-year mortality than those discharged to skilled nursing facilities.[4]

Inpatient Disorders of Consciousness Rehabilitation Programs

Proper staffing with team members trained in the care of patients with DoC is crucial to delivering the comprehensive services expected of an effective DoC rehabilitation program. Programs should be staffed by an experienced multidisciplinary team, summarized in **Table 1**, including physicians with experience or trained in brain injury medicine, psychologists, rehabilitation nursing, social workers, nutritionists, and physical, occupational and speech therapists.[,2] An attending physician should be available on-site overseeing care at least 5 days per week with accompanying on-call coverage. Furthermore, there should be access to comprehensive consultation medical services to meet specialized medical management needs of patients with DoC such as internal medicine, neurology, neurosurgery, infectious disease, pulmonology, cardiology, otolaryngology, gastroenterology, and urology. The primary rehabilitation physician should establish rapport with consulting specialists to ensure clear and prompt communication, as well as familiarity with the unique management needs of patients with DoC.

All staff members of the multidisciplinary team should be adequately trained and educated on the most up-to-date evidence-based guidelines for the assessment

Table 1 Core components of a disorders of consciousness rehabilitation program	
Discipline	**Team Members**
Medical	Rehabilitation physician with experience in brain injury medicine Consulting physicians
Therapy	Physical therapist Occupational therapist Speech therapist
Nursing	Rehabilitation nursing Wound care nursing
Psychology	Rehabilitation psychologist Neuropsychologist
Social work	Experienced social worker
Nutrition	Nutritionist

and treatment of patients with DoC. For programs looking to bolster team-member training, there are resources available through state and national organizations. The Academy of Certified Brain Injury Specialists (https://www.biausa.org/professionals/ acbis) available through the Brain Injury Association of America (https://www. biausa.org) provides dedicated coursework and a certification for any team member providing care for patients with brain injuries. Additionally, programs can be certified as a Brain Injury Specialty Program by CARF International (http://carf.org/Brain-Injury-Specialty) if all program requirements are met. Staff members should be familiar with the roles of the multidisciplinary team so that the team may effectively and efficiently address individual patient needs, such as taking swift action when a patient is identified as requiring emergent medical attention. Understanding the expertise of others on the team and having daily coordination of care (at minimum between physician, nursing, therapy, and case management) and weekly team meetings will help identify any potential discipline-specific or team-wide issues and how each role on the team will contribute to addressing those issues and maximizing patient response to rehabilitation.

Disorder of Consciousness Diagnosis

Both the AAN/ACRM recommendations and ACRM minimum competency criteria emphasize the importance of accurate diagnosis to guide prognostication. DoC are challenging to diagnose with high rates of misdiagnosis ranging from 37% to 43% in some studies.[5] Misdiagnosis can lead to inaccurate prognostication that may in turn influence how management is approached, during both acute care and inpatient rehabilitation. Comprehensive patient assessment and diagnosis should be completed upon admission to a DoC rehabilitation program.

Validated scales can be useful to assist with accurate diagnosis. Scales frequently used in assessing patients with brain injury are summarized on the Center for Outcome Measurement in Brain Injury (COMBI) website, including background information, administration guidelines, and references (https://www.tbims.org/combi/list.html). The Glasgow Coma Scale (GCS) exists as the standard diagnostic scale in the acute care initial assessment of patients with brain injuries. The GCS evaluates eye opening, motor response, and vocalization but is lacking in its ability to detect subtle behavioral signs. The Ranchos Los Amigos Scale, also known as the Ranchos Scale, is a widely accepted scale describing behavioral and cognitive characteristics in brain injury patients. The Ranchos Scale is not limited to the initial assessment and is used throughout the recovery period after brain injury with sequential progression toward higher levels signifying improvements in cognition, behavior, and level of independence.

Behavioral assessment is the standard for evaluation of patients with DoC. A 2010 systematic review by the Disorders of Consciousness Task Force of the ACRM reviewed 13 behavioral assessment scales for DoC. The Task Force concluded that the JFK Coma Recovery Scale Revised (CRS-R), Sensory Stimulation Assessment Measure (SSAM), Wessex Head Injury Matrix (WHIM), Western Neuro Sensory Stimulation Profile (WNSSP), Sensory Modality Assessment Technique (SMART), Disorders of Consciousness Scale (DOCS), and Coma/Near Coma Scale (CNC) were acceptable given their standardized administration and scoring procedures. Of these 7 behavioral assessment scales, the CRS-R was the only scale that met all criteria for accessibility, standardization, and interpretive guidelines.[6] The CRS-R is strongly recommended as the measure of choice for all studies assessing recovery in DoC.[7]

The CRS-R is a standardized assessment scale that incorporates the diagnostic criteria of coma, VS/UWS, MCS, and emergence from MCS. It consists of a 23-item scale falling under 6 subscales addressing visual, auditory, motor, oromotor, communication, and arousal categories. The CRS-R assesses emergence of consciousness with the communication and motor subscales, specifically yes/no accuracy and functional object manipulation. Conducting the CRS-R can take up to 30 to 40 minutes, and provider experience increases interrater reliability.[8] It is recommended that staff completing CRS-R assessments be trained thoroughly, either by experienced team members, workshops, instructional videos, or lectures. Furthermore, dedicated team members should be assigned to perform the CRS-R assessment of patients to maximize proficiency with the scale. Any trained team member can perform the CRS-R, but it is often performed by speech therapy, occupational therapy, or neuropsychology.

Day-to-day fluctuations between vegetative and minimally conscious states are not unusual and contribute to diagnostic instability. Furthermore, unrecognized aphasia and apraxia can also confound accurate detection of emergence from MCS. Additional contributing factors of misdiagnosis include interrater variability, sleep/wake cycle disturbance, systemic medical problems, sedating medications, and sensorimotor impairment.[6] Confounding factors should be evaluated and managed prior to establishing a diagnosis. Anticipated fluctuations in responsiveness underscore the necessity of consecutive and thorough neurobehavioral examinations. Failing to detect clinical signs of consciousness can prematurely terminate neurorehabilitative treatment, impede communication, and in severe cases lead to inappropriate decisions regarding life-sustaining treatment.[6] The European Academy of Neurology (EAN) guidelines recommend that patients be diagnosed with the "highest level of consciousness" derived from any evaluation approach. Conversely, misdiagnosing reflexive or non-purposeful behavior as signs of consciousness can evoke unrealistic expectations of recovery, extend aggressive treatment, and prevent the transition to appropriate long-term disability care.[6]

Formal assessments of consciousness should be preceded by an attempt to increase arousal. Potential confounding medical problems should be considered and addressed prior to a formal assessment of consciousness. The JFK CRS-R Arousal Facilitation Protocol is additionally recommended to prolong the amount of time a patient maintains arousal, using unilateral deep muscle pressure to the face, neck, and shoulder. The muscle should be squeezed between the examiners thumb and forefinger, and then firmly rolled between the fingertips 3 to 4 times.[9]

In the diagnostic evaluation of DoC, the possibility of covert consciousness must also be considered. When there is cognitive motor dissociation a patient may have covert consciousness, or preserved consciousness that is not detected by traditional behavioral scales.[5,10] In cases where serial neurobehavioral assessment by the JFK CRS-R is insufficient for diagnosis, emerging alternate electrophysiologic tools may be able to augment physician evaluation. These may include functional MRI (fMRI), EMG thresholds for detecting response to motor commands, EEG reactivity laser-evoked potential responses, the Perturbational Complexity Index, and odorant-dependent sniff tests.[11–14] Access to assessment tools may vary across clinical settings, with some academic medical centers using new tools to assess for covert consciousness.[15] At minimum, if a patient with a DoC admitted to inpatient rehabilitation has not had a recent MRI during their acute care stay, it is recommended that one be obtained to assess for corpus callosal lesions, dorsolateral upper brainstem injury, or corona radiata injury which may be associated with a worse prognosis for recovery. Patients with covert consciousness may have better prognosis compared to those without, underscoring the importance of making efforts to detect signs of consciousness.[16]

Prognostication for Patients with Disorders of Consciousness

Early and accurate diagnosis assists DoC care providers in providing prognostic guidance for patients and their family members. Although initial discussions with patients' family should occur early after a patient's injury, the AAN/ACRM provides a Level A recommendation against the use of statements suggesting a universally poor prognosis when clinicians discuss prognosis with family members in the first 28 days post-injury. In discussing prognosis, it is important to acknowledge the uncertainties that often surround DoC diagnosis. Care providers in a DoC program must be mindful of how their own potential biases in the interpretation of diagnoses can lead to over- or underestimation of prognosis, and how that may subsequently impact the plan of care. "Undue pessimism," a term for provider attitudes toward what appears to be poor prognosis at the time of evaluation post-injury, may lead to premature consideration for decreasing or withdrawing treatments.[5,17] Evidence supports the recommendation to avoid and be mindful of undue pessimism, with findings from a Transforming Research and Clinical Knowledge in Traumatic Brain Injury (TRACK-TBI) study demonstrating that by 12 months post-injury approximately 52% of severe TBI patients had achieved favorable outcomes as measured by the GOSE.[18] Patients progressing to MCS within 5 months of injury generally have better long-term outcomes compared to those diagnosed with VS/UWS, and traumatic etiologies of brain injury tend to have a longer course of recovery but better overall outcomes compared to non-traumatic brain injuries.[1,19] It is important to be knowledgeable of the associated prognoses in each of these categories; however, patients with any of these DoC could still make meaningful recovery even beyond 1 to 2 years post-injury.[20] This is reflected by the Aspen Neurobehavioral Conference Workgroup's recommendation to move away from the term permanent VS/UWS, and that instead VS/UWS be used in association with the cause of injury and chronicity of time since onset given the implication on interpretation of outcomes. One study demonstrated that even between 14 and 28 months, as many as 20% of patients transitioned from VS/UWS to MCS.[18,21]

Prognosis can evolve over time and the DoC program should include regular patient re-assessment including serial examinations to help determine a trajectory of recovery. Findings over time in these examinations can guide physicians in discussion of prognosis with patients' surrogate decision makers. A patient's own rate of functional change is a major predictor of the likelihood of both functional improvement and return of consciousness.[22] Although there are a variety of tools used to predict outcomes, most have wide confidence intervals, and it is important to consider the applicability of a tool to the patient's specific circumstances.[2] Time post-injury may influence the utility of an individual predictor tool and it is important to consider this in the context of regular patient reassessment for prognostication purposes. In patients with prolonged traumatic VS/UWS, several adjuncts may be useful in guiding prognosis including Disability Rating Scale (DRS) scores less than 26 at 2 to 3 months post-injury, a detectable P300 at 2 to 3 months post-injury, a reactive EEG at 2 to 3 months post-injury, and a higher-level activation of the auditory association cortex using blood oxygen level-dependent fMRI in response to a familiar voice speaking the patient's name. Furthermore, it is recommended that for patients with non-traumatic, post-anoxic VS/UWS, clinicians should perform the CRS-R and may assess somatosensory evoked potentials (SEPs) to assist in prognostication at 24 months. In patients with non-traumatic post-anoxic VS, a JFK CRS-R score of 6 or higher at more than 1 month after onset of injury could indicate increased chances of recovery of some degree of consciousness by 24 months post-injury. The presence of SEPs from bilateral median nerve stimulation is also suggestive of potential for recovery of consciousness.[1] Depending on the practice environment or geographic area, access to certain diagnostic tools may be limited and the treating team should follow published guidelines using available resources.

It is recommended that initial family meetings occur early during a patient's admission to inpatient rehabilitation to discuss overall expectations for inpatient rehabilitation, offer education on DoC and acknowledge the challenges associated with prognostication. Ongoing caregiver counseling should occur throughout the inpatient rehabilitation stay, and is discussed in further detail later in this article.

Initial Medical Evaluation and Management for Patients with Disorders of Consciousness

Severe brain injury patients frequently have pre-existing comorbidities, concomitant injuries, and secondary effects of the brain injury that can impede recovery of consciousness and limit functional improvements. Therefore, essential to rehabilitation efforts is close management of medical complexity that facilitates recovery through maintenance of overall health. Upon admission of a new patient with DoC, it is important to evaluate the acute hospitalization problem list and determine the current status of each problem. The decision should then be made on whether to resume the diagnoses as active problems during acute inpatient rehabilitation. In optimizing continuation of pharmacologic management in inpatient rehabilitation, the adverse effects (ie, sedation) and medication interactions should be recognized. If possible, alternatives should be considered for agents carrying adverse risks. Medical complications can lead to rehospitalization that causes significant interruptions in rehabilitation progress. Additionally, data suggest that medical complications in patients with DoC predict outcome, highlighting the importance of careful management.[23,24] As noted earlier, it is essential that a physician is available for daily rounding and medical review, with 24 hour physician on-call availability and nursing care, access to diagnostic resources, and supports ease of specialist involvement.

Medical management during acute inpatient rehabilitation focuses on prevention and treatment of medical complications following TBI, which can occur frequently in the early period after injury. Common medical complications include seizures, paroxysmal sympathetic hyperactivity, post-traumatic agitation, spasticity, post-traumatic hydrocephalus, hypercoagulability, pressure wounds, and infections such as pneumonia and urinary tract infection. Common medical complications by organ system are summarized in **Table 2**. A study by Whyte and colleagues[25] found that hypertonia, agitation, urinary tract infection, and sleep disturbance were the most commonly

Table 2
Body systems complications in patients with disorders of consciousness

Body System	Examples
Neurologic	Hydrocephalus Hypertonia (spasticity/rigidity) Infections (meningitis/ventriculitis) Movement disorders Peripheral nerve injuries Pneumocephalus Post-traumatic headache Seizures Visual disturbance
Cardiac	Arrhythmia Hypertension Orthostatic hypotension Paroxysmal sympathetic hyperactivity
Pulmonary	Aspiration risk Neurogenic breathing patterns Pulmonary embolism Sleep apnea, obstructive or central Tracheostomy complications
Gastrointestinal	Dysphagia Erosive gastritis GERD and peptic ulcer disease Hypomotility syndromes Neurogenic bowel Nutritional compromise Tube feeding intolerance
Genitourinary	Bladder and renal calculi Infection risk Neurogenic bladder
Neuroendocrine	Anterior/posterior pituitary dysfunction Hypothalamic dysfunction
Fluid and electrolyte	Cerebral salt wasting Dehydration Diabetes insipidus Increased aldosterone production Syndrome of Inappropriate Antidiuretic Hormone Secretion (SIADH)
Musculoskeletal	Aberrant healing/exuberant callus Difficult immobilization strategies Heterotopic ossification Myositis ossificans Pain Spasticity Undiagnosed/occult fractures
Hematologic/vascular	Anemia Coagulopathy Deep vein thrombosis
Integumentary	Pressure injuries Skin tears

reported, whereas complications such as hydrocephalus, pneumonia, paroxysmal sympathetic hyperactivity, and gastrointestinal issues other than vomiting and diarrhea were most likely to be severe. Management of environmental factors in concert with medical care is also important in optimizing recovery for the patient with DoC. Poor positioning may cause discomfort, skin-breakdown, or limit detection of purposeful movement. Ambient noise may cause overstimulation or distract patient attention, and lighting may impact sleep-wake cycles.[26] Fluctuations in level of arousal in patients with DoC may thus be influenced by both medical and environmental factors. Clinicians may find it challenging to determine when a patient's fluctuation in arousal is relatively benign or represents an acute neurologic change. In this case, discussion among the patient's care team including skilled therapies and nursing can be helpful to ascertain the time course and context of the change. When these discussions are insufficient, access to prompt neuroimaging and laboratory evaluation is critical to rule out potential complications that could result in rehospitalization.

Pain can present a challenge in patients with altered consciousness. Less obvious sources of pain in the DoC patient population such as peripheral nerve lesions, intra-abdominal pathology, increased tone, and fractures can often be missed due to a decreased level of consciousness.[,17] Potential pain generators in patients with DoC are summarized in **Box 1**. Typical subjective signs of pain such as autonomic arousal, facial grimacing, or psychomotor agitation may be due to other causes in the DoC population. There is evidence through functional brain imaging to suggest that pain is not processed cortically in patients in a VS/UWS and therefore does not reach conscious perception.[27] However, there is data to suggest that patients in MCS are able to perceive noxious stimuli.[27] Although pain should always be assessed regardless of level of consciousness, clinicians should exercise caution when deciding on the presence of pain. If clinical suspicion is increased, it is justified to investigate underlying sources of pain. In a patient experiencing episodes of paroxysmal sympathetic hyperactivity, pain should be recognized as a common trigger and investigated. Cognitive and behavioral improvements, detected through serial standardized

---

Box 1
Potential pain generators in patients with disorders of consciousness

Pain source

Headache

Central or peripheral neuropathic pain

Spasticity

Heterotopic ossification

Healing fractures

Wounds

Gastric feeding tube

Constipation

Cholelithiasis

Urinary tract infection

Nephrolithiasis

Tracheostomy

Deep vein thrombosis

neurobehavioral assessments, may increase pain perception but also allow clinicians to better identify and manage pain in patients with DoC. For the initial management of pain, mild analgesics are warranted such as nonsteroidal anti-inflammatory drugs (NSAIDs), aspirin, and acetaminophen as they are generally well-tolerated. For moderate pain, the trial of other NSAIDs such as celecoxib or acetaminophen with caffeine can be considered. Opiates should be avoided due to their unfavorable risk profile. If opiates are necessary for severe pain, one would first consider mixed opiate analgesics such as oxycodone/acetaminophen and tramadol. If initiated, medications should be given on a standing basis as patients will not reliably be able to express a need for pain medication. Additionally, if opiates are needed to manage pain for patients with DoC, they should be initiated with a plan to taper over time as most pain generators should abate in the longer term. Stimulants such as modafinil can also be considered to counter opiate-induced sedation.[27]

Amantadine has been demonstrated to accelerate functional recovery in patients with post-traumatic DoC.[28] Research demonstrates a benefit of amantadine in the 4 to 16 weeks post-injury; however, in clinical practice amantadine is often used outside of this window. If there are no medical contraindications, amantadine should be initiated early in the rehabilitation course. It is appropriate to begin with a dose of 100 mg twice daily and continue for 7 days, at which time the physician may consider an increase to 150 mg in the second week and to 200 mg twice daily in the third week. Research suggests titration to 200 mg twice daily if the Disability Rating Scale (DRS) score had not improved by at least 2 points from baseline; however, in clinical practice the CRS-R is more often used to assess improvement. Higher doses of amantadine theoretically increase seizure risk, so dosage increases past 200 mg twice daily is not recommended. Additionally, zolpidem has been demonstrated to improve level of consciousness in 5% of patients with DoC, although responders are not able to be identified in advance from non-responders.[29] High-quality conclusive evidence is lacking for behavioral improvements following neuromodulatory pharmacologic agents such as modafinil, bromocriptine, levodopa, apomorphine, and intrathecal baclofen.[30,31] There is also a lack of evidence to support increasing the number of stimulant medications. However, medications with limited evidence can still be considered to assist with medical management if the risk of use is considered to be low and the physician is actively monitoring any positive or negative medication effects.[2]

Similarly, newer nonpharmacologic therapeutic considerations such as stem cell therapy, invasive deep brain stimulation, and hyperbaric oxygen lack sufficient evidence to conclusively support or reject their use at this time. Clinicians should engage in thoughtful discussion with families seeking counsel on alternative therapies for their loved ones, recognizing their desire to maximize recovery. Clinicians caring for patients with DoC will be involved in treatment discussions during the rehabilitation process, necessitating ongoing active learning of current evidence for intervention advancements to inform discussions. Additionally, physicians caring for patients with DoC should be aware of the high cost of many novel treatments and the vulnerable position from which families may pursue these treatments.

Family Counseling and Transition from an Inpatient Disorders of Consciousness Program

Identifying patient and family preferences on admission to the DoC program and then revisiting those preferences throughout the recovery process will inform how to approach next steps in management. The patient is often unable to advocate for themselves so clear identification of the patient's personal values through family members and any preexisting legal documents will help to guide subsequent care decisions. When explaining rehabilitation care to families, time should be taken to understand patient and family preferences. Clinicians should also be prepared to sensitively navigate these conversations. The COMFORT model, supported by the Comfort Communication Project, LLC, summarizes key qualities to incorporate into conversation: simple and direct language, acknowledging gaps in knowledge and knowing when to seek further information, and never forcing the recipient to lose hope.[2] Rapport must be established and maintained with families/caregivers to help facilitate the joint decision-making process. It is also important for a DoC program to have resources available for identifying and addressing caregiver needs or caregiver burden, whether it be related to an informational deficit, instrumental need, or emotional need.[2]

When involving patients and their families in the decision-making process, leaders of the multidisciplinary team should describe the facets of the patient's recovery that remain uncertain.[5] In an appropriate level of detail for the information recipient (based on how much they want to know and what outcomes are important to them), the range of care options and possible outcomes should be presented.[2,5] The Model Systems Knowledge Translation Center provides fact sheets on the many facets of brain injury that may be helpful to share with family members and care givers (https://msktc.org/tbi/factsheets). To promote goal-concordant care throughout the rehabilitation process, the daily workflow of an effective DoC program should involve maintaining regular contact with the appointed surrogate decision-maker. Allowing the surrogate decision-maker to interact with different members of the multidisciplinary team as needed also facilitates understanding of the care the patient is receiving. Minimum competency recommendations indicate that acute rehabilitation programs should additionally establish access to ethics consults or an affiliated ethics committee when guidance is needed in navigating uncertainties associated with DoC rehabilitation.[2]

Understanding patient and family preferences is also important if clinical research is occurring in the DoC rehabilitation setting. Ongoing studies provide promising advances that could improve patient care and outcomes, such as using novel neuroimaging to help identify covert consciousness or use of new pharmacologic agents. Clinicians should weigh the risks and benefits of implementing research into patient care and maintain transparency with patients and families while making these considerations. Policies should be established for identifying situations where nonstandardized treatments described in the literature may be beneficial to maximize patient outcomes.

The likelihood of recovery in consciousness decreases as more time passes postinjury. Although a minority of patients considered to be in chronic VS/UWS could still recover consciousness later, most of these patients continue to have severe disability requiring care services.[1] For a patient entering the chronic stage of VS/UWS, prognostic counseling should be centered around planning for long-term assistive care. The clinician should discuss with surrogate decision-makers different options for long-term care, including care facilities or private residence with optional visiting services. Medical follow-up and regularly scheduled medications should be discussed as well. If applicable, over time the clinician should also assist surrogate decision-makers with determining when it may be appropriate to call upon palliative care services based on the patient's specific circumstances and goals of care. Long-term decision-making support is not standardized in the current system of care for patients with DoC, especially outside of acute and subacute care settings.[5] A dedicated DoC specialist following patients longitudinally is recommended to ensure that patients with chronic DoC continue to receive goal-concordant care that meets their long-term needs.

A DoC program should have team members who are knowledgeable in planning for long-term disability and are capable of providing guidance to families/caregivers on making proper arrangements for long-term care. In the current health care environment, patients with DoC who do not show early enough functional gains typically do not stay in high-intensity rehabilitation settings long enough for future functional improvements to be observed, despite potential for change. It is important for care providers to provide appropriate anticipatory counseling to families so they have time to make appropriate arrangements. Ideally on admission to a DoC program, guidelines should be in place for establishing code status, identifying appointed surrogate decision-maker(s) for the patient, and filling out state-specific forms regarding medical decision-making if possible.[1] The social worker or case manager can assist with application for disability benefits and provide community resources to the patient and their caregiver(s).

Transition to less intensive care settings should be considered when functional status, goals, and medical needs are unlikely to change in the near future. The care provider should formulate a structured, individualized discharge plan that aims to simplify patient care such that it may be more feasible for caregivers or facilities that are more resource-constrained.[2] In transitioning care, good communication must be maintained with outside facilities, families, and caregivers to minimize having any disruptions in the patient's care. Determining follow-ups with specialists is also an integral part of long-term care planning.

SUMMARY

Admission to a dedicated rehabilitation program for patients with DoC is important to optimize recovery, medical stability, and caregiver training and support. Many patients with DoC can regain consciousness, and a comprehensive rehabilitation program is instrumental in promoting recovery. Practice guidelines and minimum competency recommendations established by national stakeholders provide a framework for the effective implementation and management of a DOC rehabilitation program.

CLINICS CARE POINTS

- Referral to an inpatient rehabilitation program is both critical and often-overlooked for patients with DoC.
- Goals of inpatient rehabilitation for patients with DoC include accurate diagnosis, prognostication, management of medical complications following TBI, trial of neurostimulation, and family education.
- Published resources from the AAN, ACRM and NIDILRR TBI Model Systems can be helpful in establishing an effective DoC rehabilitation program.

DISCLOSURE

There are no disclosures or conflicts of interest reported by the authors. No funding was received by the authors for this work.

REFERENCES

1. Giacino JT, Katz DI, Schiff ND, et al. Practice guideline update recommendations summary: disorders of consciousness: report of the guideline development,

dissemination, and implementation subcommittee of the american academy of neurology; the american congress of rehabilitation medicine; and the national institute on disability, independent living, and rehabilitation research. Neurology 2018;91(10):450–60, published correction appears in Neurology. 2019 Jul 16;93(3):135.

2. Giacino JT, Whyte J, Nakase-Richardson R, et al. Minimum competency recommendations for programs that provide rehabilitation services for persons with disorders of consciousness: a position statement of the American congress of rehabilitation medicine and the national institute on disability, independent living and rehabilitation research traumatic brain injury model systems. Arch Phys Med Rehabil 2020;101(6):1072–89.

3. Weppner JL, Linsenmeyer MA, Wagner AK. Effects of an acute care brain injury medicine continuity consultation service on health care utilization and rehabilitation outcomes. PM R 2021;13(11):1227–36.

4. Davidson GH, Hamlat CA, Rivara FP, et al. Long-term survival of adult trauma patients. JAMA 2011;305(10):1001–7.

5. Young MJ, Bodien YG, Giacino JT, et al. The neuroethics of disorders of consciousness: a brief history of evolving ideas. Brain 2021;144(11):3291–310.

6. American Congress of Rehabilitation Medicine, Brain Injury-Interdisciplinary Special Interest Group, Disorders of Consciousness Task Force, Seel RT, Sherer M, et al. Assessment scales for disorders of consciousness: evidence-based recommendations for clinical practice and research. Arch Phys Med Rehabil 2010; 91(12):1795–813.

7. Wilde EA, Whiteneck GG, Bogner J, et al. Recommendations for the use of common outcome measures in traumatic brain injury research. Arch Phys Med Rehabil 2010;91(11):1650–60.e17.

8. Eapen BC, Georgekutty J, Subbarao B, et al. Disorders of consciousness. Phys Med Rehabil Clin N Am 2017;28(2):245–58.

9. Giacino JT, Kalmar K, Whyte J. The JFK coma recovery scale-revised: measurement characteristics and diagnostic utility. Arch Phys Med Rehabil 2004;85(12): 2020–9.

10. Schiff ND. Cognitive motor dissociation following severe brain injuries. JAMA Neurol 2015;72(12):1413–5.

11. Comanducci A, Boly M, Claassen J, et al. Clinical and advanced neurophysiology in the prognostic and diagnostic evaluation of disorders of consciousness: review of an IFCN-endorsed expert group. Clin Neurophysiol 2020;131(11):2736–65.

12. Arzi A, Rozenkrantz L, Gorodisky L, et al. Olfactory sniffing signals consciousness in unresponsive patients with brain injuries. Nature 2020;581(7809):428–33.

13. Casali AG, Gosseries O, Rosanova M, et al. A Theoretically Based Index of Consciousness Independent of Sensory Processing and Behavior. Sci Transl Med 2013;5(198):198ra05.

14. Edlow BL, Fins JJ. Assessment of covert consciousness in the intensive care unit: clinical and ethical considerations. J Head Trauma Rehabil 2018;33(6):424–34.

15. Young MJ, Edlow BL. The quest for covert consciousness: bringing neuroethics to the bedside. Neurology 2021;96(19):893–6.

16. Claassen J, Doyle K, Matory A, et al. Detection of brain activation in unresponsive patients with acute brain injury. N Engl J Med 2019;380(26):2497–505.

17. Capizzi A, Woo J, Verduzco-Gutierrez M. Traumatic brain injury: an overview of epidemiology, pathophysiology, and medical management. Med Clin North Am 2020;104(2):213–38.

18. McCrea MA, Giacino JT, Barber J, et al. Functional outcomes over the first year after moderate to severe traumatic brain injury in the prospective, longitudinal TRACK-TBI study. JAMA Neurol 2021;78(8):982–92.
19. Giacino JT, Kalmar K. The vegetative and minimally conscious states: a comparison of clinical features and functional outcome. J Head Trauma Rehabil 1997; 12(4):293–8.
20. Nakase-Richardson R, Whyte J, Giacino JT, et al. Longitudinal outcome of patients with disordered consciousness in the NIDRR TBI Model Systems Programs. J Neurotrauma 2012;29(1):59–65.
21. Estraneo A, Moretta P, Loreto V, et al. Late recovery after traumatic, anoxic, or hemorrhagic long-lasting vegetative state. Neurology 2010;75(3):239–45.
22. Giacino J, Whyte J. The vegetative and minimally conscious states: current knowledge and remaining questions. J Head Trauma Rehabil 2005;20(1):30–50.
23. Lucca LF, Lofaro D, Leto E, et al. The impact of medical complications in predicting the rehabilitation outcome of patients with disorders of consciousness after severe traumatic brain injury. Front Hum Neurosci 2020;14:570544.
24. Liuzzi P, Magliacano A, De Bellis F, et al. Predicting outcome of patients with prolonged disorders of consciousness using machine learning models based on medical complexity. Sci Rep 2022;12(1):13471.
25. Whyte J, Nordenbo AM, Kalmar K, et al. Medical complications during inpatient rehabilitation among patients with traumatic disorders of consciousness. Arch Phys Med Rehabil 2013;94(10):1877–83.
26. Giacino JT, Schnakers C, Rodriguez-Moreno D, et al. Behavioral assessment in patients with disorders of consciousness: gold standard or fool's gold? Prog Brain Res 2009;177:33–48.
27. Schnakers C, Monti MM. Disorders of consciousness after severe brain injury: therapeutic options. Curr Opin Neurol 2017;30(6):573–9.
28. Giacino JT, Whyte J, Bagiella E, et al. Placebo-Controlled Trial of Amantadine for Severe Traumatic Brain Injury. N Engl J Med 2012;366(9):819–26.
29. Whyte J, Rajan R, Rosenbaum A, et al. Zolpidem and restoration of consciousness. Am J Phys Med Rehabil 2014;93(2):101–13.
30. Georgiopoulos M, Katsakiori P, Kefalopoulou Z, et al. Vegetative state and minimally conscious state: a review of the therapeutic interventions. Stereotact Funct Neurosurg 2010;88(4):199–207.
31. Sarà M, Pistoia F, Mura E, et al. Intrathecal baclofen in patients with persistent vegetative state: 2 hypotheses. Arch Phys Med Rehabil 2009;90(7):1245–9 (Electronic)).

Evaluation and Management of Disorders of Consciousness in the Acute Care Setting

Ruth Tangonan, MD[a],*, Christos Lazaridis, MD, EDIC[a,b]

KEYWORDS

• Acute disorders of consciousness • Coma • Neurocritical care

KEY POINTS

- Acute disorders of consciousness (DOC) are impairments in arousal and awareness that occur within 28 days of an initial injury and can result from a variety of insults.
- The most important part of the clinical assessment is thorough, serial neurologic examinations with particular emphasis on the level of consciousness, brainstem reflexes, and motor responses.
- The basic evaluation of a patient with acute DOC includes laboratory evaluation, brain imaging, vessel imaging, and electrophysiology. More advanced evaluation techniques can provide information on the integrity of brain networks, covert consciousness, and early emergence of consciousness.
- Amantadine has some evidence for improving recovery of consciousness, but larger trials are needed.
- Prognostication in the acute phase of DOC must be done with caution. Frequent, ongoing conversations with families and caregivers are necessary in order for them to make the best decision they can on behalf of their loved one.

DEFINITION AND MECHANISMS

Acute disorders of consciousness (DOC) are a range of states in which an individual suffers an impairment of arousal or awareness that occurs within 28 days of an initial injury.[1] The acute period of DOC encompasses the time from when the initial injury occurs, when it is diagnosed, and when it is treated, typically at an intensive care unit, followed by monitoring in a general floor. In the United Kingdom, a recent study

[a] Neurosciences Intensive Care Unit, Department of Neurology, University of Chicago Medicine and Biological Sciences, Chicago, IL, USA; [b] Department of Neurological Surgery, University of Chicago Medicine and Biological Sciences, Chicago, IL, USA
* Corresponding author. Neurocritical Care, Department of Neurology, University of Chicago, 5841 South Maryland Avenue, MC 2030, Chicago, IL 60637-1470.
E-mail address: rtangonan@uchicagomedicine.rog

Phys Med Rehabil Clin N Am 35 (2024) 79–92
https://doi.org/10.1016/j.pmr.2023.06.013
1047-9651/24/© 2023 Elsevier Inc. All rights reserved.

based on crowd-sourced data estimates annual incidence of coma cases is 135 per 100,000 and a point prevalence of 7 per 100,000 population, whereas in the United States, the estimated incidence of coma is 258 per 100,000 with a point prevalence of 31 cases per 100,000.[2] Definitions of DOC have been refined throughout the years and can be conceptualized as occurring more on a continuum rather than as discrete states. The most profound state of DOC is the comatose state, defined as the absence of awareness, arousal to any stimuli, or clinically perceptible sleep-wake cycles.[3] The comatose state is typically not permanent and can last from 2 to 4 weeks, after which an individual enters a state of unresponsive wakefulness (UWS; formerly referred to as the vegetative state), a state which is defined by arousal with eye-opening and sleep-wake cycles, but without any evidence of awareness or volitional behavior.[3,4] Following the UWS is the minimally conscious state (MCS) wherein an individual demonstrates arousal as above, along with signs of awareness of their environment.[4] This awareness can manifest as attention to stimuli, following simple commands and/or the ability to communicate, the latter distinguishing a state of MCS+ (presence of awareness with intelligible speech or intentional communication) from a state of MCS− (presence of awareness but without speech or intentional communication).[4] The upper limit of DOC is described as the confusional state and is a period of transition whereby an individual has recovered awareness but still demonstrates impairments across multiple cognitive domains.[4] An intermediate state of DOC that is the subject of ongoing research is the state of covert consciousness (otherwise known as cognitive-motor dissociation or functional locked-in state) in which an individual displays evidence of volitional brain activity as suggested by task-based functional MRI (fMRI) and electroencephalogram (EEG) but does not display clinically evident behavioral or motor output.[1,4,5]

Mechanisms of acute DOC vary widely, with common causes including structural injuries to the brain resulting from traumatic brain injury (TBI), acute ischemic stroke, spontaneous intracranial hemorrhage (sICH), or hypoxic ischemic injury from cardiac arrest, as well as seizures, infections, or toxic-metabolic abnormalities that lead to global cerebral dysfunction. DOC in the acute phase can occur as a singular injury or because of a complex series of insults to the brain. On an anatomic level, consciousness is mediated by connections between the ascending reticular activating system (ARAS) and the cerebral hemispheres.[3,6] The ARAS is located in the paramedian tegmental region of the posterior pons and midbrain, where it runs from the rostral pons, through the midbrain, to the posterior hypothalamus, and to the thalamic reticular formation, whose reciprocal connections with the bilateral cortices form the thalamocortical network.[3,6] Bilateral hemispheric dysfunction (especially involving the mesial frontal region), large unilateral lesions to the dominant hemisphere, bilateral thalamic injury, or focal injury to the hypothalamus, midbrain, or pons can result in DOC, with its specific pathophysiology varying according to the mechanism of injury.[3,6]

In TBI, DOC can occur due to both focal and diffuse injury to the brain. Focal brain damage can occur at the initial site of impact (coup injury) and at a secondary area opposite to the initial site where the brain rebounds and strikes the skull (countercoup injury).[7] Gross injury can occur at both sites, in the form of hematomas, subdural hemorrhage, epidural hemorrhage, subarachnoid hemorrhage, and intraventricular hemorrhage. These lesions damage structures and networks important in maintaining consciousness. In addition to the primary insult, diffuse brain injury may also occur with which noncontact rapid acceleration and deceleration causing shearing and stretching to tissues.[7] This results in diffuse axonal injury (DAI) wherein tensile forces damage neuronal axons, oligodendrocytes, and vasculature causing edema, microhemorrhages, and ischemia; these injuries can insidiously cause DOC in the absence of gross lesions.[7] In pathologic studies evaluating animals with prolonged unconsciousness, axonal retraction balls, microglial clusters, and hemorrhagic injury were seen in the corpus callosum and the mesopontine junction.[3] These sites are adjacent to the free edge of the falx and the tentorium, respectively, the displacement of which places force on local tissue, resulting in necrosis and hemorrhage; this in turn causes injury to the ARAS and functional networks that mediate consciousness.[3]

In ischemic strokes, DOC usually result from large hemispheric infarctions, brainstem infarcts, or multifocal strokes affecting the bilateral medial regions or paramedian diencephalon.[8] This results in direct damage to the ARAS or disruption between its connections to the cortex, subcortical structures, and mesencephalon. In the case of large hemispheric infarctions, brain swelling and its sequelae of midline shift, raised intracranial pressure, and brain herniation result in deterioration of consciousness that can eventually lead to coma, and, if untreated, brain death.[9]

In sICH and aneurysmal subarachnoid hemorrhage (aSAH), primary injury to the brain occurs owing to tissue necrosis in the area of the hematoma, as well as mass effect on surrounding structures.[10] Secondary injury occurs from blood components that trigger inflammatory and oxidative stress pathways; this process can evolve over hours to days and contributes to further damage to surrounding tissues.[10] In both sICH and aSAH, direct damage to structures that mediate consciousness, hydrocephalus, and disruption of functional networks can lead to DOC.[11] In aSAH, delayed cerebral ischemia and vasospasm may lead to DOC within the first 2 weeks after aneurysmal rupture.[1]

In cardiac arrest, the initial and most profound insult is the loss of cerebral blood flow that occurs because of the cessation of cardiac output and oxygen delivery. This results in the loss of brain tissue viability as cells exhaust the oxygen stores necessary to maintain aerobic metabolism and generation of ATP.[12] If cerebral blood flow is restored, it may or may not be sufficient to maintain the function of neurons; furthermore, reperfusion of ischemic tissue triggers secondary injury via mitochondrial dysfunction, oxidative damage, and apoptosis, as well as activation of the inflammatory cascade, all leading to additional injury to remaining tissue.[12]

CLINICAL ASSESSMENT

Regardless of the cause, the clinical examination is the foundation of the assessment of patients with DOC in the acute setting. The neurologic examination can be performed efficiently at the bedside, repeated serially, and trended over time. It can be performed by clinicians at any level, but an assessment by an experienced clinician is necessary to ensure that subtle nuances in the examination are noted. In addition, it is imperative to consider possible confounders that can affect the neurologic examination: hypothermia and hyperthermia, hemodynamic instability, sedating medications, illicit substances, underlying infection, and profound metabolic derangements.[3]

The first part of the neurologic examination is the assessment of consciousness. To determine a patient's level of consciousness, it is necessary to assess the minimum level of stimulation necessary to arouse a patient, from verbal cues to deep noxious stimuli. It is important to apply both lateralizing stimuli (nail bed pressure, trapezius pressure) and midline stimuli (supraorbital pressure, sternal rub). A patient who is drowsy but can still arouse to verbal or light tactile stimuli can be described as lethargic or obtunded, whereas a patient who requires deep noxious stimuli to be aroused and cannot maintain arousal but can still localize toward painful stimuli is considered to be stuporous. Patients who cannot open their eyes and can only produce nonspecific motor responses (grimacing, withdrawal to stimuli) are considered comatose.[1,3]

After the assessment of consciousness, brainstem reflexes are evaluated. The pupillary light reflex tests midbrain function via CN II afferents and CN III efferents. The pupils are observed for size, symmetry, and reactivity. The pupillary light reflex has high localizing value and can aid in distinguishing metabolic from structural coma, especially when a unilateral, dilated, unreactive pupil is observed. It is therefore important to observe pupils in ambient lighting, and to use bright LED light and a magnifying glass to detect subtle pupillary reactivity. When it is available, automated pupillometry can be a useful adjunctive test to evaluate subtle anisocoria and changes in reactivity, which can be quantified and monitored over time.[1,3]

The corneal reflexes test CN V afferents and CN VII efferents and can provide information about pontine function. The optimal corneal response is achieved by drawing a cotton wisp across the cornea, closer to the edge of the iris; testing laterally on the sclera is a common mistake and can result in insufficient stimulation of the cornea and a false negative corneal response.[1,3]

As part of the evaluation of eye movements, the eyes should be passively opened in patients who are unable to spontaneously open their eyes in response to stimuli. The clinician should probe for vertical and horizontal eye movements and test for the vestibulo-ocular reflex unless there is evidence of or concern for cervical spine injury. Another recommended maneuver is the use of a mirror to diagnose visual pursuit, which is also a simple, quick way to evaluate consciousness in addition to eye movements. These maneuvers will allow for the evaluation of patients in MCS or with locked-in syndrome, bilateral ptosis, or eyelid apraxia.[1,3,13]

Other brainstem reflexes that should be assessed include the vestibulo-ocular reflex via cold calorics, and the function of the lower brainstem via the evaluation of the cough and gag reflex.[3]

The motor response should be tested in all extremities and can be described in terms of the motor subset of the Glasgow Coma Scale (GCS; obeying commands, localizing to painful stimuli, withdrawal from painful stimuli, abnormal flexion, abnormal extension, and absent motor response), which is described later in this section, and in terms of strength, symmetry, muscle tone, and presence of abnormal movements.[3]

In evaluating patients with DOC, standardized clinical assessments can be useful tools to communicate an examination between clinicians. The GCS was initially used to categorize levels of consciousness in trauma patients.[14] It is one of the most commonly used scales in clinical practice. It evaluates eye opening, verbal output, and motor response. The minimum score is 3, and the maximum score is 15; a GCS score of 8 or less is arbitrarily assigned as the definition of coma.[14] However, the GCS has several limitations, which include lack of assessment of brainstem reflexes, incomplete assessment of the verbal response (especially in intubated or aphasic patients), and possibly missing locked-in states.[15] In a recent study of 2455 patients with TBI, a wide range of GCS scores were associated with identical DOC diagnoses, with a GCS score of 4 to 14 associated with more than one DOC diagnosis; this brought the investigators to the conclusion that the total GCS score is not an accurate reflection of an individual's level of consciousness.[15] However, it remains a useful tool to succinctly and efficiently communicate a patient's level of consciousness between providers. An alternative to the GCS is the FOUR score, which evaluates a patient's eye opening, motor response, brainstem reflexes, and respiratory pattern. Unlike the GCS, the FOUR score incorporates brainstem reflexes and respiratory patterns into the examination, which can aid in localizing and detecting brainstem lesions and diagnosing a locked-in state.[16] The FOUR score has a maximum of 16 and has been shown in one study to be more predictive of in-hospital mortality in TBI compared with GCS.[16] An improvement in the FOUR score of greater than 2 is also associated with survival in cardiac arrest.[17] The most comprehensive assessment of DOC available is the Coma Recovery Scale–Revised (CRS-R), a 30- to 40-minute assessment tool that evaluates auditory, visual, motor, oromotor, communication, and arousal functions in patients with DOC.[18] This scale is more sensitive than any other scale in detecting signs of awareness, and its subscales can be used to classify states of consciousness, such as the MCS. It has been found to detect subtle volitional responses, such as eye tracking in 40% of patients thought to be in UWS.[19] However, its use is limited by the prolonged time required to administer the test, especially when it is necessary for a patient to remain off sedation. It also needs to be administered by a trained clinician in order for the results to be reliable. An alternative to using the CRS-R in its entirety is the use of CRS-R subscale scores or modified scores to diagnose UWS from MCS; a study is currently underway for the use of a fast modified version of CRS-R in the evaluating TBI patients in the intensive care unit.[20]

DIAGNOSTIC EVALUATION

Rapid and thorough diagnostic evaluation is crucial to the establishing a diagnosis, implementing interventions, and gaining prognostic information early in the course of DOC. Basic evaluation of blood counts, chemistry profiles, toxicology, and possible infectious sources is necessary to test for systemic causes of DOC.[1,3] Following this, brain imaging with a computed tomography (CT) Scan of the head is often the first diagnostic step in the evaluation of DOC. It is widely available and rapidly acquired in most settings. It is used to identify emergent intracranial pathologic conditions, including intracranial hemorrhage, large subacute infarctions, hydrocephalus, and early hypoxic injury.[1,3] It also allows for serial monitoring of lesions throughout a patient's hospital course. Along with CT head, vascular studies such as computed tomography angiography (CTA) or magnetic resonance angiography (MRA) of the head may also be necessary to elucidate the cause of DOC; specifically, it can help identify basilar artery thrombosis, large-vessel occlusions, critical arterial stenoses, and vascular abnormalities.[3] If there is clinical suspicion, venous imaging can also be obtained to evaluate for cerebral venous sinus thrombosis. In TBI, vascular imaging can also identify active extravasation or injury, which can herald expansion of hemorrhages early in a patient's course.[21] CT imaging, however, is often insufficient to detect subtle lesions that can cause DOC. MRI can detect these lesions with higher sensitivity and can characterize known lesions with higher resolution. It can help detect lesions, such as masses, small hemorrhages, diffuse axonal injury, hypoxic-ischemic injury, and infections, especially in areas such as the brainstem, which is often obscured by artifact on CT.[13]

Outside of conventional imaging, advanced techniques are also being used to evaluate injury to white matter structures and tracts in order to gain insight into how these lesions disrupt functional networks necessary to maintain consciousness. Diffusion tensor imaging (DTI) measures the direction of diffusion of water along axonal bundles and can quantify white matter injury through a measure called fractional anisotropy.[22] Early studies suggest that DTI can predict outcomes of patients in DOC secondary to cardiac arrest and TBI with increased accuracy compared with conventional imaging and clinical scoring scales.[22,23,24]

Electrophysiologic studies, such as EEG and evoked potentials, are also important studies in acute DOC that provide information about the electrical activity of the brain. EEG is important early in a patient's course to establish that a patient with DOC is not experiencing nonconvulsive seizures, defined as electrographic seizures with no apparent motor manifestations.[25,26] This has a high incidence in critically ill patients and DOC who are monitored on continuous EEG.[26] In addition to the characterization of seizures and abnormal electrographic activity, EEG monitoring also allows for evaluation of electrical background, sleep-wake cycles, and reactivity to stimuli, all of which can provide important prognostic information in the acute period.[27,28] For instance, EEG background, reactivity to visual or tactile stimuli, and presence of sleep architecture can assist in differentiating UWS and MCS. This has implications for detection of emerging consciousness as well as prognostication.[28] Decreased EEG reactivity, slower, disorganized backgrounds, and absence of reactivity have been noted as poor prognostic indicators in patients with anoxic injury.[29,30] Meanwhile, EEG reactivity, increased alpha frequencies, and the presence of sleep patterns are associated with improvement in the CRS-R and recovery of consciousness.[28]

Seizures can occur shortly after acquired brain injury and can lead to secondary brain injury. Seizures are associated with higher mortality in the acute period and can delay recovery of consciousness.[31] Myoclonic status epilepticus, in particular, has been associated with poor outcomes after cardiac arrest, more so when the EEG demonstrates suppressed or burst-suppressed backgrounds and high-amplitude polyspikes.[32]

Advanced EEG analysis can also provide clues about the status of the functional networks in the brain and their role in early recovery of consciousness. Quantitative EEG analysis evaluates spatial and temporal attributes of resting EEG, which can be used as surrogate markers for the integrity of brain networks.[27] Measures such as EEG complexity and spectral power have been shown to correlate with different states of consciousness.[27] Research is ongoing as to how these measures can be used to predict recovery of consciousness in the acute period.

Evoked potentials are another electrophysiologic study used to evaluate the connection between the peripheral sensory pathways and the somatosensory cortex in response to external stimuli.[33] The somatosensory evoked potential (SSEP) is a small-amplitude electrical signal recorded at the skull in response to an electrical signal applied to the peripheral nerves (often the median nerve).[33] The absence of bilateral, short-latency response (N20 response) has been associated with poor outcomes in patients with cardiac arrest and in TBI.[34,35]

Research is currently ongoing into interrogating consciousness beyond what is clinically apparent based on a patient's behavioral output, otherwise known as covert consciousness. Specifically, task-based fMRI and EEG are being used to investigate whether patients who appear to be in a coma or UWS have volitional capacity despite not being able to produce motor responses.[5] In these paradigms, a patient is given an instruction ("imagine opening and closing your hand") or a prompt for spatial navigation ("imagine walking through your home"); the patient's brain activity during the task is compared with their brain activity while at rest. Using these models, several small studies have detected evidence of covert consciousness in patients clinically thought to be in a coma or UWS.[5] A study by Claassen and colleagues[36] evaluated 104 patients with acute brain injury who were unresponsive to verbal commands or noxious stimuli and found that 15% of those patients demonstrated functional activity on EEG; half of these patients proceeded to follow commands before discharge. These studies have important implications for neuroprognostication and have been recommended as a possible mode of evaluation "when feasible" in the subacute to chronic DOC guidelines by the American Academy of Neurology, the US National Institute on Disability, Independent Living, and Rehabilitation Research, and the European Academy of Neurology.[13,37] However, the availability of these technologies (in particular fMRI), the medical complexity of patients with DOC, and the expertise needed to interpret these tests limit broader applicability in the clinical setting.

TREATMENT

Initial principles of management in acute brain injury focus on provision of resuscitative measures in conjunction with the treatment of the underlying cause, followed by insti-tuting measures to prevent secondary brain injury. This also includes testing to exclude all possible confounders that contribute to DOC, as well as treating medical comorbidities, such as seizures, infections, and metabolic derangements. The treat-ment of individual brain injuries that can cause DOC is beyond the scope of this article; rather, this section focuses on established and novel therapeutics that can be applied in the acute period of DOC.

The pharmacologic therapy with the best evidence in DOC is amantadine, which is thought to enhance dopaminergic activity in the mesocircuit.[38] By facilitating striatal output to the globus pallidus, increased dopamine can modulate the mesiofrontal cor-tex and increase forebrain activity.[38] In a study done by Giacino and colleagues[39] on patients with TBI in a UWS or MCS state, the investigators found that amantadine improved functional recovery compared with the control group within the first 4 weeks of treatment; no significant adverse effects were observed. Another drug with early evidence is zolpidem, which, paradoxically, may have stimulating effects on a subset of patients with TBI through its modulation of GABA-A receptors in the globus pal-lidus.[40,41] Other drugs that have been shown to have variable benefits in small studies include baclofen, midazolam, amitriptyline, desipramine, protriptyline, and modafi-nil.[42] Future areas of research in medications for acute DOC include randomized clinical trials (RCTs) on individual pharmaceuticals, testing combinations to evaluate for synergistic effects, and studying new agents (psychedelic drugs, antinarcoleptic drugs, and orexin agonists).[42]

Direct and indirect electromagnetic stimulation of the brain has been used in multiple neurologic diseases, and testing is underway to evaluate their efficacy in DOC. Of these therapies, transcranial direct current stimulation (tDCS) of the dorsolateral pre-frontal cortex has been shown to improve signs of consciousness in patients with MCS, and, to a lesser extent, UWS.[43–47] tDCS uses a weak electrical current applied to the scalp, which is hypothesized to alter neuronal membrane potential and facilitate plasticity via long-term potentiation of neurons.[42] Other electromagnetic therapies that have limited data but may be targets of potential future research include direct stimu-lation of central thalamic nuclei (the most invasive strategy), transmagnetic stimulation of the motor cortex, vagal nerve stimulation, and median nerve stimulation.[48–56]

Other therapies that have been described in case reports include the administration of low-intensity ultrasound to subcortical targets in order to stimulate neuronal tissue; sensory stimulation therapy using tactile, auditory, and vestibular stimulation to enhance neural processes, support neuroplasticity, and stimulate brainstem and thalamic projections to the cortex; and stem cell therapy using adult neural stem cells, mesenchymal bone marrow stromal cells, or umbilical cord blood.[42]

PROGNOSIS AND ETHICAL CHALLENGES

Prognostication in the acute phase is challenging especially in the absence of a clearly catastrophic injury (ie, where a patient would require testing for death by neurologic criteria). During the initial phase of brain injury, efforts are directed toward resuscita-tion, stabilization, and prevention of secondary injury. Numerous studies show that re-covery of consciousness may take up to anywhere from 3 to 12 months, depending on its cause. In patients with TBI-related DOC lasting greater than 28 days, a meta-analysis suggests that 38% of patients demonstrate recovery from DOC at 3 months, 67% at 6 months, and 78% at 12 months.[57–61] Lower rates of recovery are seen in DOC owing to nontraumatic causes, with 17% recovering consciousness at 6 months and 7.5% recovering consciousness at 24 months.[57,62,63] Patients diagnosed with MCS have better odds of improvement and less severe disability at 12 months compared with patients diagnosed with UWS, especially if injury is secondary to TBI.[57,64,65] Factors associated with better prognosis in DOC greater than 28 days include disability rating score less than 26, CRS-R scores greater than 6, reactive EEG, detectable P300 on SSEP, and increased BOLD fMRI signal in response to familiar to stimuli.[57]

The acute phase of care carries important ethical challenges, as important decisions are made during this period regarding the direction of a patient's care. This is particularly difficult, as families and caregivers depend on the clinician's experience and expertise to provide early prognostic insight that they will use to decide on the path of treatment that would be most compatible with their loved one's wishes. Often, medical stabilization and adequate time for recovery are necessary to formulate a prognosis. Early on in the acute phase, an accurate characterization of patient's state of consciousness is necessary in order to inform these crucial assessments and decisions. This can be done through assessment of covert consciousness via task-based fMRI and functional EEG, as described above. This characterization is often complicated by multiple factors, including the patient's condition (sensory and motor impairments, fluctuating level of consciousness, medical comorbidities), clinician limitations (lack of expertise or experience, individual biases, time constraints), and systemic constraints (access to specialized centers, availability of advanced diagnostics, absence of standardized guidelines, and protocols in evaluation of DOC).[5] Altogether, these result in high rates of misdiagnosis of DOC, specifically when subtle signs of consciousness are missed. To support thorough evaluation and accurate diagnosis of DOC, it is important for clinicians to have a framework with which to evaluate these patients. Recent practice guidelines by the American Academy of Neurology, European Academy of Neurology, and Royal College of Physicians recommend conducting multiple examinations done by experienced practitioners, using multimodal diagnostics in evaluating patients and avoiding delivering an overly pessimistic prognosis early on within a patient's course.[13,57,66] However, formal detailed protocols as well as concrete recommendations on the clinical examination, clinical rating scores, diagnostic evaluation, and treatment pathways, as well as the time period for evaluation, are still lacking. There is a large degree of multidimensional uncertainty affecting decision making, that has to be acknowledged by both clinicians and surrogate decision makers. This extends beyond diagnostic and prognostic, to practical, value, and moral varieties. The inability to recognize, and to some degree embrace uncertainty early on, could lead to premature decisions toward limitation of resuscitative or life-sustaining treatments.[67]

Having protocols for evaluation in place can help ensure thorough, uniform evaluation of DOC; this has important implications in the acute phase of care, as it can impact the caregivers' decision to prematurely withdraw life-sustaining treatments. This is a significant contributor to a self-fulfilling prophecy bias wherein a seemingly poor examination is taken at face value and is used to confer a poor prognosis on a patient. Although there is tremendous value in protecting an individual's dignity at the end of life (especially when artificial means of life prolongation is not within a person's wishes), it is also important for clinicians to allow, in the absence of a catastrophic injury, time for a patient's injury to be treated and stabilized before gaining a more accurate sense of their potential for recovery. Throughout this process, the clinician must help caregivers be cognizant of the possible psychological stress, physical pain, medical complications, and treatment-related trauma that a patient may experience during the acute treatment period and beyond. Recovery, even if possible, is not a benign process. To what degree a patient will recover and what level of disability they may have is another conversation with families that will evolve throughout a patient's recovery. As clinicians, it is important to recognize that individuals and families can maintain a quality of life that is acceptable to them even with some degree of disability; it is important to separate our own values on disability from that of our patients and their families.

As we consider the degree of disability that would be acceptable to patients and caregivers, it is also important to consider the emotional, psychological, and financial burden that DOC places on caregivers and families; this is in addition to the opportunity costs to caregivers who stand to lose educational, financial, and professional opportunities to care for their loved ones. It is important to have these conversations with families during the acute period of care sensitively and at regular intervals so that they can place their loved ones' medical condition—their progress, stagnation, deterioration, and complications—within a broader context.

As we expand our ability to understand, diagnose, and treat DOC, it is also important to consider the health care system's ability to care for patients with DOC. In the acute care setting, there are often limitations in personnel, ICU beds, and resources and can be seen in individual hospitals and across geographic areas, that is further exacerbated by socioeconomic and racial disparities. Equitable and just access to acute care, rehabilitation, and clinical trials should be a consideration when establishing systems of care for DOC.

SUMMARY

Acute DOC are impairments in arousal and awareness that occur within 28 days of an initial injury. These impairments occur on a spectrum of states from coma, UWS, covert consciousness, minimal consciousness, and confusional state, with each state marked by the gradual return of arousal, awareness, response to stimuli, and behavioral output. Brain injuries that can cause DOC include TBI, acute ischemic stroke, sICH, or hypoxic ischemic injury from cardiac arrest, as well as seizures, infections, or toxic-metabolic abnormalities that lead to global cerebral dysfunction. Specifically, injury to the ARAS at the level of the mesopontine region, bilateral thalamus, or hypothalamus can cause DOC, along with diffuse injury affecting bilateral hemispheres. The neurologic examination is a crucial part of the evaluation of DOC in the acute phase and includes evaluation of consciousness and a thorough assessment of brainstem reflexes. Particular attention should be paid to the level of consciousness, ensuring that adequate stimulation is provided to the patient, as well as the eye examination, taking care to closely evaluate pupillary reactivity, corneal reflexes, and eye movements. Clinical rating scales, such as the GCS, FOUR score, and the CRS-R, are also important tools for the evaluation and monitoring of patients with DOC. Further evaluation of DOC patients is done with laboratory evaluations, imaging (CT head, MRI), and electrophysiology (EEG, SSEP) to evaluate the cause of DOC as well as to provide prognostic information. If available, advanced imaging and electrophysiologic techniques, such as fMRI, DTI, diffusion MRI tractography, and quantitative EEG analysis, can provide information on the integrity of brain networks and early emergence of consciousness. Task-based fMRI and EEG, in particular, have evidence supporting the detection of covert consciousness. The treatment of acute DOC is focused on resuscitation and treatment of the underlying cause, followed by prevention of secondary injury. Amantadine has some evidence in improving functional recovery in DOC. Other experimental treatments that are being investigated include direct and indirect electromagnetic stimulation, low-intensity ultrasound, sensory stimulation, and stem cell therapy. Prognostication in the acute phase of DOC is done with caution unless there is a clear catastrophic injury. Otherwise, efforts are directed toward stabilization and prevention of secondary injury. Better outcomes are seen in DOC related to trauma and in patients diagnosed with MCS. It is important to have frequent, ongoing conversations with caregivers and families about the status of their loved one with DOC, so that they can anticipate what to expect during a patient's clinical course and make decisions that would be most consistent with their loved one's wishes. As our ability to diagnose and treat DOC evolves, health care systems must expand as well in order to provide equitable access to care for patients at all stages of DOC.

CLINICS CARE POINTS

- In the acute period of disorders of consciousness, it is important to perform thorough, serial neurologic examinations with particular emphasis on the level of consciousness, brainstem reflexes, and motor response.
- The Glasgow Coma Scale is the commonly used clinical rating scale, but use of the FOUR score or the Coma Recovery Scale-Revised can provide more meaningful information about brainstem function and in-depth evaluation of consciousness, respectively.
- The basic evaluation of a patient with acute disorders of consciousness includes laboratory evaluation, brain imaging (computed tomography, MRI), vessel imaging (CTA, MRA), and electrophysiology (electroencephalogram, somatosensory evoked potential).
- More advanced evaluation techniques, such as functional MRI, diffusion tensor imaging, diffusion MRI tractography, and quantitative electroencephalogram, can provide information on the integrity of brain networks and early emergence of consciousness. Task-based fMRI and electroencephalogram, specifically, can help detect covert consciousness.
- Aside from treatment of the underlying condition, therapeutic interventions for acute disorders of consciousness are largely experimental. Amantadine has some evidence in improving recovery of consciousness, but larger trials are needed.
- Prognostication in the acute phase of disorders of consciousness must be done with caution, and every effort must be made to thoroughly assess the patient's level of consciousness before delivering a prognosis. Frequent, ongoing conversations with families and caregivers are necessary in order for them to make the best decision they can on behalf of their loved one.

DISCLOSURE

The authors reported no conflicts of interest.

REFERENCES

1. Edlow BL, Claassen J, Schiff ND, et al. Recovery from disorders of consciousness: mechanisms, prognosis and emerging therapies. Nat Rev Neurol 2021; 17(3):135–56.

2. Kondziella D, Amiri M, Othman MH, et al. Incidence and prevalence of coma in the UK and the USA. Brain Commun 2022;4. https://doi.org/10.1093/braincomms/fcac188.

3. Posner J, Saper C, Schiff N, Plum F. Plum & Posner's Diagnosis of Stupor and Coma.; 2007.

4. Young MJ, Bodien YG, Giacino JT, et al. The neuroethics of disorders of consciousness: A brief history of evolving ideas. Brain 2021;144(11):3291–310. https://doi.org/10.1093/brain/awab290.

5. Edlow BL, Fins JJ. Assessment of covert consciousness in the intensive care unit: clinical and ethical considerations. J Head Trauma Rehabil 2018;33(6):424–34.

6. Brazis PW, Masdeu JC, Biller J. Localization in clinical Neurology. Wolters Kluwer Health/Lippincott Williams & Wilkins; 2011.

7. Ng SY, Lee AYW. Traumatic Brain Injuries: Pathophysiology and Potential Therapeutic Targets. Front Cell Neurosci 2019;13. https://doi.org/10.3389/fncel.2019.00528.

8. Dostović Z, Smajlović D, Dostović E, et al. Stroke and disorders of consciousness. Cardiovasc Psychiatry Neurol 2012. https://doi.org/10.1155/2012/429108. Published online.

9. Li J, Zhang P, Wu S, et al. Impaired consciousness at stroke onset in large hemisphere infarction: incidence, risk factors and outcome. Sci Rep 2020;10(1). https://doi.org/10.1038/s41598-020-70172-1.

10. Madangarli N, Bonsack F, Dasari R, et al. Intracerebral hemorrhage: Blood components and neurotoxicity. Brain Sci 2019;9(11). https://doi.org/10.3390/brainsci9110316.

11. Jang SH, Chang CH, Jung YJ, et al. Relationship between Impaired Consciousness and Injury of Ascending Reticular Activating System in Patients with Intracerebral Hemorrhage. Stroke 2019;50(8):2234–7.

12. Sandroni C, Cronberg T, Sekhon M. Brain injury after cardiac arrest: pathophysiology, treatment, and prognosis. Intensive Care Med 2021;47(12):1393–414.

13. Kondziella D, Bender A, Diserens K, et al. European Academy of Neurology guideline on the diagnosis of coma and other disorders of consciousness. Eur J Neurol 2020;27(5):741–56.

14. Teasdale G, Maas A, Lecky F, et al. The Glasgow Coma Scale at 40 Years: Standing the Test of Time. Lancet Neurol 2014;13(8):844–54. www.thelancet.com/neurology.

15. Bodien YG, Barra A, Temkin NR, et al. Diagnosing Level of Consciousness: The Limits of the Glasgow Coma Scale Total Score. J Neurotrauma 2021;38(23):3295–305. https://doi.org/10.1089/neu.2021.0199.

16. Wijdicks EFM, Bamlet WR, Maramattom Bv, et al. Validation of a new coma scale: The FOUR score. Ann Neurol 2005;58(4):585–93.

17. Fugate JE, Rabinstein AA, Claassen DO, et al. The FOUR score predicts outcome in patients after cardiac arrest. Neurocrit Care 2010;13(2):205–10.

18. Lucca LF, Lofaro D, Pignolo L, et al. Outcome prediction in disorders of consciousness: The role of coma recovery scale revised. BMC Neurol 2019;19(1). https://doi.org/10.1186/s12883-019-1293-7.

19. Schnakers C, Vanhaudenhuyse A, Giacino J, et al. Diagnostic accuracy of the vegetative and minimally conscious state: Clinical consensus versus standardized neurobehavioral assessment. BMC Neurol 2009;9. https://doi.org/10.1186/1471-2377-9-35.

20. Bodien Y, Bergin MV. Validation and Feasibility of the Coma Recovery Scale-Revised for Accelerated Standardized Assessment (CRSR-FAST): a Brief,

Standardized Assessment Instrument to Monitor Recovery of Consciousness in the Intensive Care Unit. Ongoing study https://clinicaltrials.gov/study/NCT03549572.

21. Tunthanathip T, Phuenpathom N, Sae-Heng S, et al. Traumatic cerebrovascular injury: Clinical characteristics and illustrative cases. Neurosurg Focus 2019; 47(5). https://doi.org/10.3171/2019.8.FOCUS19382.

22. Velly L, Perlbarg V, Boulier T, et al. Use of brain diffusion tensor imaging for the prediction of long-term neurological outcomes in patients after cardiac arrest: a multicentre, international, prospective, observational, cohort study. Lancet Neurol 2018;17(4):317–26.

23. Galanaud D, Perlbarg V, Puybasset L. Assessment of White Matter Injury and Outcome in Severe Brain Trauma. Anesthesiology 2012;117:1300–10. Available at: http://www.csie.ntu.edu.tw/~cjlin/libsvm/.

24. Wang J, Bakhadirov K, Abdi H, et al. Longitudinal Changes of Structural Connectivity in Traumatic Axonal Injury From the Department of Cognition and Neuroscience (Supplemental Data at Www.Neurology.Org Supplemental Data Editorial, Page 810.; 2011. www.neurology.org.

25. Claassen J, Mayer SA, et al. Detection of Electrographic Seizures with Continuous EEG Monitoring in Critically Ill Patients. Neurology 2004;62(10):1743–8.

26. Towne A, Waterhouse E, Boggs J, et al. Prevalence of Nonconvulsive Status Epilepticus in Comatose Patients. Neurology 2000;54(2):340–5.

27. Comanducci A, Boly M, Claassen J, et al. Clinical and advanced neurophysiology in the prognostic and diagnostic evaluation of disorders of consciousness: review of an IFCN-endorsed expert group. Clin Neurophysiol 2020;131(11):2736–65.

28. Estraneo A, Loreto V, Guarino I, et al. Standard EEG in diagnostic process of prolonged disorders of consciousness. Clin Neurophysiol 2016;127(6):2379–85.

29. Rossetti AO, Tovar Quiroga DF, Juan E, et al. Electroencephalography Predicts Poor and Good Outcomes after Cardiac Arrest: A Two-Center Study. Crit Care Med 2017;45(7). https://doi.org/10.1097/CCM.0000000000002337.

30. Rossetti AO, Rabinstein AA, Oddo M. Neurological prognostication of outcome in patients in coma after cardiac arrest. Lancet Neurol 2016;15(6). https://doi.org/10.1016/S1474-4422(16)00015-6.

31. Pascarella A, Trojano L, Loreto V, et al. Long-term outcome of patients with disorders of consciousness with and without epileptiform activity and seizures: a prospective single centre cohort study. J Neurol 2016;263(10):2048–56.

32. Elmer J, Rittenberger JC, Faro J, et al. Clinically distinct electroencephalographic phenotypes of early myoclonus after cardiac arrest. Ann Neurol 2016;80(2):175–84.

33. Cloostermans MC, Horn J, van Putten MJAM. The SSEP on the ICU: Current applications and pitfalls. Netherlands Journal of Critical Care 2013;17(1).

34. Carter BG, Butt W. Review of the use of somatosensory evoked potentials in the prediction of outcome after severe brain injury. Crit Care Med 2001;29(1). https://doi.org/10.1097/00003246-200101000-00036.

35. Rothstein TL. SSEP retains its value as predictor of poor outcome following cardiac arrest in the era of therapeutic hypothermia. Crit Care 2019;23(1). https://doi.org/10.1186/s13054-019-2576-5.

36. Claassen J, Doyle K, Matory A, et al. Detection of Brain Activation in Unresponsive Patients with Acute Brain Injury. N Engl J Med 2019;380(26). https://doi.org/10.1056/nejmoa1812757.

37. Giacino JT, Katz DI, Schiff ND, et al. Practice Guideline Update Recommendations Summary: Disorders of Consciousness: Report of the Guideline Development,

Dissemination, and Implementation Subcommittee of the American Academy of Neurology; the American Congress of Rehabilitation Medicine; and the National Institute on Disability, Independent Living, and Rehabilitation Research. Arch Phys Med Rehabil 2018;99. https://doi.org/10.1016/j.apmr.2018.07.001.

38. Schiff ND. Recovery of consciousness after brain injury: a mesocircuit hypothesis. Trends Neurosci 2010;33(1). https://doi.org/10.1016/j.tins.2009.11.002.

39. Giacino JT, Whyte J, Bagiella E, et al. Placebo-Controlled Trial of Amantadine for Severe Traumatic Brain Injury. N Engl J Med 2012;366(9). https://doi.org/10.1056/nejmoa1102609.

40. Tucker C, Sandhu K. The Effectiveness of Zolpidem for the Treatment of Disorders of Consciousness. Neurocrit Care 2016;24(3). https://doi.org/10.1007/s12028-015-0227-5.

41. Sutton JA, Clauss RP. A review of the evidence of zolpidem efficacy in neurological disability after brain damage due to stroke, trauma and hypoxia: A justification of further clinical trials. Brain Inj 2017;31(8). https://doi.org/10.1080/02699052.2017.1300836.

42. Edlow BL, Sanz LRD, Polizzotto L, et al. Therapies to Restore Consciousness in Patients with Severe Brain Injuries: A Gap Analysis and Future Directions. Neurocrit Care 2021;35:68–85.

43. Wu M, Yu Y, Luo L, et al. Efficiency of repetitive transcranial direct current stimulation of the dorsolateral prefrontal cortex in disorders of consciousness: A randomized sham-controlled study. Neural Plast 2019;2019. https://doi.org/10.1155/2019/7089543.

44. Thibaut A, Wannez S, Donneau AF, et al. Controlled clinical trial of repeated prefrontal tDCS in patients with chronic minimally conscious state. Brain Inj 2017;31(4). https://doi.org/10.1080/02699052.2016.1274776.

45. Martens G, Lejeune N, O'Brien AT, et al. Randomized controlled trial of home-based 4-week tDCS in chronic minimally conscious state. Brain Stimul 2018;11(5). https://doi.org/10.1016/j.brs.2018.04.021.

46. Thibaut A, Bruno MA, Ledoux D, et al. TDCS in patients with disorders of consciousness: Sham-controlled randomized double-blind study. Neurology 2014;82(13). https://doi.org/10.1212/WNL.0000000000000260.

47. Cavinato M, Genna C, Formaggio E, et al. Behavioural and electrophysiological effects of tDCS to prefrontal cortex in patients with disorders of consciousness. Clin Neurophysiol 2019;130(2). https://doi.org/10.1016/j.clinph.2018.10.018.

48. Noé E, Ferri J, Colomer C, et al. Feasibility, safety and efficacy of transauricular vagus nerve stimulation in a cohort of patients with disorders of consciousness. Brain Stimul 2020;13(2). https://doi.org/10.1016/j.brs.2019.12.005.

49. Corazzol M, Lio G, Lefevre A, et al. Restoring consciousness with vagus nerve stimulation. Curr Biol 2017;27(18). https://doi.org/10.1016/j.cub.2017.07.060.

50. Lei J, Wang L, Gao G, et al. Right median nerve electrical stimulation for acute traumatic coma patients. J Neurotrauma 2015;32(20). https://doi.org/10.1089/neu.2014.3768.

51. Liu JT, Wang CH, Chou IC, et al. Regaining consciousness for prolonged comatose patients with right median nerve stimulation. Acta Neurochir Suppl 2003;87. https://doi.org/10.1007/978-3-7091-6081-7_3.

52. Peri Cv, Shaffrey ME, Farace E, et al. Pilot study of electrical stimulation on median nerve in comatose severe brain injured patients: 3-month outcome. Brain Inj 2001;15(10). https://doi.org/10.1080/02699050110065709.

53. Cooper JB, Jane JA, Alves WM, et al. Right median nerve electrical stimulation to hasten awakening from coma. Brain Inj 1999;13(4). https://doi.org/10.1080/026990599121638.
54. Cincotta M, Giovannelli F, Chiaramonti R, et al. No effects of 20 Hz-rTMS of the primary motor cortex in vegetative state: A randomised, sham-controlled study. Cortex 2015;71. https://doi.org/10.1016/j.cortex.2015.07.027.
55. Yamamoto T. Deep brain stimulation therapy for a persistent vegetative state. Acta Neurochir Suppl 2001;79. https://doi.org/10.1007/978-3-7091-6105-0_18.
56. Yamamoto T, Katayama Y, Kobayashi K, et al. Deep brain stimulation for the treatment of vegetative state. Eur J Neurosci 2010;32(7). https://doi.org/10.1111/j.1460-9568.2010.07412.x.
57. Giacino JT, Katz DI, Schiff ND, et al. Comprehensive systematic review update summary: Disorders of consciousness: Report of the Guideline Development, Dissemination, and Implementation Subcommittee of the American Academy of Neurology; The American Congress of Rehabilitation Medicine; And the National Institute on Disability, Independent Living, and Rehabilitati. Neurology 2018; 91(10):461–70.
58. Bagnato S, Minafra L, Bravatà V, et al. Brain-derived neurotrophic factor (Val66-Met) polymorphism does not influence recovery from a post-traumatic vegetative state: A blinded retrospective multi-centric study. J Neurotrauma 2012;29(11). https://doi.org/10.1089/neu.2011.2184.
59. Sarà M, Pistoia F, Pasqualetti P, et al. Functional isolation within the cerebral cortex in the vegetative state: A nonlinear method to predict clinical outcomes. Neurorehabil Neural Repair 2011;25(1). https://doi.org/10.1177/1545968310378508.
60. Cavinato M, Freo U, Ori C, et al. Post-acute P300 predicts recovery of consciousness from traumatic vegetative state. Brain Inj 2009;23(12). https://doi.org/10.3109/02699050903373493.
61. Bagnato S, Boccagni C, Sant'Angelo A, et al. Longitudinal Assessment of Clinical Signs of Recovery in Patients with Unresponsive Wakefulness Syndrome after Traumatic or Nontraumatic Brain Injury. J Neurotrauma 2017;34(2). https://doi.org/10.1089/neu.2016.4418.
62. Mateen FJ, Niu JW, Gao S, et al. Causes and outcomes of persistent vegetative state in a Chinese versus american referral hospital. Neurocrit Care 2013;18(2). https://doi.org/10.1007/s12028-012-9789-7.
63. Sazbon L, Zagreba F, Ronen J, et al. Course and outcome of patients in vegetative state of nontraumatic aetiology. J Neurol Neurosurg Psychiatry 1993;56(4). https://doi.org/10.1136/jnnp.56.4.407.
64. Kotchoubey B, Lang S, Mezger G, et al. Information processing in severe disorders of consciousness: Vegetative state and minimally conscious state. Clin Neurophysiol 2005;116(10). https://doi.org/10.1016/j.clinph.2005.03.028.
65. Giacino JT, Kalmar K. The vegetative and minimally conscious states: A comparison of clinical features and functional outcome. J Head Trauma Rehabil 1997; 12(4). https://doi.org/10.1097/00001199-199708000-00005.
66. Turner-Stokes L, Wade DT, Playford D, et al. Prolonged disorders of consciousness following sudden onset brain injury. National Clinical Guidelines.; 2020.
67. Lazaridis C. Withdrawal of Life-Sustaining Treatments in Perceived Devastating Brain Injury: The Key Role of Uncertainty. Neurocrit Care 2019;30(1). https://doi.org/10.1007/s12028-018-0595-8.

Special Considerations in Behavioral Assessments for Disorders of Consciousness

Katherine O'Brien, PhD[a,b,c],*, Bei Zhang, MD, MSc[d],
Elizabeth Anderl, PT, DPT[a], Sunil Kothari, MD[a,c]

KEYWORDS

- Disorders of consciousness (DoCs) • Behavioral assessment • Mindset • Bias
- Qualitative assessment • Quantitative assessment • Therapist • Rehabilitation

KEY POINTS

- Rehabilitation clinicians must be mindful of potential biases in assessing a patient's level of consciousness and how those biases can compromise the accuracy of assessments.
- Assessments should be performed under conditions that maximize the possibility of detecting signs of consciousness; the patient should be "set up for success."
- Qualitative behavioral observations can be as informative as the use of standardized measures.
- All therapy disciplines (physical therapy/occupational therapy/speech language pathology) have a significant role in assessments of consciousness. Nursing staff and family members should also be encouraged to share their observations.
- The individualized quantitative behavioral assessment can provide information that is not otherwise obtainable.

INTRODUCTION

Behavioral assessment remains the cornerstone of the clinical evaluation of disorders of consciousness (DoCs). Although rapidly developing technologies hold great promise (see article "Technological Modalities in the Assessment and Treatment of

[a] TIRR Disorders of Consciousness Program, TIRR Memorial Hermann Hospital, 1333 Moursund Street, Houston, TX 77030, USA; [b] Department of Physical Medicine and Rehabilitation, McGovern Medical School, University of Texas Health Science Center at Houston, Houston, USA; [c] H. Ben Taub Department of Physical Medicine and Rehabilitation, Baylor College of Medicine, Houston, TX 77030, USA; [d] Division of Physical Medicine and Rehabilitation, Department of Neurology, Texas Tech University Health Sciences Center, 3601 4th Street, STOP 8321, Lubbock, TX 79430, USA
* Corresponding author. TIRR Memorial Hermann, 1333 Moursund Street, Houston, TX 77030.
E-mail address: Katherine.OBrien@memorialhermann.org
Twitter: @BeiZhangMD (B.Z.)

Phys Med Rehabil Clin N Am 35 (2024) 93–108
https://doi.org/10.1016/j.pmr.2023.07.007

Disorders of Consciousness" in this issue), especially in the context of severe cognitive-motor dissociation (CMD), their limited availability means that most clinicians still rely almost exclusively on bedside behavioral assessments to determine a patient's level of consciousness. Yet, studies have repeatedly found that there is a high rate of misdiagnosis with clinical assessments of consciousness.[1–6] Because the basic use of DoC behavioral assessment scales have been reviewed elsewhere,[7] in this article, we would want to focus on topics that may be less familiar to clinicians working with patients with DoC. These include (1) recognizing the influence of mindset and unconscious bias; (2) understanding the nuances of obtaining evidence of consciousness, whether qualitative or quantitative; (3) recognizing the unique role of therapists, neuropsychologists, and other team members in the assessment of DoC; and (4) being able to design and implement an individualized quantitative behavioral assessment (IQBA) to detect and interpret observations that may be missed by more standardized assessments. We think that an appreciation of all of these points can significantly improve the quality and accuracy of behavioral assessments of DoC.

MINDSETS AND BIASES IN THE ASSESSMENT OF DISORDERS OF CONSCIOUSNESS

Mindsets are mental frameworks that direct an individual's attention and motivation toward specific sets of associations and expectations.[8] The term is most commonly used to refer to "pre-evidential" beliefs of what is likely to be the case. In this context, mindsets refer to the unavoidable assumptions and expectations we bring to all situations, before we are able to assess the facts or data that allow us to form more objective—*"post-evidential"*—beliefs. Ideally, a pre-evidential mindset serves as a starting hypothesis that is then confirmed or revised based on the neutral acquisition of objective information. However, it is now known that these pre-evidential mindsets often serve as "biases" that can affect the collection and interpretation of the information itself, thereby compromising the neutrality of the process of belief formation. These biases have been extensively described in the medical literature; the most common ones are described below.[9–11]

Anchoring Bias (First Impression Bias)

Anchoring bias occurs when a clinician relies too heavily on any initial information obtained (the "anchor").[12,13] For example, a rehabilitation physician admitting a patient with a DoC may have been told by the referring physician that the patient is in a vegetative state; the physician may then rely too heavily on this initial information in assessing the patient, anchoring on the idea that the patient is unconscious and thereby potentially missing subtle signs of consciousness.

Confirmation Bias

Confirmation bias occurs when clinicians selectively gather and interpret evidence in ways that confirm existing beliefs and discount evidence that contradicts them.[12,14,15] Clinicians (unconsciously) "see what they want to see." For example, thinking a patient to be unconscious, a clinical team may discount the possibility that the ambiguous movements they see are intentional. Even when using a standardized scale, a patient may not be "given credit" when a response is unclear or equivocal, thereby potentially underestimating the patient's level of consciousness.

Salience Bias

Salience bias describes our tendency to focus on information that is more prominent or emotionally striking (and ignore information that is not).[16] For example, a patient's brain imaging may demonstrate a significant amount of damage (eg, **Fig. 1** A–C). A physician may find the patient's scan so striking that they may invest less effort in the clinical assessment and/or discount ambiguous findings that might have represented the presence of consciousness.

Representativeness Bias

The representativeness bias refers to our tendency to judge the likelihood or frequency of an event by comparing it to an existing prototype or paradigm in our mind.[11,17,18] For example, if the clinician's mental prototype of a patient with an anoxic brain injury is someone who is experiencing almost always in an unresponsive wakefulness syndrome (UWS), they may tend to overlook or discount evidence that would indicate a patient is conscious.

Diagnostic Momentum

Although not an actual bias, diagnostic momentum refers to a phenomenon that can, similar to the biases described above, compromise the objectivity and neutrality of evaluations. It refers to an inclination to continue with a diagnosis once it is made, leading to the overlooking or discounting of contrary evidence.[19] The bias amplifies as more clinicians accept the initial diagnosis, leading to a potential (mis)diagnosis being passed on to other clinicians.[12] This phenomenon is likely common in patients with a DoC who have been in several other facilities before reaching the current clinicians; a

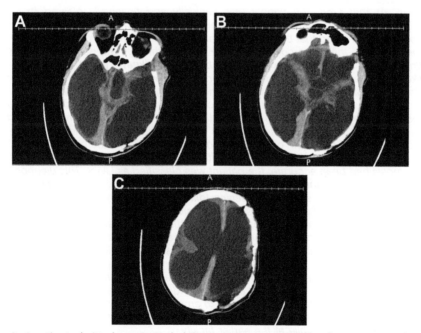

Fig. 1. A patient admitted to a DoC rehabilitation program 8 months after a traumatic brain injury. CT head showed extremely enlarged ventricles (*black areas* in the calvarium) and compressed brain parenchyma (*gray areas* in the middle of the calvarium in [A] and [B] and the inner periphery of the calvarium in [C]). The images are so striking that clinicians may wonder how a person with these findings could possibly be conscious. In reality, the patient was able to read, do simple math, and answer yes/no questions.

diagnosis (or label) of UWS may "follow the patient," even though the patient may have improved during the time that has elapsed.

Rosenthal (Pygmalion) Effect

An example of how mindsets can function as self-fulfilling biases was reported by Weaver and colleagues in a study of performance evaluation in sports.[20] In this study, coaches were given false expectations about the basketball shooting ability of players whom they had not yet met. It was found that the coaches allocated more shooting opportunities to players for whom the false expectation was favorable and fewer shots to players for whom the false expectation was unfavorable. In turn, players who were allocated more shots made a higher percentage of them, thereby confirming their coaches' expectations about their shooting ability. This phenomenon of higher expectations leading to better performance is referred to as the Pygmalion or Rosenthal effect and has long been observed in education and management.[21–24] It is possible that a similar effect might be operative in the assessment of patients with DoC: that the expectation or presumption that someone is conscious may increase the likelihood of detecting actual signs of consciousness (see "setting the patient up for success" section).

AN ILLUSTRATIVE REAL-LIFE SCENARIO

A young man sustained an anoxic brain injury after a cardiac arrest requiring prolonged resuscitation. Several weeks after the incident, he opened his eyes but remained unresponsive, even after being weaned off of all sedating medications. At that time, the patient was clinically and financially cleared to be admitted to an inpatient rehabilitation facility. Before admission, the rehabilitation clinicians heard that this was a "vegetative patient" (diagnostic momentum); they came to the same conclusion after reading through the patient's records immediately after admission (anchoring bias). They "knew" that it was very unlikely that the patient was conscious after such a severe hypoxic-ischemic event (representativeness bias). The team did not find any behavioral evidence of consciousness despite repeated evaluations (including frequent standardized testing) during several months (confirmation bias). However, the family reported several times that they had seen "things" that led them to think their loved one was conscious but their opinion was discounted by the team (confirmation bias). After several months, the rehabilitation team concluded that their initial diagnosis had been accurate: the patient was classified as UWS. This diagnosis was agreed on by the entire team: all of the rehabilitation clinicians, neurologists, and internal medicine physicians (diagnostic momentum). Not agreeing with the team, the family requested a transfer to another DoC program. The new program endorsed a philosophy of "setting the patient up for success" (see the next section) and quickly discovered that the patient was fully conscious (Rosenthal effect?). The patient was completely paralyzed except for trace movements in their head/neck; these movements were leveraged to create a low-tech communication system and the patient immediately answered a series of questions with 100% accuracy and soon was able to spell out full sentences. The diagnosis was changed to emergence from minimally conscious state (eMCS). The patient had reported that he had regained consciousness many weeks earlier while at the earlier facility.

Mindsets Acting as Biases

The potential of mindsets acting as biases is highest in situations of limited available information and/or where the available information is ambiguous. Both criteria apply to the assessment of patients with DoC, when evidence for consciousness is infrequent, inconsistent, and ambiguous. Because of this, the mindset that clinicians bring to their evaluations likely plays an outsized role in determining the results of their assessments. Indeed, it is possible that the reported high rate of misdiagnosis of patients experiencing DoC is as much due to the biases of the evaluating clinicians as it is to the actual processes of evaluation. Given the significant influence biases can have on the assessment of patients with DoC, it is important for clinicians to take steps to minimize their influence.

The first step in this regard is simply to acknowledge the risk of bias and to recognize the different forms it can take. Clinicians should also cultivate a reflective and reflexive attitude, regularly asking themselves whether they are accounting for the influence of potential biases.[12,25,26] There is evidence to suggest that raising awareness of bias-related diagnostic errors can improve the diagnostic performance of clinicians.[27] With regard to DoC assessments, there may be specific questions that clinicians can ask themselves to help screen and compensate for potential biases (**Table 1**). Finally, because almost all biases we have described are likely to result in the underestimation of a patient's level of consciousness, an approach that explicitly attempts to maximize the likelihood of detecting signs of consciousness should be adopted. We will discuss such a strategy in the next section.

SETTING THE PATIENT UP FOR SUCCESS

The clinical assessment of consciousness begins with 2 core assumptions.

1. Behavioral evidence of consciousness can be infrequent, inconsistent, and subtle and
2. Underestimating someone's true level of consciousness can have life-changing (and even life-ending) consequences.

Given these facts, we think that all DoC assessments should always aim to *set the patient up for success*. That is, assessments should always be structured and executed in such a way as to maximize the possibility of detecting evidence that reflects the patient's highest level of consciousness. During every step of the assessment process, clinicians should ask themselves, "are we collecting information under conditions that best allow the patient to demonstrate their current level of consciousness?" In what follows, we will discuss specific ways in which clinicians can operationalize this attitude of "setting the patient up for success."

As discussed in the previous section, the first step is to recognize the impact that mindset and unconscious biases can have on the assessment of consciousness. An approach that may be helpful is for the clinical team to begin with *a presumption of the presence of consciousness*. That is, the team could assume that all patients are fully conscious and that the role of the assessment is to find evidence to support the truth of the assumption. The starting hypothesis would be that "all patients are conscious until proven otherwise." We think that approaching assessments in this manner reduces the chance of missing signs of consciousness or emergence. As with a detective or prosecutor looking to support their case, the team would be making an *active* effort to look for "relevant evidence." Another analogy might be playing a "Spot the Difference" game. If one quickly skims through the 2 similar pictures, one may not notice any differences between them. However, if one is specifically instructed to identify the subtle ways in which the 2 pictures differ (ie, starting with the presumption that there *are* differences), one will make an active effort to locate them.

Table 1
Debiasing strategies

	Potential Biases	Thought Modifications	Preferred Mindset
Initial chart review	Anchoring bias Salience bias	*"The prior evaluation may or may not be accurate."* *"Although the image does not look good, the person might still be conscious and able to do well. I will keep an open mind."* *"I will develop creative assessment paradigms, aiming to identify voluntary movements."*	Open mindset: • Embrace all possibilities • Open to new ideas/concepts • Collaborative Flexible mindset: • Persist in setbacks • Try multiple approaches • Counterfactual thinking
First and recurrent assessments	Anchoring bias Confirmation bias Salience bias	*"XXX does not make sense, which warrants further investigation."* *"How can we make the movements faster and more consistent?"* *"What are the confounders?"* *"How could we better assess this behavior?"* *"Let us try XXX."* *"Did I miss something?"*	Creative mindset: • Think outside of the box • Try new approaches • Use useful criticism
Making a clinical determination of the level of consciousness	Anchoring bias Representativeness bias	*"Am I overconfident in my conclusion?"* *"How could I obtain more information?* *"Is it possible it is because of XXX?"*	

Of course, it could be argued that such an approach is itself biased (although in the positive direction). Although technically correct, we think that, for several reasons, this is not a significant issue. First, unlike unconscious biases, the *presumption of consciousness* we are advocating is deliberately chosen. This allows it to be consciously reflected on and modified as evidence is collected. Second, the presumption of consciousness is a starting assumption, not a fixed conclusion. Finally, given the current high rate of underestimation of the level of consciousness, a "positive" bias may be more likely to reduce the rate of "false negatives" (ie, missed signs of consciousness or emergence). Perhaps, paradoxically, a presumption of a patient being conscious may yield more accurate diagnoses than an assessment that focuses purely on being standardized and "objective."

From a more practical point of view, *setting the patient up for success* means ensuring that assessments are, as much as possible, performed under conditions that maximize the possibility of detecting signs of consciousness or emergence. These conditions include (but are not limited to):

Address Confounds and Reversible Causes of Impaired Consciousness

At the outset, it is important to identify and address all reversible causes of impaired consciousness (conditions that may directly affect arousal and awareness) as well as confounders (conditions such as aphasia that do not affect consciousness itself but compromise its assessment).

Perform Serial Assessments

Given that behavioral manifestations of consciousness are infrequent and inconsistent, assessments (whether qualitative or quantitative) should be performed as often as possible. With regard to formal assessments with standardized scales, studies have suggested that at least 5 assessments using the Coma Recovery Scale-Revised (CRS-R) during 2 weeks increased the diagnostic accuracy.[28] Serial assessments were also endorsed by the 2018 AAN/ACRM/NIDLRR DoC guidelines.[29] In addition, it should be kept in mind that the amount of time spent on observation can significantly increase the likelihood of obtaining relevant findings.

With Multiple Examiners

Each team member brings different skills and experience to the assessment and may therefore be able to observe or elicit behaviors that others cannot. All team members should be involved in selecting stimuli, behaviors to look for, and proper patient positioning for the assessments.

At Different Times of the Day

Patients' level of consciousness may vary at different times of the day. This may be due to normal circadian rhythms with superimposed disturbances of the sleep–wake cycle. It may also be a result of the effects of medications. For example, patients may have diminished arousal after being administered sedating medications; conversely, their arousal may be better for a period after taking a stimulant. Given this variability, it is important to evaluate the patient at different times of the day and, ideally, to target those times that the patient seems most alert.

Under Conditions of Maximal Arousal

Evaluating a patient when they are underaroused can result in significant underestimation of their level of consciousness. Therefore, evaluations should ideally take place during periods of maximal arousal. In addition, the clinician can enhance the level of arousal at the time of evaluation through various interventions (eg, administering a stimulant medication before the evaluation, performing the assessment with the patient in a standing position, and so forth).

Including the Upright Position

Both everyday experience and studies suggest that the supine position is more often associated with diminished arousal, which decreases the likelihood that patients will be able to demonstrate their true level of consciousness. Additionally, movements in a supine position can be more challenging due to the resistance from gravity or friction from sheets/pillows. Therefore, as much as possible, assessments should take place with the patient in a sitting or even standing position (eg, using a tilt-table or standing frame). It is noted that a subset of patients may perform better in a supine position because they may be uncomfortable in other positions.

Recognizing the Role (and Limitations) of Standardized Scales

Although the emphasis on standardized assessments in DoCs is appropriate, it is important to realize that they are a means to an end. Their primary purpose is to identify (and quantify) signs of consciousness and emergence. Although these scales are an important tool, clinicians should recognize that relevant information can also be obtained through careful (nonstandardized) observation, whether at the bedside or in therapies. If one is attempting to determine whether a patient can follow commands, it is irrelevant whether they do so during the administration of a standardized scale or during an informal bedside assessment. The point is for clinicians to use *all tools* available to them to collect data: standardized assessments, focused qualitative evaluations, serendipitous observations, and so forth.

Seeking the Observations of Families

Among the most valuable sources of information are the observations of family members. Unfortunately, DoC clinicians frequently undervalue and even discount the reports made by families. The presumption is that family members do not have the knowledge to properly interpret behaviors (eg, to be able to distinguish reflexive from nonreflexive movement) or that a family's hope may cause them to "see what they want to see." It is unlikely that these attitudes (biases) on the part of clinicians are justified. Not only do family members often spend far more time with the patient than the clinical team (and thus have much more opportunity to observe important behaviors); studies have also shown that patients with DoCs seem to respond better to family members (eg, by following a command when given by a family member but not when given by a clinician).[30] Therefore, clinicians should always solicit the observations of families to help with the investigation of signs of consciousness or emergence.

Finally, it is important to keep in mind that, as in other areas of medicine, "lack of evidence" is not the same as "evidence of lack." Rather than concluding that a patient is definitely unconscious in these situations, a more accurate conclusion would be that "we (the clinical team) have not been able to detect any behavioral signs of consciousness in this patient."

THE ROLE OF REHABILITATION CLINICIANS

The behavioral evaluation of consciousness should be a holistic process, using the experience and skills of all team members. This includes disciplines that may not always be thought to be directly involved with assessing consciousness such as physical therapy (PT) and occupational therapy (OT). Frequently, those disciplines are thought to only (or primarily) deal with the patient's body but not their mind. Not only is the distinction between "mind" and "body" problematic but, as discussed below, all therapy disciplines play a crucial role in the direct assessment of DoCs.

Speech-Language Pathology

The role of the speech language pathologist (SLP) in the assessment of consciousness is widely recognized. They have training in both cognition as well as communication and thus play a central role in these evaluations. Examples of their contributions to the assessment process include (1) identifying possible expressive and/or receptive language deficits that may act as confounds, (2) recognizing the presence of oral apraxia that may limit the patient's ability to respond verbally, (3) detecting possible auditory and visual deficits that may confound the assessment and complicate the patient's ability to interact, and (4) advising the team on how head and neck position might influence the patient's ability to use movement of these parts of the body to communicate. Regardless of the location of any residual movement (eg, head, arm, leg, and so forth), the SLP plays a leading role in transforming those movements into a viable communication system, with or without the aid of technology.

Physical and Occupational Therapy

It is being increasingly recognized that many patients with DoCs have significant CMD.[31] In these situations, the patient's ability to manifest their level of consciousness is limited by profound motor impairments. Thus, an accurate assessment of consciousness is contingent on identifying and compensating for these impairments. Because of their training in neuromusculoskeletal anatomy and biomechanics, physical and occupational therapists are ideally situated to (1) identify parts of the body that may have the capacity for movement, however minimal; (2) identify barriers to movement such as biomechanical disadvantage, spasticity, and so forth; (3) position the body in such a way as to maximize the potential for movement; (4) address intrinsic barriers to movement such as spasticity, contractures, and so forth, either by accommodating for them (eg, through splinting) or by directly treating them; and (5) where possible, implement means to amplify any residual movement that is present. The behavioral expression of consciousness can only occur through motor output. Thus, it is imperative that the team invest the time, energy, and expertise to ensure that the patient's motor capacities are optimized. In situations where the patient demonstrates minimal to no responsiveness, the evaluation cannot be considered accurate (or even adequate) unless both the physical and occupational therapists have participated in the assessment. Thus, in all cases of possible or confirmed significant CMD, *the active participation of physical and occupational therapists in the assessment of consciousness should be considered mandatory.*

Often, the identification of residual movement, however subtle and weak, can mean the difference between a patient being considered unconscious (ie, UWS) or conscious (and even fully emerged/eMCS). Such an identification, based on our clinical experience, commonly occurs in therapy sessions when the patient is up, stretched, and comfortable, as well as instructed to perform and observed closely. Physical and occupational therapists can improve the sensitivity of the assessment of consciousness through their ability to enhance the arousal of patients via stimulation and, especially, mobilization. Verticalization, whether through sitting or standing, should be considered obligatory for all patients who seem to be unresponsive or minimally responsive. Preliminary data from our center (not yet published) have revealed that patients' arousal level and performance on the CRS-R were significantly worse when lying in bed than when sitting at the edge of the mat or in a wheelchair. Physical and occupational therapists play a crucial role in addressing bodily barriers (eg, spasticity, contractures, weakness, and so forth), enabling mobilization, and facilitating patients' performance in assessments.

Neuropsychology

It is sometimes thought that neuropsychologists have a limited role to play in the assessment of consciousness because their training has traditionally focused on more downstream forms of cognition such as memory, visuospatial skills, executive functioning, and so forth. However, their training and skill set are actually well suited to aid in the evaluation of consciousness. Neuropsychologists are educated and experienced in standardized assessments and psychometrics allowing them to help the team in the collection and interpretation of behavioral information. Their knowledge of neuroanatomy and psychomotor function can also be crucial in correlating the patient's presentation with the location and extent of their brain injury. Neuropsychologists thus often play a central role on the DoC team, communicating with the staff and families to collate observed evidence, helping interpret ambiguous behaviors, collaborating with the team to design assessment paradigms, and working with the physician in interpreting the patient's response to psychoactive medications such as neurostimulants.[32]

AN ILLUSTRATIVE REAL-LIFE SCENARIO (*CONTINUED*)

The patient—who had been diagnosed as being in a UWS at an earlier DoC program—was discovered on postadmission evaluations to have slight but definite head/neck movements when the effect of gravity was minimized (through head support) and the neck muscles were sufficiently stretched. The team also determined that the patient had to be inclined at a specific angle in his tilt-in-space wheelchair to allow for the head/neck movements. Once placed at a biomechanical advantage through positioning, the patient's voluntary head movements, although minimal, were able to be joined to a low-tech communication system (a laser pointer affixed to a head band), and the patient was immediately able to answer questions accurately. In this case, it was the ability of the therapists (SLP/OT/PT) along with the neuropsychologist to detect, maximize, and leverage very subtle movements that led to the diagnosis of eMCS rather than UWS. In addition, the expertise of the PT and OT also enabled, in collaboration with the SLP and neuropsychologist, the creation of a viable communication method.

Other Team Members

Although we have focused on the role of therapists and neuropsychologists in the evaluation of consciousness, it should be kept in mind that *every* team member has a role to play. This is especially true of the nursing staff (including nursing aides) who, by virtue of the time they spend directly with the patient, have the opportunity to identify signs of consciousness or communication that may not have been seen by the rest of the team. Moreover, the nursing staff is often stimulating the patient (through bed positioning, transfers, personal hygiene, and so forth), which can frequently result in behaviors that may not occur at other times. Therefore, the nursing staff should be trained (and expected) to look for potential signs of consciousness and communication. Additionally, as discussed previously, family and other caregivers should also be a part of the assessment process. The family often spends much more time with the patient than other team members, allowing them opportunities to detect signs of consciousness, especially at times that most of the rest of the team is gone (eg, evenings and nights). Moreover, because families are often able to elicit responses from patients that other team members cannot, even with identical stimuli,[30] consideration should be given to requesting the family members' direct participation in the team's assessments (eg, by being asked to give a verbal command to the patient, as directed by the team).

INDIVIDUALIZED QUANTITATIVE BEHAVIORAL ASSESSMENT (IQBA)

Sometimes behaviors can be so ambiguous and inconsistent that even careful observation according to the suggestions discussed above will not be enough to definitively establish their presence. These situations are characterized by a low "signal-to-noise" ratio. For example, attempting to determine whether a patient with frequent spontaneous myoclonus is following motoric commands. In this situation, there is so much "noise" (background spontaneous movement) that it is difficult to determine whether the movements seen after command are random or true attempts to comply with the examiner's instructions. Other situations may be characterized by low "signal strength" (rather than excessive "noise"). For example, determining whether a patient with severe motor deficits is following commands when the movement requested occurs infrequently. In this situation, the fact that the movement only occurs rarely after command raises doubts about whether the patient is actually following the examiner's instructions.

An IQBA can be a powerful tool in these situations.[33,34] An IQBA is not a scale but an *approach* that, as the name implies, is specific to an individual patient. Rather than relying on a few observations, it pools a large number of them and then subjects this large set of observations to simple quantitative analysis. As with a clinical trial, increasing the sample size (by collecting a large number of observations) significantly increases the "power" of the assessment to identify meaningful differences. In this way, a "signal" that might otherwise be missed, due to either a high background noise and/or a low signal strength, can be more confidently confirmed. The general workflow of an IQBA is illustrated in **Fig. 2**. However, the actual steps required to design and execute an IQBA are best understood through examples; therefore, we will illustrate its use in a "high background noise" scenario (the Appendix provides a "low signal strength" scenario).

Scenario

A patient developed diffuse myoclonus in the head/neck and limbs after hypoxic ischemic brain injury. The team is struggling to differentiate purposeful voluntary movements from involuntary myoclonic movements.

Step 1: Identify a Questionable Behavior

The team is questioning if a movement in the patient's arm is really to command because it is hard to differentiate from the frequent myoclonic movements. Therefore, the question might be as follows: can the patient follow a verbal command to move their right arm?

Step 2: Setup and Specifications

After information about the patient's presentation is collected from all team members, the IQBA team leader establishes a setup plan and response specifications. It is noted that even though each protocol is individualized, the actual assessment paradigm should be standardized as much as possible to guard against observer bias and coincidental responses.[33] Once the team agrees to all specifications and the setup plan, an IQBA form is created (**Fig. 3**) and placed in the patient's room for each team member to fill out.

Step 3: Data Collection

Trained personnel, including clinicians and families, perform the assessments and record the data. The leader supervises the process for coordination and troubleshooting. Occasionally, more than one assessment could be done per session (eg, before and during standing). The team continues to collect data until instructed to discontinue by the leader.

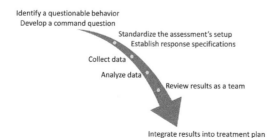

Fig. 2. The workflow of an IQBA to investigate a suspected voluntary movement.

Patient: _____
Date/Time: _____
Examiner: _____
Position: _____

Pt seated in WC with lap tray on. Arm resting on pillow case on lap tray with shoulder at neutral and palm facing down. Stand directly in front of patient looking at patient in the eyes. DO NOT LOOK DIRECTLY AT ARM. Pt has 10 seconds to respond. Give command 2x total during 10 seconds. Arm must move at least the width (bottom edge) of hospital badge to be considered movement.

Command	Moved Right Arm	DID NOT Move Right Arm	Comments
Observation			
Move your right arm			
Hold Still			
Move your right arm			
Observation			
Hold Still			
Observation			
Move your right arm			
Hold Still			

Total Positive Response to Command (Pt moved right arm to command)	
Total False Positives (Pt moved right arm when asked to HOLD still)	
Total Movements Observation (Pt moved right arm during 10 second observation)	

TO ADMINISTER:
Follow order and be clear and specific with your commands (no extra words).

Comments:

Fig. 3. An example of an IQBA form.

Step 4: Data Analysis

The leader is responsible for compiling all IQBA data. The data are then condensed into a table (**Table 2**). As seen in the table, due to their myoclonus, the patient frequently moves their RUE regardless of whether they are asked to (and even when asked to hold still). However, it is noted that the patient moves their RUE more often in the command condition. To determine whether the difference in frequency is due to chance or actually represents command-following, 2×2 chi-square statistics were performed comparing the different conditions. The following results are shown[a]:

Command versus contra-command
The chi-square statistical is 9.9646. The P value is .0016; thus, there is a statistically significant difference between the number of times the patient moved their RUE when asked to (command) versus when they were asked to "hold still" (contra-command).

Command versus observation
The chi-square statistical is 7.9398. The P value is .0048; thus, there is a statistically significant difference between the number of times the patient moved their RUE

---

[a] Please note that due to multiple comparisons, an adjusted and more stringent alpha level needs to be achieved for statistical significance to minimize Type I error. For example, by using the Bonferroni method, the new alpha level is adjusted to 0.0167 for 3 comparisons performed (rather than setting alpha at 0.05). If any box contains a number less than 5, Fisher's exact test needs to be adopted.

Table 2		
Example of IQBA data (*see text for details*)		
	Patient Moved Right Arm	Patient Did Not Move Right Arm
Command (*Move your right arm*)	46	20
Contra-command (*Hold still*)	28	38
Observation only	30	36

when asked to (command) versus when no command was given and the patient was just quietly observed (observation).

Contra-command versus observation

The chi-square statistical is 0.1230. The *P* value is .7258; thus, there is *no* statistically significant difference between the number of times the patient moved their RUE when asked to hold still (contra-command) versus when no command was given and the patient was just quietly observed (observation).

The team can stop performing the IQBA when there are sufficient data to reach a conclusion.

Step 5: Review Results as a Team

The team identifies that the patient clearly moves their arm more in the command condition compared with the contra-command and observation-only conditions. The differences are statistically significant. Given the findings, the team concludes the patient is able to understand and follow verbal commands to move their arm.

A practice case, using a "low signal strength" scenario, is available in the Appendix.

CLINICS CARE POINTS

- Raising awareness of bias-related diagnostic errors can improve the diagnostic performance of clinicians.
- Assessments, whether qualitative or quantitative, should be performed as often as possible.
- The behavioral evaluation of consciousness should be a holistic process, incorporating the experience and skills of all rehabilitation team members.
- Patients with DoC may respond better to family members.
- Individualized Quantitative Behavioral Assessment (IQBA) is a powerful tool for detecting ambiguous and inconsistent behaviors in a scientific manner. It is an assessment approach specific to an individual patient that could be informative in addition to other standardized approaches.

DISCLOSURE

The authors have nothing to disclose.

REFERENCES

1. Porcaro C, Nemirovsky IE, Riganello F, et al. Diagnostic Developments in Differentiating Unresponsive Wakefulness Syndrome and the Minimally Conscious State. Front Neurol 2022;12. https://doi.org/10.3389/FNEUR.2021.778951.

2. Schnakers C, Vanhaudenhuyse A, Giacino J, et al. Diagnostic accuracy of the vegetative and minimally conscious state: Clinical consensus versus standardized neurobehavioral assessment. BMC Neurol 2009;9(1):1–5. https://doi.org/10.1186/1471-2377-9-35/TABLES/2.

3. Zhang B, Woo J, O'Brien K. What Happens to the Small Number of Referrals That Make it to a Disorders of Consciousness (Doc) Rehabilitation Program. Arch Phys Med Rehabil 2020;101(11):e58–9. https://doi.org/10.1016/j.apmr.2020.09.175.

4. Childs NL, Mercer WN, Childs HW. Accuracy of diagnosis of persistent vegetative state. Neurology 1993;43(8):1465–7. https://doi.org/10.1212/WNL.43.8.1465.

5. Andrews K, Murphy L, Munday R, et al. Misdiagnosis of the vegetative state: retrospective study in a rehabilitation unit. BMJ 1996;313(7048):13–6. https://doi.org/10.1136/BMJ.313.7048.13.

6. Wang J, Hu X, Hu Z, et al. The misdiagnosis of prolonged disorders of consciousness by a clinical consensus compared with repeated coma-recovery scale-revised assessment. BMC Neurol 2020;20(1). https://doi.org/10.1186/S12883-020-01924-9.

7. Seel RT, Sherer M, Whyte J, et al. Assessment Scales for Disorders of Consciousness: Evidence-Based Recommendations for Clinical Practice and Research. Arch Phys Med Rehabil 2010;91(12):1795–813. https://doi.org/10.1016/J.APMR.2010.07.218.

8. Crum A, Zuckerman B. Changing Mindsets to Enhance Treatment Effectiveness. JAMA 2017;317(20):2063. https://doi.org/10.1001/JAMA.2017.4545.

9. Blumenthal-Barby JS, Krieger H. Cognitive biases and heuristics in medical decision making: a critical review using a systematic search strategy. Med Decis Making 2015;35(4):539–57. https://doi.org/10.1177/0272989X14547740.

10. Walston Z, Whelehan DF, O'Shea N. Clinical decision making in physical therapy - Exploring the "heuristic" in clinical practice. Musculoskelet Sci Pract 2022;62. https://doi.org/10.1016/J.MSKSP.2022.102674.

11. Whelehan DF, Conlon KC, Ridgway PF. Medicine and heuristics: cognitive biases and medical decision-making. Ir J Med Sci 2020;189(4):1477–84. https://doi.org/10.1007/S11845-020-02235-1.

12. Doherty TS, Carroll AE. Believing in Overcoming Cognitive Biases. AMA J ethics 2020;22(9):773–8. https://doi.org/10.1001/AMAJETHICS.2020.773.

13. Anchoring Bias - The Decision Lab. https://thedecisionlab.com/biases/anchoring-bias. Accessed April 22, 2023.

14. Nickerson RS. Confirmation Bias: A Ubiquitous Phenomenon in Many Guises. 1998;2(2):175-220. doi:10.1037/1089-2680.2.2.175.

15. Confirmation Bias - The Decision Lab. Available at: https://thedecisionlab.com/biases/confirmation-bias. Accessed April 22, 2023.

16. Salience Bias - The Decision Lab. Available at: https://thedecisionlab.com/biases/salience-bias. Accessed April 22, 2023.

17. Representativeness Heuristic - The Decision Lab. Available at: https://thedecisionlab.com/biases/representativeness-heuristic. Accessed July 16, 2023.

18. Saposnik G, Redelmeier D, Ruff CC, et al. Cognitive biases associated with medical decisions: a systematic review. BMC Med Inform Decis Mak 2016;16(1):1–14.

19. Satya-Murti S, Lockhart J. Recognizing and reducing cognitive bias in clinical and forensic neurology. Neurol Clin Pract 2015;5(5):389.

20. Weaver J, Moses JF, Snyder M. Self-Fulfilling Prophecies in Ability Settings. J Soc Psychol 2016;156(2):179–89.

21. Eden D. Leadership and expectations: Pygmalion effects and other self-fulfilling prophecies in organizations. Leadersh Q 1992;3(4):271–305.
22. Murphy D, Campbell C, Garavan TN. The Pygmalion effect reconsidered: Its implications for education, training and workplace learning. J Eur Ind Train 1999; 23(4–5):238–51.
23. Pygmalion in Management. https://hbr.org/2003/01/pygmalion-in-management. Accessed April 22, 2023.
24. Rosenthal R, Jacobson L. Pygmalion in the classroom. Urban Rev 1968;3(1): 16–20.
25. Sassenberg K, Winter K, Becker D, et al. Flexibility mindsets: Reducing biases that result from spontaneous processing. 2021;33(1):171-213.
26. Pelaccia T, Tardif J, Triby E, et al. An analysis of clinical reasoning through a recent and comprehensive approach: the dual-process theory. Med Educ Online 2011;16(1). https://doi.org/10.3402/MEO.V16I0.5890.
27. Croskerry P. The importance of cognitive errors in diagnosis and strategies to minimize them. Acad Med 2003;78(8):775–80.
28. Wannez S, Heine L, Thonnard M, et al. The repetition of behavioral assessments in diagnosis of disorders of consciousness. Ann Neurol 2017;81(6):883–9.
29. Giacino JT, Katz DI, Schiff ND, et al. Practice guideline update recommendations summary: Disorders of consciousness: Report of the Guideline Development, Dissemination, and Implementation Subcommittee of the American Academy of Neurology; the American Congress of Rehabilitation Medicine; and the National Institute on Disability, Independent Living, and Rehabilitation Research. Neurology 2018;91(10):450.
30. Sattin D, Giovannetti AM, Ciaraffa F, et al. Assessment of patients with disorder of consciousness: do different Coma Recovery Scale scoring correlate with different settings? J Neurol 2014;261(12):2378–86.
31. Edlow BL, Claassen J, Schiff ND, et al. Recovery from disorders of consciousness: mechanisms, prognosis and emerging therapies. Nat Rev Neurol 2020; 17(3):135–56.
32. Zhang B, O'Brien K, Woo J, et al. Specialized intensive inpatient rehabilitation is crucial and time-sensitive for functional recovery from disorders of consciousness. Front Neurol 2023;14:1126532.
33. Whyte J, DiPasquale MC, Vaccaro M. Assessment of command-following in minimally conscious brain injured patients. Arch Phys Med Rehabil 1999;80(6): 653–60.
34. Day KV, DiNapoli MV, Whyte J. Detecting early recovery of consciousness: a comparison of methods. Neuropsychol Rehabil 2018;28(8):1233–41.

APPENDIX: AN IQBA PRACTICE CASE

Case example: The team is questioning if a movement in the patient's arm is to command as it happens very rarely, and team members have divided opinions.

1. Identify a questionable behavior: "Can the patient follow verbal command to move the arm?"
2. IQBA setup and specifications: Please follow the instructions in the main text and refer to the sample IQBA form.
3. Data collection: Please follow the instructions in the main text.
4. Data analysis: The data are presented in **Supplement Table 1**. The patient has a very low response rate to command, only about one-third of the time (25/ (25 + 67)). It is also noted that the patient moves their right arm more when they

Supplement Table 1
Example of IQBA data

	Patient Moved Right Arm	Patient did Not Move Right Arm
Command (*Move your right arm*)	25	67
Contra-command (*Hold still*)	20	72
Observation only	6	86

receive verbal input (both command and contra-command conditions) than without verbal input (observation only). When running 2 × 2 chi-square statistics on the data comparing different conditions, one finds the following results:

Command versus Contra-command: The chi-square statistical is 0.7354. The *P* value is .3911, not significant.

Command versus Observation: The chi-square statistical is 14.0046. The *P* value is .0002, significant.

Contra-command versus Observation: The chi-square statistical is 8.7790. The *P* value is .0030, significant.

5. Review results as a team: The team identifies that the patient is clearly moving their arm more when verbal input is provided regardless of the content. It is also clear that there is no statistical difference between the command and contra-command conditions. This suggests that the patient did not differentiate between these 2 conditions. Given the findings, the team concludes the patient may have language comprehension deficits.

6. Integrate into treatment plan: In further interactions/interventions, the team is to provide multimodal input for instructions, for example, verbal, visual, tactile, and hand-over-hand demonstration. The family can also be shown the data and informed of the findings. This would allow them to also modify their interactions with the patient to include more prosody and intonation as well as gestures to assist with communication.

Technological Modalities in the Assessment and Treatment of Disorders of Consciousness

Gang Liu, MD, PhD[a], Bradley Chi, MD[b],*

KEYWORDS

- Disorders of consciousness (DoC) • Medical technology • Diagnostic modalities
- Therapeutic modalities

KEY POINTS

- There have been recent advances in the development of technological modalities that show promise in the diagnosis and treatment of patients with disorder of consciousness (DoC).
- Although most of these modalities are still only appropriate for research use, some should be considered in the clinical care of patients with DoC.
- Decisions about which modalities to use in clinical practice should be based on considerations of evidential support, risk, cost, and availability.

BACKGROUND

In the past 10 years, there has been a rapid advancement in the development of technologies that can be used in the diagnosis and treatment of people with a disorder of consciousness (DoC).[1,2] In what follows, we will review these modalities, beginning with technologies used in assessment and concluding with technological treatments, both noninvasive and invasive. It is noted that the role of neuroimaging is treated in a separate article (Linda B. Xu and colleagues' article, "Neuroimaging in Disorders of Consciousness and Recovery," in this issue) and so will not be discussed here.

ASSESSMENTS
Neurophysiology

Standard electroencephalography
The application of standard electroencephalography (EEG) in the diagnosis and assessment of acute DoC has a long history. The most common EEG waveforms

[a] Department of Rehabilitation Medicine, Huashan Hospital, Fudan University, No 12 Wulumuqi Middle Road, Shanghai 200040, China; [b] H. Ben Taub Department of Physical Medicine and Rehabilitation, Baylor College of Medicine, 7200 Cambridge Street, Houston, TX 77030, USA
* Corresponding author. 7200 Cambridge Street, Suite 10C, Houston, TX 77030.
E-mail address: bradley.chi@BCM.edu

Phys Med Rehabil Clin N Am 35 (2024) 109–126
https://doi.org/10.1016/j.pmr.2023.07.005
1047-9651/24/© 2023 Elsevier Inc. All rights reserved.

observed in patients with acute DoC include the disappearance of alpha rhythm, which is usually replaced by continuous irregular slow (theta or delta) waves, and decreased brain electrical reactivity.[3] To quantitatively reflect the severity of coma, several EEG grading criteria have been proposed, including the Synek (1988) and Young (1997) EEG grading systems. These criteria are based on characteristic EEG waveforms (such as triphasic waves, spindle waves, burst-suppression patterns, epileptiform activity) and the reactivity of the EEG to stimuli.[4] The higher the grade, the worse the prognosis is.[4]

Quantitative electroencephalography

To facilitate the analysis of EEG, quantitative electroencephalogram (qEEG) plots the raw EEG signals into intuitive trend maps. These techniques enable clinicians, who are not specialized or trained in neurophysiology, to perform and analyze EEGs at bedside.[3] The following sections review application of qEEG in diagnosis of patients with DoC.

Spectral power. Multiple studies demonstrate differences in power of frequency bands between DoC and healthy controls (HC). Evidence is most supportive of characteristically increased delta activity and decreased alpha activity in DoC. When comparing patients with minimally conscious state (MCS) and unresponsive wakefulness syndrome (UWS), the increase in delta power is more pronounced in UWS. Similarly, decrease in alpha power is significantly more pronounced in UWS; MCS has higher alpha activity. A study also demonstrated higher theta power in MCS than UWS. Gamma power appears lower in patients with DoC compared with HC, while evidence on beta activity pattern is inconclusive. Finally, there is a positive correlation between CRS-R score with power ratio and peak frequency of the spectrum.[3]

Nonlinear dynamics. Brain electrical activity measured by EEG is complex and displays nonlinear dynamic properties. Therefore, analysis using a nonlinear dynamic approach may be advantageous compared with traditional linear approaches.

When focused on time domains, several studies consistently demonstrate decreased EEG complexity in patients with DoC relative to HC. Patients with MCS have moderately lower complexity while those with UWS have even lower complexity. Two indices capturing EEG complexity are most studied in the DoC population: (1) approximate entropy (ApEn) and (2) permutation entropy. ApEn is lower in DoC relative to HC, with UWS consistently lower than MCS. Lower ApEn is correlated with death or poor recovery.[5] Permutation entropy is significantly lower in UWS relative to MCS making it promising in differentiating between the 2 states.[6,7]

Similar to the time domain, when focused on frequency domains, spectral entropy is lower in patients with DoC relative to HC with UWS lower than MCS.[8,9] Patients with MCS seem to have a characteristic periodic fluctuation in spectral entropy that is not present in patients with UWS. Lesser studied indices in DOC such as state entropy,[10] reaction entropy,[10] and bispectral index[10,11] have been shown to differentiate MCS and UWS (sensitivity 89%, specificity 90%).[10]

Brain networks. EEG signals have been used to estimate brain connectivity through mapping of brain networks known as functional connectivity. Studies show characteristic changes to functional connectivity in patients with DoC which are positively correlated with the level of consciousness.[12,13] Compared with non-DoC severe neurocognitive disorders, patients with MCS were characterized by impaired connectivity between frontal and parietal–occipital regions[14] as well as between temporal and parietal–occipital regions.[15] Differences in connectivity between MCS and UWS have also been demonstrated.[12,16,17] A study has also shown biocoherence, as measured by quadratic phase self-coupling in delta, theta, and alpha bands, is correlated with CRS-R score.[18] Finally, certain treatments have been shown to produce changes to connectivity including transcranial direct current stimulation (tDCS),[19–21] transcranial alternating current stimulation (tACS),[22] and spinal cord electrical stimulation (SCS).[23]

Another approach called graph theory analysis, which quantifies features of functional neural networks, has been used with DoC patients. Compared with HC, patients with DoC demonstrate decreased network integration (global information processing) and increased network isolation (local information processing).[24,25] The level of consciousness was positively correlated with network integration[24] and negatively correlated with network isolation.[26] MCS has characteristically more robust frontoparietal networks compared with UWS and these differences have been shown to predict clinical misdiagnosis of UWS.[27] For example, a support vector machine (SVM) trained on these characteristics (alpha participation coefficient and delta band power) could diagnose UWS, MCS (−), and MCS (+) with 74%, 100%, and 71% accuracy, respectively.[27] Other network characteristics such as path length and clustering coefficient have also been shown to distinguish MCS from UWS.[28]

Finally, a trial evaluated EEG microstates in a DoC cohort. The number and diversity of microstates seem to be positively correlated with state of consciousness. Furthermore, the investigators found alpha band microstates may actually play a role in formation of consciousness. Alpha band microstates have also been shown to differentiate MCS from UWS.[28]

Sleep patterns. Clinical trials show disturbances in sleep-stage-dependent EEG patterns in patients with DoC compared with HC. In particular, sleep spindles and slow-wave oscillations are positively correlated with state of consciousness. In one study, patients with MCS did not demonstrate the day–night variation in these sleep EEG patterns seen in HC.[29] Others have found that slow-wave sleep characteristics are significantly correlated with CRS-R scores and can distinguish MCS from UWS.[30–32] Of note, studies of patients with UWS have found conflicting results regarding the presence[33,34] vs. lack[35] of sleep EEG patterns leading to some debate over whether sleep EEG patterns are present in patients with UWS.

Electroencephalographic reactivity. EEG reactivity is a measure of the change in baseline activity with external stimuli. EEG reactivity was shown to be positively correlated with CRS-R scores.[36] Another prospective cohort study found that the type of stimulus evoking EEG reactivity affected the ability to differentiate MCS from UWS.[37] EEG reactivity evoked by eye opening/closing, auditory, and intermittent photic stimulation had high specificity for identifying MCS from UWS while EEG reactivity evoked by pain and tactile stimulation was not useful in differentiating MCS from UWS.[37]

Evoked potentials

Evoked potentials (EPs) measure brain electrical activity after specific stimuli, therefore reflecting the perception and processing of environmental stimuli in the cerebral cortex after sensory input.[38,39] They may also reflect the presence of conscious processing in patients with DoC.[38,39] The most studied EPs are auditory EPs (AEPs) where there are characteristic differences distinguishing UWS, MCS, and HC. A few studies have evaluated somatosensory evoked potentials (EP) and visual EP (VEP) showing important differentiators in patients with DoC. Multimodal approaches combining multiple markers are likely most beneficial diagnostically. The following sections summarize key findings from the literature related to each type of EP.

Auditory evoked potentials. Most MCS and some UWS patients have preserved cortical response to auditory stimulation, therefore many studies evaluating EP response to auditory stimulation are available.[40,41] Most commonly studied is the use of the oddball paradigm for auditory stimulation (ie, comparing the subject's own name vs. another first name).[42] When evaluating the P300 wave, a response was detected in most MCS patients but was not detected in most UWS patients.[43] Similarly, patients with MCS demonstrate a higher and wider spatial distribution in P300 response between active and passive task conditions compared to patients with UWS.[44,45] In comparison, the N400 response is not detected in most DoC patients and does not reliably distinguish MCS from UWS.[46,47] Another marker, mismatch negativity, an EP component regarded as an indicator of pre-attentive sensory memory processes, was shown to differentiate patients with DoC from conscious patients with traumatic brain injury (TBI) but did not differentiate patients with UWS from patients with MCS.[8,48] The late positive component (P600) marker is only seen in MCS and conscious patients,[49] while the natural speech envelope (NSE) marker was shown to be significantly delayed in patients with DoC (UWS and MCS).[50] In the same study, they found that the NSE in behaviorally diagnosed DoC patients with intact communicative function on functional MRI (fMRI) was not different than the NSE in HC, suggesting a potential role for the NSE in detecting cognitive motor dissociation. Auditory stimulation has also been used as part of multidimensional evaluation of consciousness and cognitive domains in DoC.[51]

Somatosensory evoked potentials. A small clinical trial evaluating vibrotactile stimulation as a marker for consciousness in patients with DoC found that the presence of P3a, a marker of bottom-up attention orienting, was predictive of command following.[52] Specifically, all DoC patients (3 MCS, 2 UWS) with P3a demonstrated command following (measured either behaviorally or via fMRI). Conversely, most (5 of 6) patients without P3a did not show command following.[52]

Visual evoked potentials. Flash VEPs are smaller with longer latency in DoC compared with HC, but use can be limited due to the need for active patient cooperation.[53] A novel approach to circumventing this challenge used a combination of transcranial magnetic stimulation (TMS) with visual stimulation through transorbital ACS to evaluate visuomotor integration (VMI) and visual P300 patterns, markers that reflect sensory–motor integration.[54] They found preserved VMI and P300 in patients with MCS, but nearly all patients with UWS did not show significant VMI.

Brain–computer interface

Brain–computer interface (BCI)'s translate brain activity to an external device allowing command following without muscle activation. A recent systematic review on the use of EEG-based BCI for DoC included 27 clinical trials.[55] Most studies (n = 26) focused on assessment of consciousness, with all but one trial finding significant classification accuracy. The most common BCI paradigm used was oddball (vibrotactile, visual, auditory, or audiovisual)[56–61] although motor action,[62] motor imagery,[63–66] and passive emotion recognition[67] were also used. Of the studies testing a P300-based BCI for CRS-R assessment (n = 6), classification accuracy above chance ranged from 30.8% to 78.6% showing the ability of BCI to detect abilities not detected on behavioral CRS-R assessment. CRS-R items evaluated by BCI included visual pursuit,[57,68] object recognition,[69] auditory startle,[70] sound localization,[58] and communication.[71] Importantly, across studies, BCI detected all cases with a positive CRS-R behavioral response with the exception of 2 patients where visual fixation was appreciated on behavioral CRS-R assessment but not BCI assessment.[68] A study found repeat BCI assessment to significantly improve classification accuracy (10 of 20 with first session, 20 of 20 after all sessions).[60] Furthermore, classification accuracy with BCI seems to be correlated with clinical prognosis at 3 [59] and 6 months.[72]

Machine learning
A few studies have evaluated machine learning algorithms to predict level of consciousness in patients with DoC. The 2 main models used were SVMs[8,27] and multivariate pattern analysis (MVPA).[6] These studies all showed machine learning models outperforming clinical behavioral assessment. The largest of these studies is a prospective nonrandomized trial evaluating an EEG biomarker-trained machine learning algorithm in the diagnosis of DoC.[6] They used 28 EEG biomarkers comparing univariate vs. MVPA machine learning to predict state of consciousness. The multivariate analysis outperformed almost all individual biomarkers regardless of changes in EEG configuration. Additionally, a 2017 study's machine model had comparable predictive accuracy to expert assessment using positron emission tomography (PET) imaging.[27]

Transcranial magnetic stimulation
Transcranial magnetic stimulation–electroencephalography. TMS–EEG involves applying TMS to specific brain regions during routine EEG testing, allowing real-time observation of brain electrical activity and reactivity under stimulation.[73,74] A small clinical trial used TMS–EEG on DoC patients to evaluate changes in cortical effective connectivity acutely and longitudinally.[75] They found TMS stimulated a simple, local response in UWS similar to patterns seen in sleep or general anesthesia. Conversely, in MCS the response was complex, distant, bilateral activation, similar to patterns seen in locked-in syndrome and other conscious patients.[75] In a longitudinal study of 3 UWS patients that recovered to eMCS, they demonstrated the characteristic EEG patterns changed from simple, local to complex, distant as patients clinically recovered.[54] Similar findings were found in chronic DoC patients where cortical reactivity and connectivity were severed impaired in UWS, but preserved with abnormal features in MCS.[76]

Another index of TMS–EEG, known as the perturbational complexity index (PCI), reflects the brain's ability to maintain stability and complexity in its functional networks after being perturbed.[77,78] It provides insight into overall brain functional connectivity and diversity.[77,78] Two clinical trials have evaluated TMS–EEG on patients with DoC using PCI as the primary outcome. The larger of these 2 studies (n = 81) compared the test population to a benchmark population including both conscious and unconscious conditions.[79,80] They derived an empiric cutoff PCI (PCI*) from the benchmark population that differentiated consciousness and unconsciousness with 100% sensitivity and 100% specificity. When applied to the test population, this PCI* was 94.7% sensitive in detecting MCS. They also identified 4 out of 9 UWS patients with PCI consistent with the conscious state based on PCI*, suggesting the possibility of behavioral misdiagnosis.[80] Existing research suggests that a higher PCI value is associated with a better prognosis of DoC.

Transcranial magnetic stimulation–electromyography. TMS has also been combined with electromyography (EMG) to detect motor-EPs and evaluate the corticospinal tract. A study treated DoC patients with a single-session of TMS-EMG to evaluate corticospinal excitability and its relationship to CRS-R scores.[81] They found significant differences in measures of cortical excitability/inhibition in DoC compared with HC. Specifically, resting threshold intensity was elevated in UWS compared with HC but not significantly different between MCS and HC. Stimulus/response curves were decreased in UWS compared with MCS and HC. Short afferent inhibition (SAI) was decreased in UWS and MCS compared with HC but no different between UWS and MCS. These findings suggest decreased cortical excitability and inhibitory activity in patients with DoC. Additionally, they found SAI in UWS and MCS was correlated with CRS-R total score.

Autonomic nervous system
A prospective nonrandomized trial compared changes in autonomic cardiac markers and EEG after auditory stimuli in patients with DoC. Cardiac markers were measured indirectly using independent component analysis of EEG recordings. Baseline heart rate and heart rate variability were similar between UWS and MCS participants but there was a significant difference in cardiac cycle modulation (decreased R wave peak latency) after global auditory stimuli with MCS. No cardiac cycle modulation was noted in UWS or with local auditory stimulation. The authors concluded that the cardiac cycle was an independent predictor of consciousness and when used with EEG characteristics, enhanced predictive value.[82]

TREATMENT
Noninvasive Technologies

Transcranial direct current stimulation
tDCS is a technique that involves applying a constant, low-intensity (usually ≤2 mA) direct current to the neurons of the cerebral cortex, thereby producing a subthreshold stimulation to the neuronal membrane and modulating cortical excitability.[83]

Common stimulation modes include anode-tDCS (a-tDCS), cathode-tDCS (c-tDCS), and dual-tDCS. In a-tDCS, the anode electrode is placed at the target area of stimulation, while the cathode electrode is placed on the contralateral orbit, resulting in excitatory effects over the stimulated region.[83] In c-tDCS, the cathode electrode is placed at the target area, while the anode electrode is placed on the contralateral orbit, leading to local neuronal inhibition.[83] Dual-tDCS refers to the simultaneous application of both anodal and cathodal stimulation.[83]

Increasing evidence suggests that tDCS could improve the level of consciousness in patients with chronic DoC and the use of multiple sessions (≥20) may optimize response.[84–86] A recent meta-analysis pooled 15 randomized controlled trials (RCTs) that assessed behavioral changes in patients with DoC after treatment with tDCS.[87] They found CRS-R scores significantly increased with tDCS compared with controls. Analysis of subgroups showed CRS-R improvement in MCS but not in UWS. When evaluating stimulation dose subgroups, only the studies using greater than 20 tDCS session demonstrated significantly increased CRS-R scores. The preferred treatment regimen involves a-tDCS targeting the left dorsolateral prefrontal cortex (DLPFC).[88] However, having an intact DLPFC and associated cortices and subcortical structures may be a prerequisite for the therapeutic effects of tDCS. Research on new stimulation targets primarily involves the posterior parietal cortex and the left primary sensorimotor cortex, but currently lacks valid evidence from larger sample sizes.

Oscillating transcranial direct current stimulation. Typical brain activity has an oscillatory natural neural rhythm. Oscillating tDCS (o-tDCS) produces an oscillating current that matches the intrinsic frequencies of these natural neural rhythms. This is proposed to improve cerebral function beyond the excitatory effect seen with traditional tDCS. A small blinded RCT compared treatment of DoC with a single session o-tDCS vs. sham. They found transient significant increases in CRS-R motor and arousal subscales and trending improvement in auditory and oromotor subscales in MCS patients. They also demonstrated extensive frontoparietal networks h and c power modulation and coherence increase which were correlated with CRS-R changes. There was no change of CRS-R or electrophysiologic measures in patients with UWS.[19]

High-definition transcranial direct current stimulation. Traditional tDCS delivers current through relatively large electrodes while high-definition tDCS (HD-tDCS) is an alternative using arrays of smaller, specially designed electrodes. This technique improves spatial targeting of stimulation and was shown to increase stimulus intensity and prolong after-effects. In a nonrandomized clinical trial, 28 patients with DoC were treated with HD-tDCS for 14 days. Although most (86%) participants showed improvement in total CRS-R scores, only the patients with MCS had significant improvement.[89]

Transcranial alternating current stimulation

tACS is a noninvasive method of modulating the cerebral cortex using alternating electrical current.[90] It involves applying low-intensity sinusoidal currents to specific regions of the brain, thereby synchronizing the electrical activity of neuronal populations in the target brain area in line with the frequency of the applied alternating current.[91] The stimulation intensity used in tACS is generally smaller than that in tDCS, ranging from 0.25 to 1 mA, and the duration is relatively shorter, typically around 2 to 5 minutes. The mechanism of tACS may involve promoting neural oscillatory activity in specific frequency bands, enhancing cortical neuroplasticity and connectivity, and facilitating large-scale cortical–subcortical network interactions.

Some studies used tACS to modulate gamma-band neural oscillatory patterns in the right DLPFC in patients with DoC. The results showed that tACS could selectively modulate large-scale cortical connectivity and excitability in all patients with MCS and some patients with vegetative state (VS)/UWS. However, no significant changes were observed in the CRS-R scores before and after single session tACS intervention.[22]

Transcranial pulsed-current stimulation

Transcranial pulsed-current stimulation (tPCS) uses a unidirectional pulsed flow of current compared with the continuous flow used in tDCS. Studies have demonstrated modification of electrical activity in cortical and subcortical structures and improved functional tasks such as speech comprehension and arithmetic tasks in healthy subjects. The mechanism underlying its effect may be modulation of neuronal membrane polarization. A pilot RCT treated DoC patients with a single session of tPCS, tDCS, and sham in a crossover design. Although behavioral improvement and electrophysiologic changes were seen with tDCS, they did not find any effect with tPCS or sham.[92]

Transcranial random noise stimulation

Transcranial random noise stimulation (tRNS) utilizes white noise, a multi-frequency electrical oscillatory spectrum, which has been shown to produce long-lasting increases in cortical excitability when applied to the motor cortex or DLPFC. Functionally, tRNS was found to improve performance on visuoperceptual learning and facial identity tasks in healthy subjects. The first study to apply tRNS to the DoC population was a small prospective blinded, sham-controlled RCT where patients with subacute UWS were given 5 sessions of tRNS targeting the bilateral DLPFC. They did not find a significant difference in CRS-R or electrophysiologic measures between tRNS and sham groups.[93] No studies have evaluated tRNS as a primary treatment of MCS patients at this time.

Transcranial magnetic stimulation

TMS is a noninvasive technique that involves generating a time-varying magnetic field using an electrically powered coil. This magnetic field can penetrate the scalp and skull, inducing electric currents in the cortical tissue and exerting a neuromodulatory effect. The mechanisms of TMS include altering ion channel activity, depolarizing or hyperpolarizing neuronal membrane, modulating synaptic plasticity, and stimulating synchronized oscillations in the cerebral cortex. These mechanisms allow for the modulation of cortical excitability.[94]

TMS modes include single pulse transcranial magnetic stimulation (spTMS), paired pulse transcranial magnetic stimulation (ppTMS), paired associative stimulation (PAS), repetitive transcranial magnetic stimulation (rTMS), and theta burst stimulation (TBS). Among them, spTMS, ppTMS, and PAS are commonly used as evaluation tools, while rTMS and TBS are often used as therapeutic methods.[95]

Multiple studies including 2 recent class I RCTs[96,97] and a meta-analysis from 2020[98] support the ability of rTMS to improve consciousness in DoC. Despite this evidence, an effective TMS paradigm, including treatment protocol and patient selection, in the treatment of DoC has not been identified. The most common targets for rTMS are the primary motor cortex or DLPFC. Some consistent findings in the literature include patients with MCS benefit more than patients with UWS both in response rate and magnitude. Additionally, multiple (≥ 10) treatment sessions are needed for optimal response.

The 2 largest class 1 RCTs, by Fan and colleagues (n = 40) and Chen and colleagues (n = 50), both treated subacute–chronic DoC patients with high-intensity rTMS targeting the left DLPFC.[96,97] Fan and colleagues treated patients with 20 Hz rTMS for 4 weeks while Chen and colleagues used 10 Hz rTMS for 6 weeks. Both studies found CRS-R improved postintervention in rTMS and sham groups but the rTMS group had significantly greater improvement compared with the sham group. Despite this, Fan and colleagues[96] found no significant difference in emergence at follow-up between the groups (rTMS 45%, sham 35%). Chen and colleagues[97] also collected simultaneous electrophysiologic evaluation with SEP and brainstem AEP grades, which responded to rTMS and were correlated with clinical changes on CRS-R. Finally, a systematic review/meta-analysis from 2020 with 10 pooled studies found that MCS (71.4%) was more likely than UWS (22.9%) to respond to rTMS and MCS improved more than UWS on CRS-R.[98] In 2019, the International Federation of Clinical Neurophysiology released rTMS treatment guidelines, which identified high-frequency stimulation of the DLPFC or M1 as a promising approach for DoC.[95]

Median nerve stimulation

The median nerve innervated muscle groups dominate a relatively large area in the brain's representational cortex. When the sensory pathway is intact, stimulating the median nerve can transmit sensory signals to a large cortical area, forming the theoretical basis for its stimulating mechanism. Compared with bilateral median nerve stimulation (MNS), right MNS seems to be a more effective stimulation method.[99] The conventional treatment parameters include a current intensity at 10 to 20 mA (with slightly visible movement of the thumb being optimal), a frequency of 40 to 70 Hz, a pulse width of 300 ms, and a treatment duration of 3 to 8 hours per day, for 2 weeks.[100]

Previous studies found that MNS could improve the Glasgow Coma Scale scores, EEG patterns, cerebral blood flow, and other indicators in comatose patients.[100] Its potential mechanisms include increasing the release of neurotransmitters (such as norepinephrine in the arousal system), increasing cerebral blood flow, activating consciousness-related nuclei, maintaining excitability between the reticular system and the cortex, and promoting functional connectivity between the primary somato-sensory cortex and widespread cortical networks, including the frontoparietal association cortex.[101] Although some studies have suggested benefits, the efficacy of MNS in treating DoC has not been confirmed. However, considering its noninvasiveness, simplicity in application, and minimal adverse effects, MNS remains a modality worth trialing in conjunction with other treatments.

Novel approaches

Near-infrared low-level laser and transcranial shock wave therapy. Near-infrared low-level laser therapy (N-LT) involves application of transcranial low-power lasers, which have been shown to have photobiomodulatory effects including cerebral oxygenation and oxidative stress. Transcranial focused shock wave therapy (F-SWT) involves use of acoustic waves that carry energy. The biomechanical effect on tissue is proposed to improve neuroplasticity. A prospective trial treated chronic DoC patients with a 4 week course of either N-LT or F-SWT. The primary outcome of CRS-R showed improvement in both groups ($\sim$4 points) with sustained benefit at 12 weeks follow-up. There was no difference in CRS-R outcomes between N-LT and F-SWT. Patients with low initial CRS-R and global damage secondary to cerebral hypoxia performed poorly. One patient in the F-SWT treatment group had a focal seizure with secondary generalization 32 hours following the last stimulation.[102]

Low-intensity focused ultrasound pulsation. Low-intensity focused ultrasound pulsation (LIFUS) can stimulate deep brain nuclei similar to other neuromodulatory techniques but has benefits including being noninvasive and having better penetration depth than tDCS. A single case report has demonstrated use of LIFUS for noninvasive direct thalamic stimulation in a young male with acute DoC in MCS. After thalamic LIFUS, there was a 4 point increase on CRS-R. Three days post-LIFUS the behavioral assessment was consistent with emergence from MCS and 5 days post-LIFUS, the patient attempted to walk.[103] A larger feasibility trial (NCT02522429) that is recruiting both acute and chronic DOC patients is underway and has completed data collection.

Caloric vestibular stimulation. During the caloric reflex, afferent vestibular nerve stimulation leads to downstream responses in the distal frontal-parietal and striatal networks associated with arousal. Therefore, caloric vestibular stimulation (CVS) could potentially benefit patients with DoC. A single 2017 case series treated 2 chronic MCS (−) patients using an alternating cross-over active stimulation vs. sham design over 16 to 18 weeks. Both patients demonstrated improvement in voluntary behaviors, measured by the Wessex Head Injury Matrix, with changes temporally correlated with CVS. Total CRS-R and arousal subscale increased with sustained benefit at 4 weeks follow-up in 1 out of 2 individuals, with behavior consistent with MCS plus.[104]

Brain computer interface. In addition to diagnostic uses, BCI has potential therapeutic efficacy, although this has not yet been established, by allowing DoC patients to regain the ability perform goal-directed behavior. A study using EEG-based BCI showed improvement in CRS-R scores after 10 sessions suggesting the potential for improvement with repetitive BCI training.[60]

Invasive Technologies

Deep brain stimulation

Deep brain stimulation (DBS) involves the surgical implantation of fine needle electrodes in specific locations of the brain to deliver electrical pulses and modulate neural activity. Multiple small nonrandomized clinical trials have evaluated the treatment of DoC with DBS and demonstrated some clinical benefit, including sustained improvement on CRS-R scores, in both UWS and MCS patients.[105–109] In these studies, the most common DBS target was thalamic intralaminar nuclei, although some studies specifically target the centromedian parafasicular nuclei, or mesencephalic reticular formation.

The optimal patient population and target for DBS is unclear at this time, although evidence suggests patients with retained neurophysiologic activity such as somato-sensory/auditory evoked-potentials and desynchronized activity on EEG may be better candidates. Considering the spontaneous recovery after brain injury and the significant risks associated with surgical interventions, DBS should be reserved for chronic DoC. Before considering surgery, conventional treatments should be exhausted. Family members should be fully informed about the rationale of proceeding with the treatment and provided with clear explanations regarding potential risks and benefits.[110]

Spinal cord electrical stimulation

SCS is a surgical procedure in which electrodes are placed in the extradural space of the spinal cord at the C2–C4 level. After surgery, the spinal cord is stimulated using different parameters of pulsed electrical currents. The patient's response to the stimulation, as well as changes in the EEG or fNIRS signals, are monitored. Parameters that increase high-frequency signals in the brain's electrical spectrum without causing sympathetic reflexes are preferred. The typical stimulation frequencies are 5 or 70 Hz, with a voltage range of 1 to 5 V. The daily stimulation duration is 8 to 12 hours, consisting of 8 to 15 minutes of stimulation followed by 8 to 15 minutes of rest periods.[111]

Although high-quality studies are still lacking, recent studies found that SCS could improve the level of consciousness in some patients with DoC.[112,113] The effectiveness varies greatly between different studies, but overall, patients with MCS may benefit more from this treatment than those with UWS.[23] The mechanism of SCS in treating DoC is not yet clear. It is speculated that electrical stimulation can enhance brain blood flow in critical areas relating to consciousness by activating the ascending reticular activating system and subcortical activation system, thereby improving information transmission in the reticular-thalamo-cortical pathway. It may also enhance the induction of impulses relating to consciousness, leading to increased electrical activity and metabolic rate in the brain.[7] Compared with DBS, SCS has the relative advantage of being less invasive and complicated to perform than DBS. Under strict adherence to the indications, SCS may have efficacy in improving DoC; however, more large-scale studies are needed.

Vagus nerve stimulation

Vagus nerve stimulation (VNS) has been approved for various conditions, such as drug-resistant epilepsy, depression, migraines.[114] In 2017, VNS was first used to treat patients with DoC and achieved some promising results. General visceral sensory fibers of the vagus nerve relay information through the solitary tract nucleus and project to the hypothalamus, limbic system, amygdala, prefrontal cortex, and other cortical areas, bonding with the ascending reticular activating system and higher cortical areas. This provides an anatomical basis for VNS in the treatment of DoC.[115,116]

Although most studies targeting VNS have used noninvasive approaches, a case report from 2017 described the use of surgically implanted VNS on a patient with chronic UWS due to TBI. They found that the CRS-R score improved from 5 to 10 and was consistent with improvement to MCS. Concurrent EEG and PET demonstrated increased theta band power most significantly in centro-parietal regions and increased metabolic activity respectively.[115]

More recently, noninvasive VNS has become possible. Advantages to a noninvasive approach include elimination of surgical and postoperative complications while still maintaining the neuromodulatory effects that make application to DoC patients promising. Two noninvasive VNS approaches, transauricular VNS (tA-VNS) and vagus nerve magnetic modulation (VNMM), have been trialed on patients with DoC.

A small prospective trial treated DoC patients with tA-VNS.[117,118] Patients were grouped into responsive (rAS) vs. nonresponsive to auditory stimuli (nAS) based on pretreatment CRS-R auditory function subscale. A significant improvement in total CRS-R and each subscale was seen posttreatment in the rAS group. Furthermore, functional outcomes improved (Glascow outcome scale [GOS] > 3) posttreatment. There was no improvement in CRS-R or GOS in the nAS group.

VNMM utilizes rTMS for extracranial VNS. A feasibility trial using VNMM on DoC patients demonstrated significant increase in CRS-R after VNMM treatment.[119] MCS patients improved more than patients in UWS and coma. All CRS-R subscales significantly improved except for oromotor function. Behavioral classification of UWS and MCS also improved with 3 out of 4 UWS recovering to MCS (-) and 6 out of 11 MCS (-) recovering to MCS (+)(2) or eMCS (4).

CLINICS CARE POINTS

- Research into use of technological modalities in the assessment and treatment of patients with a DoC is expaning rapidly and demonstrates promising results.
- Clinical application of these technological modalities is reasonable in select settings as long as family members/surrogate decision makers are fully informed about the rationale, goals, risks, benefits, and alternatives.

DISCLOSURE

The authors have nothing to disclose.

REFERENCES

1. Edlow BL, Claassen J, Schiff ND, et al. Recovery from disorders of consciousness: mechanisms, prognosis and emerging therapies. Nat Rev Neurol 2021; 17(3):135–56.
2. Thibaut A, Schiff N, Giacino J, et al. Therapeutic interventions in patients with prolonged disorders of consciousness. Lancet Neurol 2019;18(6):600–14.
3. Bai Y, Lin Y, Ziemann U. Managing disorders of consciousness: the role of electroencephalography. J Neurol 2021;268(11):4033–65.
4. Kempny AM, James L, Yelden K, et al. Patients with a severe prolonged Disorder of Consciousness can show classical EEG responses to their own name compared with others' names. NeuroImage Clin 2018;19:311–9.
5. Wu DY, Cai G, Yuan Y, et al. Application of nonlinear dynamics analysis in assessing unconsciousness: a preliminary study. Clin Neurophysiol 2011;122(3): 490–8.
6. Engemann DA, Raimondo F, King JR, et al. Robust EEG-based cross-site and cross-protocol classification of states of consciousness. Brain 2018;141(11): 3179–92.

7. Wang Y, Bai Y, Xia X, et al. Spinal cord stimulation modulates complexity of neural activities in patients with disorders of consciousness. Int J Neurosci 2020; 130(7):662–70.

8. Sitt JD, King JR, El Karoui I, et al. Large scale screening of neural signatures of consciousness in patients in a vegetative or minimally conscious state. Brain 2014;137(8):2258–70.

9. Piarulli A, Bergamasco M, Thibaut A, et al. EEG ultradian rhythmicity differences in disorders of consciousness during wakefulness. J Neurol 2016;263(9): 1746–60.

10. Gosseries O, Schnakers C, Ledoux D, et al. Automated EEG entropy measurements in coma, vegetative state/unresponsive wakefulness syndrome and minimally conscious state. Funct Neurol 2011;26(1):25–30.

11. Schnakers C, Ledoux D, Majerus S, et al. Diagnostic and prognostic use of bispectral index in coma, vegetative state and related disorders. Brain Inj 2008; 22(12):926–31.

12. Cavinato M, Genna C, Manganotti P, et al. Coherence and consciousness: study of fronto-parietal gamma synchrony in patients with disorders of consciousness. Brain Topogr 2015;28(4):570–9.

13. Wu DY, Cai G, Zorowitz RD, et al. Measuring interconnection of the residual cortical functional islands in persistent vegetative state and minimal conscious state with EEG nonlinear analysis. Clin Neurophysiol 2011;122(10):1956–66.

14. Leon-Carrion J, Leon-Dominguez U, Pollonini L, et al. Synchronization between the anterior and posterior cortex determines consciousness level in patients with traumatic brain injury (TBI). Brain Res 2012;1476:22–30.

15. Pollonini L, Pophale S, Situ N, et al. Information communication networks in severe traumatic brain injury. Brain Topogr 2010;23(2):221–6.

16. Lehembre R, Bruno MA, Vanhaudenhuyse A, et al. Resting-state EEG study of comatose patients: a connectivity and frequency analysis to find differences between vegetative and minimally conscious states. Funct Neurol 2012; 27(1):41–7.

17. Naro A, Bramanti A, Leo A, et al. Shedding new light on disorders of consciousness diagnosis: the dynamic functional connectivity. Cortex 2018;103:316–28.

18. Bai Y, Xia X, Wang Y, et al. Electroencephalography quadratic phase self-coupling correlates with consciousness states and restoration in patients with disorders of consciousness. Clin Neurophysiol 2019;130(8):1235–42.

19. Naro A, Russo M, Leo A, et al. Cortical connectivity modulation induced by cerebellar oscillatory transcranial direct current stimulation in patients with chronic disorders of consciousness: a marker of covert cognition? Clin Neurophysiol 2016;127(3):1845–54.

20. Bai Y, Xia X, Wang Y, et al. Fronto-parietal coherence response to tDCS modulation in patients with disorders of consciousness. Int J Neurosci 2018;128(7): 587–94.

21. Cavinato M, Genna C, Formaggio E, et al. Behavioural and electrophysiological effects of tDCS to prefrontal cortex in patients with disorders of consciousness. Clin Neurophysiol 2019;130(2):231–8.

22. Naro A, Bramanti P, Leo A, et al. Transcranial alternating current stimulation in patients with chronic disorder of consciousness: a possible way to cut the diagnostic gordian knot? Brain Topogr 2016;29(4):623–44.

23. Bai Y, Xia X, Li X, et al. Spinal cord stimulation modulates frontal delta and gamma in patients of minimally consciousness state. Neuroscience 2017;346: 247–54.

24. Rizkallah J, Annen J, Modolo J, et al. Decreased integration of EEG source-space networks in disorders of consciousness. NeuroImage Clin 2019; 23(April):101841.

25. Cai L, Wang J, Guo Y, et al. Altered inter-frequency dynamics of brain networks in disorder of consciousness. J Neural Eng 2020;17(3):036006.

26. Cacciola A, Naro A, Milardi D, et al. Functional brain network topology discriminates between patients with minimally conscious state and unresponsivewakefulness syndrome. J Clin Med 2019;8(3). https://doi.org/10.3390/jcm8030306.

27. Chennu S, Annen J, Wannez S, et al. Brain networks predict metabolism, diagnosis and prognosis at the bedside in disorders of consciousness. Brain 2017; 140(8):2120–32.

28. Stefan S, Schorr B, Lopez-Rolon A, et al. Consciousness indexing and outcome prediction with resting-state EEG in severe disorders of consciousness. Brain Topogr 2018;31(5):848–62.

29. Wislowska M, Del Giudice R, Lechinger J, et al. Night and day variations of sleep in patients with disorders of consciousness. Sci Rep 2017;7(1):1–11.

30. Rossi Sebastiano D, Visani E, Panzica F, et al. Sleep patterns associated with the severity of impairment in a large cohort of patients with chronic disorders of consciousness. Clin Neurophysiol 2018;129(3):687–93.

31. Malinowska U, Chatelle C, Bruno MA, et al. Electroencephalographic profiles for differentiation of disorders of consciousness. Biomed Eng Online 2013;12(1). https://doi.org/10.1186/1475-925X-12-109.

32. Zieleniewska M, Duszyk A, Różański P, et al. Parametric description of EEG profiles for assessment of sleep architecture in disorders of consciousness. Int J Neural Syst 2019;29(03):1850049.

33. Oksenberg A, Gordon C, Arons E, et al. Phasic activities of rapid eye movement sleep in vegetative state patients. Sleep 2001;24(6):703–6.

34. Isono M, Wakabayashi Y, Fujiki MM, et al. Sleep cycle in patients in a state of permanent unconsciousness. Brain Inj 2002;16(8):705–12.

35. Landsness E, Bruno MA, Noirhomme Q, et al. Electrophysiological correlates of behavioural changes in vigilance in vegetative state and minimally conscious state. Brain 2011;134(8):2222–32.

36. Bagnato S, Boccagni C, Sant'Angelo A, et al. EEG predictors of outcome in patients with disorders of consciousness admitted for intensive rehabilitation. Clin Neurophysiol 2015;126(5):959–66.

37. Estraneo A, Loreto V, Guarino I, et al. Standard EEG in diagnostic process of prolonged disorders of consciousness. Clin Neurophysiol 2016;127(6):2379–85.

38. Pruvost-Robieux E, Marchi A, Martinelli I, et al. Evoked and event-related potentials as biomarkers of consciousness state and recovery. J Clin Neurophysiol 2022;39(1):22–31.

39. Kotchoubey B. Evoked and event-related potentials in disorders of consciousness: a quantitative review. Conscious Cogn 2017;54:155–67.

40. Kotchoubey B, Lang S, Mezger G, et al. Information processing in severe disorders of consciousness: vegetative state and minimally conscious state. Clin Neurophysiol 2005;116(10):2441–53.

41. Fischer C, Luaute J, Morlet D. Event-related potentials (MMN and novelty P3) in permanent vegetative or minimally conscious states. Clin Neurophysiol 2010; 121(7):1032–42.

42. Perrin F, Schnakers C, Schabus M, et al. Brain response to one's own name in vegetative state, minimally conscious state, and locked-in syndrome. Arch Neurol 2006;63(4):562–9.

43. Li R, Song WQ, Du JB, et al. Connecting the P300 to the diagnosis and prognosis of unconscious patients. Neural Regen Res 2015;10(3):473–80.

44. Schnakers C, Perrin F, Schabus M, et al. Voluntary brain processing in disorders of consciousness. Neurology 2008;71(20):1614–20.

45. Risetti M, Formisano R, Toppi J, et al. On ERPs detection in disorders of consciousness rehabilitation. Front Hum Neurosci 2013;7(NOV):1–10.

46. Erlbeck H, Real RGL, Kotchoubey B, et al. Basic discriminative and semantic processing in patients in the vegetative and minimally conscious state. Int J Psychophysiol 2017;113:8–16.

47. Beukema S, Gonzalez-Lara LE, Finoia P, et al. A hierarchy of event-related potential markers of auditory processing in disorders of consciousness. NeuroImage Clin 2016;12:359–71.

48. Qin P, Di H, Yan X, et al. Mismatch negativity to the patient's own name in chronic disorders of consciousness. Neurosci Lett 2008;448(1):24–8.

49. Rohaut B, Faugeras F, Chausson N, et al. Probing ERP correlates of verbal semantic processing in patients with impaired consciousness. Neuropsychologia 2015;66:279–92.

50. Braiman C, Fridman EA, Conte MM, et al. Cortical Response to the Natural Speech Envelope Correlates with Neuroimaging Evidence of Cognition in Severe Brain Injury. Curr Biol 2018;28(23):3833–9.e3.

51. Sergent C, Faugeras F, Rohaut B, et al. Multidimensional cognitive evaluation of patients with disorders of consciousness using EEG: A proof of concept study. NeuroImage Clin 2017;13:455–69.

52. Gibson RM, Chennu S, Fernández-Espejo D, et al. Somatosensory attention identifies both overt and covert awareness in disorders of consciousness. Ann Neurol 2016;80(3):412–23.

53. Wijnen VJM, Eilander HJ, de Gelder B, et al. Visual processing during recovery from vegetative state to consciousness: Comparing behavioral indices to brain responses. Neurophysiol Clin 2014;44(5):457–69.

54. Naro A, Leo A, Buda A, et al. Do you see me? The role of visual fixation in chronic disorders of consciousness differential diagnosis. Brain Res 2016; 1653(June):59–66.

55. Galiotta V, Quattrociocchi I, D'Ippolito M, et al. EEG-based brain-computer interfaces for people with disorders of consciousness: features and applications. A systematic review. Front Hum Neurosci 2022;16. https://doi.org/10.3389/fnhum.2022.1040816.

56. Lulé D, Noirhomme Q, Kleih SC, et al. Probing command following in patients with disorders of consciousness using a brain-computer interface. Clin Neurophysiol 2013;124(1):101–6.

57. Xiao J, Xie Q, Lin Q, et al. Assessment of visual pursuit in patients with disorders of consciousness based on a brain-computer interface. IEEE Trans Neural Syst Rehabil Eng 2018;26(6):1141–51.

58. Xiao J, He Y, Yu T, et al. Toward assessment of sound localization in disorders of consciousness using a hybrid audiovisual brain–computer interface. IEEE Trans Neural Syst Rehabil Eng 2022;30:1422–32.

59. Pan J, Xie Q, Qin P, et al. Prognosis for patients with cognitive motor dissociation identified by brain-computer interface. Brain 2020;143(4):1177–89.

60. Murovec N, Heilinger A, Xu R, et al. Effects of a Vibro-Tactile P300 based brain-computer interface on the coma recovery scale-revised in patients with disorders of consciousness. Front Neurosci 2020;14(April):1–11.

61. Pan J, Xie Q, He Y, et al. Detecting awareness in patients with disorders of consciousness using a hybrid brain-computer interface. J Neural Eng 2014;11(5). https://doi.org/10.1088/1741-2560/11/5/056007.

62. Eliseyev A, Jerome I, Le A, et al. Development of a brain-computer interface for patients in the critical care setting. PLoS One 2021;16(1 January):1–13.

63. Höller Y, Bergmann J, Thomschewski A, et al. Comparison of EEG-features and classification methods for motor imagery in patients with disorders of consciousness. PLoS One 2013;8(11). https://doi.org/10.1371/journal.pone.0080479.

64. Guger C, Heilinger A, Ortner R, et al. MindBEAGLE — A new system for the assessment and communication with patients with disorders of consciousness and complete locked-in syndrom. In: 2017 IEEE International Conference on Systems, Man, and Cybernetics (SMC). IEEE; 2017:3008-3013. doi:10.1109/SMC.2017.8123086.

65. Chatelle C, Spencer CA, Cash SS, et al. Feasibility of an EEG-based brain-computer interface in the intensive care unit. Clin Neurophysiol 2018;129(8):1519–25.

66. Coyle D, Stow J, McCreadie K, et al. Sensorimotor modulation assessment and brain-computer interface training in disorders of consciousness. Arch Phys Med Rehabil 2015;96(3):S62–70.

67. Huang H, Xie Q, Pan J, et al. An EEG-based brain computer interface for emotion recognition and its application in patients with disorder of consciousness. IEEE Trans Affect Comput 2021;12(4):832–42.

68. Xiao J, Pan J, He Y, et al. Visual fixation assessment in patients with disorders of consciousness based on brain-computer interface. Neurosci Bull 2018;34(4):679–90.

69. Wang F, He Y, Qu J, et al. A brain-computer interface based on three-dimensional stereo stimuli for assisting clinical object recognition assessment in patients with disorders of consciousness. IEEE Trans Neural Syst Rehabil Eng 2019;27(3):507–13.

70. Xiao J, Xie Q, He Y, et al. An auditory BCI system for assisting CRS-R behavioral assessment in patients with disorders of consciousness. Sci Rep 2016;6(June):1–13.

71. Wang F, He Y, Qu J, et al. Enhancing clinical communication assessments using an audiovisual BCI for patients with disorders of consciousness. J Neural Eng 2017;14(4). https://doi.org/10.1088/1741-2552/aa6c31.

72. Spataro R, Heilinger A, Allison B, et al. Preserved somatosensory discrimination predicts consciousness recovery in unresponsive wakefulness syndrome. Clin Neurophysiol 2018;129(6):1130–6.

73. Bensaid S, Modolo J, Merlet I, et al. COALIA: a computational model of human EEG for consciousness research. Front Syst Neurosci 2019;13:59.

74. Lee M, Baird B, Gosseries O, et al. Connectivity differences between consciousness and unconsciousness in non-rapid eye movement sleep: a TMS-EEG study. Sci Rep 2019;9(1):5175.

75. Rosanova M, Gosseries O, Casarotto S, et al. Recovery of cortical effective connectivity and recovery of consciousness in vegetative patients. Brain 2012;135(4):1308–20.

76. Ragazzoni A, Pirulli C, Veniero D, et al. Vegetative versus minimally conscious states: a study using TMS-EEG, sensory and event-related potentials. PLoS One 2013;8(2). https://doi.org/10.1371/journal.pone.0057069.

77. Sinitsyn DO, Poydasheva AG, Bakulin IS, et al. Detecting the potential for consciousness in unresponsive patients using the perturbational complexity index. Brain Sci 2020;10(12). https://doi.org/10.3390/brainsci10120917.

78. Colombo MA, Comanducci A, Casarotto S, et al. Beyond alpha power: EEG spatial and spectral gradients robustly stratify disorders of consciousness. Cereb cortex 2023;33(11):7193–210.

79. Casali AG, Gosseries O, Rosanova M, et al. A theoretically based index of consciousness independent of sensory processing and behavior. Sci Transl Med 2013;5(198). https://doi.org/10.1126/scitranslmed.3006294.

80. Casarotto S, Comanducci A, Rosanova M, et al. Stratification of unresponsive patients by an independently validated index of brain complexity. Ann Neurol 2016;80(5):718–29.

81. Lapitskaya N, Gosseries O, De Pasqua V, et al. Abnormal corticospinal excitability in patients with disorders of consciousness. Brain Stimul 2013;6(4):590–7.

82. Raimondo F, Rohaut B, Demertzi A, et al. Brain–heart interactions reveal consciousness in noncommunicating patients. Ann Neurol 2017;82(4):578–91.

83. Lefaucheur J-P, Antal A, Ayache SS, et al. Evidence-based guidelines on the therapeutic use of transcranial direct current stimulation (tDCS). Clin Neurophysiol 2017;128(1):56–92.

84. Zhang Y, Song W. Transcranial direct current stimulation in disorders of consciousness: a review. Int J Neurosci 2018;128(3):255–61.

85. Aloi D, della Rocchetta AI, Ditchfield A, et al. Therapeutic use of transcranial direct current stimulation in the rehabilitation of prolonged disorders of consciousness. Front Neurol 2021;12(April). https://doi.org/10.3389/fneur.2021.632572.

86. Han J, Chen C, Zheng S, et al. Functional connectivity increases in response to high-definition transcranial direct current stimulation in patients with chronic disorder of consciousness. Brain Sci 2022;12(8):1095.

87. Ma H, Zhao K, Jia C, et al. Effect of transcranial direct current stimulation for patients with disorders of consciousness: a systematic review and meta-analysis. Front Neurosci 2023;16(January). https://doi.org/10.3389/fnins.2022.1081278.

88. Liu S, Gao Q, Guan M, et al. Effectiveness of transcranial direct current stimulation over dorsolateral prefrontal cortex in patients with prolonged disorders of consciousness: a systematic review and meta-analysis. Front Neurol 2022; 13. https://doi.org/10.3389/fneur.2022.998953.

89. Cai T, Xia X, Zhang H, et al. High-definition transcranial direct current stimulation modulates neural activities in patients with prolonged disorders of consciousness. Brain Stimul 2019;12(6):1619–21.

90. Feng Y, Zhang J, Zhou Y, et al. Noninvasive brain stimulation for patients with a disorder of consciousness: a systematic review and meta-analysis. Rev Neurosci 2020;31(8):905–14.

91. Riddle J, Frohlich F. Targeting neural oscillations with transcranial alternating current stimulation. Brain Res 2021;1765:147491.

92. Barra A, Rosenfelder M, Mortaheb S, et al. Transcranial pulsed-current stimulation versus transcranial direct current stimulation in patients with disorders of consciousness: a pilot, sham-controlled cross-over double-blind study. Brain Sci 2022;12(4). https://doi.org/10.3390/brainsci12040429.

93. Mancuso M, Abbruzzese L, Canova S, et al. Transcranial random noise stimulation does not improve behavioral and neurophysiological measures in patients with subacute Vegetative-Unresponsive Wakefulness State (VS-UWS). Front Hum Neurosci 2017;11(November):1–10.

94. Somaa FA, de Graaf TA, Sack AT. Transcranial magnetic stimulation in the treatment of neurological diseases. Front Neurol 2022;13. https://doi.org/10.3389/fneur.2022.793253.

95. Lefaucheur J-P, Aleman A, Baeken C, et al. Evidence-based guidelines on the therapeutic use of repetitive transcranial magnetic stimulation (rTMS): An update (2014–2018). Clin Neurophysiol 2020;131(2):474–528.

96. Fan J, Zhong Y, Wang H, et al. Repetitive transcranial magnetic stimulation improves consciousness in some patients with disorders of consciousness. Clin Rehabil 2022;36(7):916–25.

97. Chen JM, Chen QF, Wang ZY, et al. Influence of high-frequency repetitive transcranial magnetic stimulation on neurobehavioral and electrophysiology in patients with disorders of consciousness. Neural Plast 2022;2022. https://doi.org/10.1155/2022/7195699.

98. O'Neal CM, Schroeder LN, Wells AA, et al. Patient outcomes in disorders of consciousness following transcranial magnetic stimulation: a systematic review and meta-analysis of individual patient data. Front Neurol 2021;12(August):1–13. https://doi.org/10.3389/fneur.2021.694970.

99. Wu X, Zhang C, Feng J, et al. Right median nerve electrical stimulation for acute traumatic coma (the Asia Coma Electrical Stimulation trial): study protocol for a randomised controlled trial. Trials 2017;18(1):311.

100. Wang P, Cao W, Zhou H, et al. Efficacy of median nerve electrical stimulation on the recovery of patients with consciousness disorders: a systematic review and meta-analysis. J Int Med Res 2022;50(12). https://doi.org/10.1177/03000605221134467. 030006052211344.

101. Feller D, Vinante C, Trentin F, et al. The effectiveness of median nerve electrical stimulation in patients with disorders of consciousness: a systematic review. Brain Inj 2021;35(4):385–94.

102. Werner C, Byhahn M, Hesse S. Non-invasive brain stimulation to promote alertness and awareness in chronic patients with disorders of consciousness: Low-level, near-infrared laser stimulation vs. focused shock wave therapy. Restor Neurol Neurosci 2016;34(4):561–9.

103. Monti MM, Schnakers C, Korb AS, et al. Non-invasive ultrasonic thalamic stimulation in disorders of consciousness after severe brain injury: a first-in-man report. Brain Stimul 2016;9(6):940–1.

104. Vanzan S, Wilkinson D, Ferguson H, et al. Behavioural improvement in a minimally conscious state after caloric vestibular stimulation: Evidence from two single case studies. Clin Rehabil 2017;31(4):500–7.

105. Yamamoto T, Katayama Y, Obuchi T, et al. Deep brain stimulation and spinal cord stimulation for vegetative state and minimally conscious state. World Neurosurg 2013;80(3–4):S30.e1–9.

106. Schiff ND, Giacino JT, Kalmar K, et al. Behavioural improvements with thalamic stimulation after severe traumatic brain injury. Nature 2007;448(7153):600–3.

107. Schiff ND. Central thalamic contributions to arousal regulation and neurological disorders of consciousness. Ann N Y Acad Sci 2008;1129:105–18.

108. Magrassi L, Maggioni G, Pistarini C, et al. Vegetative state patients. J Neurosurg 2016;125(October):1–10.

109. Chudy D, Deletis V, Almahariq F, et al. Deep brain stimulation for the early treatment of the minimally conscious state and vegetative state: experience in 14 patients. J Neurosurg 2018;128(4):1189–98.

110. Vanhoecke J, Hariz M. Deep brain stimulation for disorders of consciousness: systematic review of cases and ethics. Brain Stimul 2017;10(6):1013–23.

111. Zhuang Y, Yang Y, Xu L, et al. Effects of short-term spinal cord stimulation on patients with prolonged disorder of consciousness: a pilot study. Front Neurol 2022;13. https://doi.org/10.3389/fneur.2022.1026221.
112. Yang Y, He Q, Xia X, et al. Long-term functional prognosis and related factors of spinal cord stimulation in patients with disorders of consciousness. CNS Neurosci Ther 2022;28(8):1249–58.
113. Yang Y, He Q, He J. Short-term spinal cord stimulation in treating disorders of consciousness monitored by resting-state fMRI and qEEG: The first case report. Front Neurol 2022;13. https://doi.org/10.3389/fneur.2022.968932.
114. Farmer AD, Albu-Soda A, Aziz Q. Vagus nerve stimulation in clinical practice. Br J Hosp Med (Lond) 2016;77(11):645–51.
115. Corazzol M, Lio G, Lefevre A, et al. Restoring consciousness with vagus nerve stimulation. Curr Biol 2017;27(18):R994–6.
116. Wang Y, Zhan G, Cai Z, et al. Vagus nerve stimulation in brain diseases: therapeutic applications and biological mechanisms. Neurosci Biobehav Rev 2021;127:37–53.
117. Yu Y-T, Yang Y, Wang L-B, et al. Transcutaneous auricular vagus nerve stimulation in disorders of consciousness monitored by fMRI: The first case report. Brain Stimul 2017;10(2):328–30.
118. Yu Y, Yang Y, Gan S, et al. Cerebral hemodynamic correlates of transcutaneous auricular vagal nerve stimulation in consciousness restoration: an open-label pilot study. Front Neurol 2021;12(July):1–9.
119. Wang L, Wu Q, Yang Z, et al. Preliminary study of vagus nerve magnetic modulation in patients with prolonged disorders of consciousness. Neuropsychiatr Dis Treat 2022;18(September):2171–9.

Medical, Neurologic, and Neuromusculoskeletal Complications

Jean E. Woo, MD[a,b,*], Abana Azariah, MD[a,c], Eboni A. Reed, MD[b],
Nicholas Gut, MD[c]

KEYWORDS

- Disorders of consciousness • Paroxysmal sympathetic hyperactivity • Seizure
- Hydrocephalus • Spasticity • Movement disorders • Infection
- Neuroendocrine disturbances

KEY POINTS

- Medical, neurologic, and neuromuscular complications in DoC population are very common and often present in more severe forms.
- Treating those complications not only stabilizes their medical disturbances, but also minimizes confounding factors that interfere with accurate diagnosis for level of consciousness, maximizes their recovery, and prevents further complications.
- When weighing the risks and benefits of invasive interventions such as intrathecal baclofen pump and venticuloperitoneal shunt, the risks of the procedures should also be weighed against the risks of not pursuing any intervention and not giving the patients the best chance of improving their function.

INTRODUCTION

Medical, neurologic, and neuromuscular complications in the disorders of consciousness (DoC) population are very common and often present in more severe forms than in patients with less severe brain injury.[1–4] As a result, patients with DoC tend to be medically complex and fragile, especially in the acute rehabilitation setting.[1–4] These complications take on added significance in these patients because, in addition to threatening bodily integrity and function, they can interfere with the assessment of the patient's actual level of consciousness, either by impairing the level of

a TIRR Memorial Hermann, 1333 Moursund Street, Houston, TX 77030, USA; b H. Ben Taub Department of Physical Medicine and Rehabilitation, Baylor College of Medicine, 7200 Cambridge Street, Houston, TX 77030, USA; c Department of Physical Medicine and Rehabilitation, McGovern Medical School, The University of Texas Health Science Center at Houston, 1333 Moursund Street, Houston, TX 77030, USA
* Corresponding author.
E-mail address: Jean.woo@bcm.edu

Phys Med Rehabil Clin N Am 35 (2024) 127–144
https://doi.org/10.1016/j.pmr.2023.06.024
1047-9651/24/© 2023 Elsevier Inc. All rights reserved.

consciousness itself (for example, an infection) or by preventing the patient from being able to demonstrate their level of consciousness (for example, spasticity). Unfortunately, these complications are often not treated aggressively in the DoC population compared to patients with less severe brain injury, due to overly negative assumptions about the prognosis of DoC. In this article, we will review the diagnosis and management (and, if applicable, prevention) of the most common complications encountered in the care of patients with DoC. In addition to addressing the medical aspects of these complications in this population, we will emphasize the ways in which their presence intersects with larger questions about the assessment and enhancement of the level of consciousness.

PAROXYSMAL SYMPATHETIC HYPERACTIVITY
Background

Paroxysmal sympathetic hyperactivity (PSH), also referred to as "neurostorming," is a common complication after a severe brain injury characterized by increased sympathetic activity. Although not fully understood, it is thought to be an exaggerated, allodynic response to noxious and non-noxious stimuli due to decreased inhibitory input from the cortex. PSH is more commonly seen in the earlier stages after a severe brain injury and in patients with a traumatic etiology.[5] Peak symptoms are seen within 2 weeks after injury.[6]

Diagnosis

Clinical signs of PSH include tachypnea, hypertension, tachycardia, diaphoresis, hyperthermia, and dystonic posturing. PSH is a diagnosis of exclusion given its nonspecific symptoms, and other medical complications that have similar presentations (such as infection, pain, and so forth), need to be explored. The time of onset, duration, and frequency of the episodes vary greatly among patients. There are no specific diagnostic tests for PSH. In 2014, the Paroxysmal Sympathetic Hyperactivity Assessment Measure (PSH-AM) tool was designed to help with early diagnosis and assess treatment response.[7] This tool is composed of two parts: the Clinical Feature Scale (CFS) and the Diagnostic Likelihood Tool (DLT) (**Table 1**).

Treatment

Management of PSH includes both environmental modification and pharmacologic interventions. The goals are symptom relief as well as prevention. The first step is eliminating any noxious stimuli, such as infection, pain source (eg, heterotopic ossification, venous thromboembolism, occult fractures, serial casting, decubitus ulcers), constipation, and bladder distension.[8] Simple measures such as repositioning, changing the wet brief, and taking off the cast/splint may alleviate the symptoms.

Several pharmacologic agents are available for PSH. While there are no consensus treatment guidelines, the general strategies in medication selection are to target the predominant symptoms and then add other agents as needed (**Table 2**).[9,10] Among those agents, benzodiazepines and opioids can be used as abortive therapy that should be limited to severe PSH episodes, while other agents with less sedating effects can be used routinely as maintenance therapy. There is a fine balance between patients' comfort and function that clinicians need to weigh.[4] Empirical pain management can not only minimize a patient's insidious suffering, but reduce PSH episodes. Scheduling non-opioids (eg, acetaminophen) or low-dose opioids (eg, oxycodone 2.5-5mg two to three times per day) in severe PSH cases is reasonable as patients with

Table 1
Paroxysmal sympathetic hyperactivity assessment measure (PSH-AM)[7]

A: Clinical feature scale (CFS) score

	0	I	2	3
Heart rate (beats per min)	<100	100–119	120–139	≥140*
Respiratory rate (breaths per min)	<18	18–23	24–29*	≥30
Systolic blood pressure (mm Hg)	<140	140–159*	160–179	≥180
Temperature (°C)	<37.0*	37.0–37.9	38.0–38.9	≥39.0
Sweating	Absent	Mild	Moderate*	Severe
Posturing during episodes	Absent	Mild	Moderate	Severe*

B: Diagnosis likelihood tool (DLT): one point per feature present

Antecedent acquired brain injury
Clinical features occur simultaneously*
Episodes are paroxysmal in nature*
Sympathetic over-reactivity to normally non-noxious stimuli*
Absence of parasympathetic features during episodes
Features persist for >3 consecutive days*
Features persist for >2 wk post-brain injury
Two or more episodes daily*
Absence of other presumed causes of features*
Features persist despite treatment of alternative differential diagnosis
Medication administered to decrease sympathetic features*

C: Interpretation of scores

CFS subtotal	Sum of CFS scores for each of the six features (0–3 points for individual features; maximum subtotal = 18)
CFS subtotal severity scores	0 = nil; 1–6 = mild; 7–12 = moderate; 13 = severe
OLT subtotal	Sum of points for each feature present (one point per feature; maximum subtotal% 11)
PSH-AM	CFS subtotal + DLT subtotal
PSH-AM score	<8 = PSH unlikely; 8–16 = PSH possible; ≥17 = PSH probable

Paroxysmal Sympathetic Hyperactivity Assessment Measure (PSH-AM). The Clinical Feature Scale (CFS) scores the severity of clinical features. A score of zero is considered within normal limits. 1-6 = mild symptoms, 7-12 = moderate symptoms, ≥13 = severe symptoms. The Diagnostic Likelihood Tool (DLT) assesses the occurrence of commonly observed features estimating the likelihood of PSH. Each feature present is scored one point. The score of the CFS and DLT are combined to assess the likelihood of PSH. A combined score of <8 = unlikely, 8-16 = possible, and ≥17 probable. (Reprinted with permission from Elsevier. The Lancet Neurology, Sep 2017, 16 (9), 721-729.)

DoC have no or minimal ability to report discomfort. For refractory PSH, intrathecal baclofen therapy needs to be considered.[11]

It is worth noting that PSH is usually a temporary condition. Once PSH seems to have resolved, the abovementioned agents should be gradually weaned. Many DoC patients are maintained on multiple anti-PSH medications due to a history of PSH. As neural recovery progresses, their level of consciousness could be affected and underestimated by those medications. To better understand the necessity of each medication, a stepwise approach is recommended - one change at a time followed by close observation of one's arousal, pain, vital signs, and therapy tolerance.

Table 2
Medications for paroxysmal sympathetic hyperactivity[9,10]

Medication	Medication Class	Targeted Symptom Profile	Side Effects
Propranolol Labetalol	Beta blocker	Tachycardia, diaphoresis, hypertension	Hypotension, bradycardia
Gabapentin	Anticonvulsant	Allodynia, spasticity	Sedation
Clonidine	Alpha-2 agonist	Hypertension, tachycardia	Hypotension, bradycardia, sedation
Bromocriptine	Dopamine receptor agonist	Hyperthermia, rigidity, diaphoresis; may exert additional benefits as a neurostimulant	Dyskinesia, hypotension, nausea, confusion
Dantrolene	Skeletal muscle relaxant Ryanodine receptor antagonist	Posturing, spasticity	Hepatotoxicity, respiratory depression
Baclofen	Antispasmodic GABA-B receptor agonist	Spasticity	Sedation
Morphine Fentanyl	Opioid mu-receptor agonist	Allodynia, hypertension, tachycardia, tachypnea	Respiratory depression, sedation, constipation
Diazepam Lorazepam Midazolam	Benzodiazepine GABA-A receptor agonist	Agitation, hypertension, tachycardia, posturing	Sedation, respiratory depression

Clinicians can select medications to wean based on their side effect profiles. For example, if a patient experiences orthostatic hypotension during verticalization (ie, sitting up, standing up in a tilt table), alpha agonists can be weaned first.

HYDROCEPHALUS
Background

Hydrocephalus (HCP) is defined as an active distension of the ventricular system within the brain related to an imbalance between cerebral spinal fluid (CSF) production and absorption, and/or impaired CSF circulation.[12] HCP can be classified as normal- or high-pressure depending on the opening pressure during a lumbar puncture. The normal range of opening pressure on lumbar puncture in adults is 6 to 25 cmH$_2$O.[13] However, as there is a considerable individual variability, the measurements must be interpreted in the clinical context.[13] High-pressure HCP is commonly seen after a subarachnoid hemorrhage or intraventricular hemorrhage where the blood blocks the villi causing impaired CSF absorption and subsequent accumulation of CSF within a fixed space. This high pressure expands the ventricles and causes CSF extravasation into the brain parenchyma.

In normal pressure hydrocephalus (NPH), it is thought that, after an initial period of volume expansion and elevated pressure, the pressure normalizes.[14] This is analogous to a balloon which requires higher pressure to inflate initially but less pressure to continue expanding or stay expanded. When there is an inciting event such as a brain injury preceding the development of NPH, it is termed secondary NPH. HCP can also be divided into communicating and non-communicating HCP. Communicating HCP develops due to an imbalance of CSF production versus absorption affecting the entire ventricular and cistern system[13] and is the most common form of HCP seen after traumatic brain injury (TBI). Non-communicating HCP is due to obstruction within the CSF ventricular system itself (ie, mass effect).[13]

Regardless of the type (high pressure vs normal pressure, communicating vs non-communicating), HCP can have a profoundly negative impact on a patient's neurologic status and potential for recovery. Indeed, HCP can, in and of itself, be responsible for a patient being in DoC. Therefore, identifying and treating HCP is of the utmost importance in patients with DoC.

Diagnosis

The primary challenge in diagnosis is distinguishing true HCP from compensatory ventricular enlargement after extensive cerebral injury. That is because ventriculomegaly can be caused by both true HCP and *hydrocephalus ex vacuo*, which is enlargement of CSF spaces caused by cerebral atrophy. There are multiple schools of thought for how to distinguish the two on imaging, although the proposed parameters remain controversial (**Table 3**).[15]

The diagnostic difficulty is compounded in DoC. Under normal circumstances, clinicians can rely on certain neurologic changes (eg, gait disturbances, urinary incontinence, and cognitive dysfunction) and ventriculomegaly seen on neuroimaging to diagnose idiopathic NPH. However, identifying clinical changes in patients who already have profound cognitive and motoric deficits can be very challenging.[16] Moreover, it is difficult for clinicians to know to what extent a patient's deficits are due to underlying HCP or the brain injury itself. Therefore, clinicians need to rely on several different sources of information to assist with diagnosing HCP: patient's overall clinical presentation, imaging studies, and CSF diversion. CSF diversion, such as a large-volume lumbar puncture ("tap test") and external lumbar drainage, can be a useful tool to

Table 3
Radiographic features to differentiate normal pressure hydrocephalus versus hydrocephalus ex vacuo

Parameters	Normal Pressure Hydrocephalus	Hydrocephalus ex vacuo
Callosal angle[a] (Angle between lateral ventricles in the coronal plane)	Smaller (average 87.36)	Greater (average 110.94)
Height of the Sylvian fissure[a] (Average of heights measured in 5 coronal planes from where midbrain emerges)	Greater (average 27.19mm)	Smaller (average 25.41mm)
Narrowing of superior parietal sulci[a] (At high convexity and medial parafalcine measured on the coronal plane)	Present	Absent
Perihippocampal fissure (PHF) dilatation	Absent	Present
Width of temporal horn (Average of the max width of right and left temporal horns on transverse plane)	Greater (average 9.01mm)	Smaller (average 8.34mm)
Evan's index (Frontal horn diameter divided by inner skull diameter from a transverse section	Higher (average 0.38)	Lower (average 0.39)

[a] Indicates statistically significant difference.

Adapted from Kim M, Park SW, Lee JY, et al. Differences in Brain Morphology between Hydrocephalus Ex Vacuo and Idiopathic Normal Pressure Hydrocephalus. Psychiatry Investig. 2021;18(7):628-635. https://doi.org/10.30773/pi.2020.0352

identify a shunt-responsive HCP. During a tap test, about 30 to 50 mL of CSF is drained. If patients demonstrate clinical improvement after the test, usually within 2-4 hours, it is considered positive.[17] Tap test is specific but not sensitive in diagnosing shunt-responsive HCP, meaning that a lack of positive response does not preclude response to a shunt (because patients may respond better to a more sustained shunting mechanism).[18] For this reason, a lumbar drain or serial lumbar punctures for several days might be considered in order to gain greater sensitivity and a higher positive predictive value.[18]

In idiopathic NPH, the most prominent improvement is seen in gait disturbances after a tap test.[17] As this is not applicable in the DoC population, assessment should focus on a patient's overall clinical presentation such as level of arousal, initiation, muscle tone, movement coordination, command following, head/trunk control, swallowing, and so forth. If their clinical improvement dissipates several hours or a day after the tap test, it can further validate that the test was positive.

Decision-Making for Shunt Placement

Although shunting is an invasive intervention that carries risks, it should be kept in mind that there is a significant risk to not intervening, namely that the patient's level of consciousness may remain permanently impaired. Therefore, even if the diagnosis of HCP is not certain, shunt placement should be strongly considered, especially in patients in the subacute or chronic phase who have had little change in their clinical status. When it comes to decision-making for shunt placement, several factors should be considered: (1) the likelihood of HCP based on etiology, neurologic status, rate of recovery, results from diagnostic testing, (2) risks and benefits of the intervention, including the risk of no intervention; (3) the patient's previous beliefs and values, if known.

The decision-making process should involve clear communications among physiatrists, neurosurgeons, and the patient's health care surrogates. Potential benefits and risks as well as limitations in the current understanding of HCP need to be clearly presented and discussed for fully informed consent. As mentioned above, as time since injury passes with limited functional improvement and exhaustion of other treatment options, the benefits of a shunt placement may well outweigh the risks. It should be kept in mind that earlier shunting was correlated with better rehabilitation outcome.[19,20]

SPASTICITY AND CONTRACTURE
Background

Spasticity is an upper motor neuron sign that results from disinhibited tonic stretch reflexes from extensive damage to the motor pathways, exacerbated by prolonged immobility, disuse, and poor positioning. It is one of the most frequent complications after severe brain injury, with a prevalence of 59% to 95% in patients with a DoC.[21,22] Timely and effective spasticity management allows patients to maintain or regain motoric abilities, promoting their demonstration of signs of consciousness and establishment of nonverbal communication.[23] It can also improve patients' quality of life. For example, achieving safe wheelchair positioning from successful spasticity management allows transportation via wheelchair-accessible vehicles. Otherwise, their transportation would be limited to a stretcher in an ambulance, which is not available for non-medical excursions (eg, going out for trips with family). Clinicians should be familiar with the benefits of effective spasticity management to optimize DoC patients' opportunities for recovery and quality of life (**Box 1**).

Assessment

Spasticity in DoC tends to be more severe and diffuse.[22] The Modified Ashworth Scale (MAS) and Tardieu scale remain the most commonly used measures for spasticity, mostly in a static setting. Assessing for concomitant hypertonias (eg, dystonia, paratonia, rigidity) and movement disorders (eg, myoclonus, chorea) is critical for effective treatment. In those cases, a more qualitative, syntaxic assessment may be needed. A comprehensive evaluation should include how the spasticity affects a patient's comfort level, tolerance to stretching, sleep, positioning in bed/sitting/standing, transfers, command following, functional use of the limbs, swallowing, and caregiver burden. Therapists commonly see patients in different positions and activities, and they are more likely to notice abnormal tone that is not captured at rest, making them a valuable information source.

Treatment

Clinicians should start by looking for underlying medical conditions that can worsen spasticity, such as constipation, urinary retention, infection, pain, shunt malfunction, and so forth. Treatment options include conventional measures (eg, passive range of motion (PROM), stretching, serial casting, splints, standing program), enteral antispasmodic agents, chemodenervation, chemoneurolysis, and intrathecal baclofen. Newer interventions, such as cryoneurotomy and transcranial direct current stimulation that are under development are out of the scope of the article.

> **Box 1**
> **Benefits of effective spasticity treatment**
>
> Enhance the accuracy of assessments of level of consciousness
> - Improved accuracy and reliability of assessment by enabling patient's motoric response
>
> Improve quality of life
> - Decreased pain
> - Improved positioning
> - Increased volitional/functional movement
> - Nonverbal communication
>
> Minimize complications
> - Contractures
> - Skin breakdown
>
> Reduce caregiver burden
> - Ease with hygiene, dressing, bathing, transfers

Conventional measures are the "bread and butter" in spasticity management, which cannot be emphasized more in routine clinical practice. Enteral antispasmodic agents (eg, baclofen, tizanidine, dantrolene, benzodiazepines) are less favored due to their sedative effects. However, they can still be considered for diffuse mild spasticity given their systemic effectiveness. Among those agents, dantrolene works peripherally and may be prioritized.

Focal spasticity can be better managed with local injections using botulinum neurotoxin (BoNT), phenol/alcohol, or a combination of both. Subsequent aggressive stretching and PROM are critical. Phenol/alcohol causes neurolysis that takes effect immediately and can reach peak effect in about a week.[24] Its effect tends to last longer than BoNT. Chemoneurolysis can be more effective in managing spasticity in larger muscle groups based on the nerve's innervation. Paresthesia/allodynia may occur after injecting mixed motor and sensory nerves (as opposed to motor branches or motor point blocks). During procedure planning, it is important not to compromise volitional movements that are functionally being used. For example, for a patient who uses elbow flexion for "yes," and extension for "no," for non-verbal communication even if the elbow flexors or extensors are spastic, they need to be managed cautiously to avoid compromising the communication system.

Intrathecal baclofen (ITB) therapy is an ideal option for diffuse severe spasticity, especially in lower limbs. An ITB trial is usually performed to test responsiveness prior to the pump implantation. Besides improvement in spasticity, post-trial assessment should include positions at rest/in wheelchair/during transfers, head and trunk control, volitional movement, command following, tolerance to stretching, and overall initiation. Once deemed appropriate, clinicians should work closely with surgeons to determine the optimal catheter tip location, pump size, starting dose, and delivery mode. Even with an ITB pump, patients may still require further management for upper body spasticity, preferrably with chemodenervation or chemoneurolysis. With ITB and focal injections, enteral antispasmodic agents may be weaned off in attempt to improve patients' arousal and cognitive function. There have been case reports and observational studies on chronic DoC patients whose level of consciousness significantly improved following ITB therapy.[25–27] Some of the improvements appeared to be independent of spasticity reduction, raising the possibility that ITB may have a direct effect on cognition in selected patients.[26] It is important for a clinician to have a comprehensive discussion with the patient's

---

Box 2
Intrathecal baclofen therapy education for families

- Risks and benefits of ITB therapy
  - Risks
    - Gastroparesis
    - Constipation
    - Urinary retention
    - Drowsiness
  - Benefits of ITB therapy
    - Fewer systemic side effects
    - More effective than injections in treating diffuse spasticity
    - Potential to be weaned off enteral antispasmodic medications

- Signs and symptoms of baclofen withdrawal and overdose
  - Baclofen withdrawal
    - Increased tone, itching without rash, irritability, fever, seizures, coma
  - Baclofen overdose
    - Flaccid tone, drowsiness, nausea/vomiting, respiratory depression, hypothermia, seizures, coma
  - If concerned for withdrawal, enteral baclofen should be administered as a rescue and medical attention should be sought

- Post-pump implant precautions (usually for 6–8 weeks)
  - No flexion at the hips greater than 90°
  - No twisting
  - No direct pressure on the pump
  - Can participate in therapy within the precautions

- ITB dose titration

- ITB pump maintenance
  - Pump refills
  - Pump replacement for battery life

- Importance of compliance with follow-up appointments

- Reliable transportation

- Identified physician to manage the pump

- Safety
  - Types of pump alarms: non-critical and critical alarms
  - Avoid activities with significant atmospheric pressure change such as scuba diving, skydiving, hyperbaric oxygen therapy
  - Need for interrogation after magnetic exposure (eg MRI)

---

health care surrogates to explain the rationale, set up appropriate expectations, and answer their questions (**Box 2**).

Contractures are irreversible with the abovementioned interventions. With a contracted joint, even if a patient has voluntary muscle contractions, their movement can be confined by the limited ROM. Surgical interventions become the only option to restore ROM and reveal their motor abilities. Surgical release of a contracted joint may be significant and meaningful enough for them to demonstrate their level of consciousness, develop a non-verbal communication system, or participate in standing program/therapeutic gait training. The beneficence and maleficence of "extraordinary measures" in DoC need to be reconsidered in certain cases. Continued management of underlying spasticity following the surgery is crucial in preventing recurrent contractures. All things considered, primary prevention of contractures in the early course of DoC is extremely important.

CRITICAL ILLNESS POLYNEUROPATHY AND MYOPATHY

While upper motor deficits such as spasticity are quite familiar to DoC clinicians, the impact of lower motor neuron deficits in these patients is not widely recognized. However, conditions such as critical illness polyneuropathy and/or myopathy (CIPM), seen in critically ill patients, can also profoundly diminish a patient's motor abilities.[28] Those patients develop significant muscle weakness and paralysis which can confound the assessment of their level of consciousness. Thus, it is important that DoC clinicians recognize CIPM and account for its presence in interpreting assessments of consciousness that depend on motor responses.

CIPM should be suspected in DoC patients with lower motor neuron symptoms such as diffuse areflexia/hyporeflexia, hypotonia, and muscle atrophy who have had prolonged or complicated hospital stays.[29,30] Electromyography (EMG) can be used to diagnose the condition and predict outcomes, but it should be noted that the clinical value of EMG is partially compromised in DoC patients (who cannot cooperate with active muscle recruitment during testing). Although recovery is primarily a function of time, there is some evidence that early aggressive mobilization and electrical muscle stimulation can lead to favorable outcomes.[31]

MOVEMENT DISORDERS

Although uncommon, several movement disorders may arise as a consequence of acquired brain injury (**Table 4**).[32–36] Movement disorders often have a delayed onset and occur in the acute rehabilitation setting. Both hyperkinetic and hypokinetic movement disorders can significantly impair patients' voluntary motor control. Reversible causes such as medications, metabolic/endocrine derangements, HCP, and epidural/subdural hemorrhage should be addressed first.[33,37] Trials of medications and injections could be attempted along with assistive devices and therapies for functional gains, although with unknown efficacy.[33] Many medications that are effective in movement disorders (eg, antiepileptic drugs, benzodiazepines, non-selective beta blockers, and neuroleptics) can cause cognitive side effects. The Abnormal Involuntary Movement Scale (AIMS) can be used to quantify the severity of movement disorders and efficacy of treatment. In certain cases, stereotactic brain surgery and deep brain stimulation (DBS) might be considered. In hypoxic-ischemic brain injury, post-hypoxic movement disorder (PMD) and chronic post-hypoxic myoclonus (CPM) presented an unexpected favorable prognosis with remission rates $\geq$ 50%.[37] Seder and colleagues noted that cardiac arrest survivors with myoclonus had good functional outcomes when there was no associated epileptiform activity, and that the presence of myoclonus should not be considered a sign of futility.[38] Catatonia, although not a movement disorder, is a psychomotor disorder that can present similar to DoC. Patients who remain in DoC should be considered for a trial with benzodiazepines for diagnostic and therapeutic purposes.[39]

SEIZURES
Background

Acquired brain injuries are associated with an increased risk of seizures with an estimated prevalence of 27%. Epileptic abnormalities are found in 41% of patients with a prolonged DoC (ie, lasting $\geq$ 28 days).[40] Detecting seizures in patients with DoC is challenging due to their altered state of consciousness at baseline.[41] Subclinical seizures and post-ictal state are reversible causes of decreased level of consciousness, which is imperative to identify and treat. Additionally, distinguishing aberrant

Table 4
Movement disorders that may be seen in patients with disorders of consciousness[33-36]

Hyperkinetic Movement	Characteristics	Frequently Associated Brain Lesion	Treatment
Tremor	Rhythmic oscillations Resting tremor: seen at rest Postural: seen with steady tonic contraction Action: seen with smooth movement Intentional tremor: terminal exacerbation of action tremor	Basal ganglia Cerebellum Thalamus	Propranolol, benzodiazepines, primidone, levetiracetam, levodopa/carbidopa, botulinum toxin, stereotactic brain surgery, deep brain stimulation (DBS)
Dystonia	Slow, sustained contractions leading to twisting movement or abnormal posturing	Basal ganglia Thalamus	Benzodiazepines, tizanidine, baclofen, botulinum toxin, intrathecal baclofen, stereotactic surgery, DBS
Myoclonus	Brief muscle contractions (positive myoclonus) or inhibition of muscle contractions (negative myoclonus) leading to jerking movements Lance Adams syndrome (chronic post-hypoxic myoclonus)	No specific neuroanatomic association – can be cortical or subcortical	Levetiracetam, clonazepam, valproate, piracetam, ITB
Chorea	Non-rhythmic, dance-like movements	Overactive basal ganglia with excess dopamine	Neuroleptics (risperidone, olanzapine), diazepam, ITB, cyclobenzaprine, stereotactic surgery
Ballismus	Rapid, aggressive, non-suppressible movements of proximal joints producing wild, flinging, high-amplitude movements of the extremity	Thalamus	Neuroleptics, tetrabenazine, ITB, stereotactic surgery
Athetosis	Slow, non-rhythmic, writhing movements with alternating postures in the limbs	Overactive basal ganglia with excess dopamine	Neuroleptics

Hypokinetic Movement	Characteristics	Associated Brain Lesion	Treatment
Bradykinesia	Slowness or poverty of movement	Basal ganglia	Levodopa/carbidopa, amantadine
Akinetic rigidity	Increase in resistance to slow passive movement which is not velocity-dependent	Basal ganglia	Levodopa/carbidopa

Other Abnormal Movement	Characteristics	Associated Brain Lesion	Treatment
Catatonia	Immobility with muscular rigidity or waxy flexibility, "frozen"	Medial orbitofrontal cortex	Benzodiazepine (lorazepam), electroconvulsive therapy, memantine
Paratonia	Facilitatory: actively assisting passive movement or involuntary cooperation. Oppositional "Gegenhalten": involuntary resistance. The degree of paratonia is proportional to the amount of force applied	Frontal lobe	Passive movement therapy, botulinum toxin, harmonic techniques, stabilizing cushion, massage have been trialed without clear benefit

movements from seizures can be challenging. Many DoC patients present with twitches, jerks, convulsions, and abnormal ocular movements that are not epileptic in origin.[42,43] Nevertheless, they are often treated with antiepileptic drugs (AEDs), which can negatively affect arousal and cognition.

Diagnosis

Electroencephalogram (EEG) can be ordered to assess epileptic or epileptiform activities. However, a routine EEG may not capture short-lived epileptic activities. If seizures are strongly suspected but the initial EEG is negative, a prolonged EEG should be considered to increase the likelihood of capturing the episodes. Additionally, elevation in serum prolactin levels may help differentiate epileptic from nonepileptic seizures, with a high specificity and low sensitivity; however, its utilization remains in question.[44]

Treatment

AEDs are the first-line treatment for epilepsy. Considering their cognitive and behavioral profiles, newer AEDs such as levetiracetam, lacosamide, lamotrigine may be better choices. It is important to monitor metabolic abnormalities related to the use of certain AEDs as they can also alter the level of consciousness. Other treatment options include vagus nerve stimulation and surgical resection of the seizure focus.

The Challenge: Antiepileptic Drugs or No Antiepileptic Drugs

As mentioned above, AEDs have cognitive side effects. However, undetected and suboptimally treated seizures can also lead to decreased one's arousal and cognitive ability.[41,45] It is important to weigh probabilities of epileptic seizures as well as the risks and benefits of the use of AEDs in the clinical context. Sometimes, AEDs were started in acute care for prophylaxis but were never discontinued during transitions of care; high-dose AEDs may be started purely for abnormal movements when some patients never had a clearly captured seizure episode clinically or in any EEG studies. In those cases, AEDs may be weaned as tolerated. The general strategies are to attempt it slowly and monitor the patients closely. It is important to recognize seizure risks based on the etiology of the brain injury, time since injury, and history of seizures. Usually, there is an increased risk for seizures with penetrating injury, intracranial hemorrhage, cortical contusions, and a history of late seizures.[46,47] Certain commonly used medications can decrease the seizure threshold, such as fluoroquinolones and tramadol.

Prophylaxis

Studies have shown that AEDs are effective in reducing early (ie, within 1 week) post-traumatic seizures (PTS).[48] Therefore, seizure prophylaxis is recommended for the first 7 days following TBI. There is no evidence that AEDs reduce late PTS, or prevention of early seizures affects mortality and morbidity, or prophylactic use of AEDs reduce seizures in non-TBI.[48]

NEUROENDOCRINE DISTURBANCES
Background

Endocrine-metabolic abnormalities in DoC may also affect outcomes.[49–51] Metabolic abnormalities, such as electrolyte dysregulation, increased creatinine clearance, abnormal liver function panel, hyperglycemia, were seen in almost all patients, mostly transient and reversible.[4] Reportedly, up to 68% of patients have neuroendocrine dysfunction after TBI, which often go undetected and thus untreated. They could be reversible causes of impaired consciousness.[50]

Table 5
Anterior pituitary deficiency

Hormone	Clinical Manifestations	Work up	Treatment
Growth hormone (GH)	Cognitive dysfunction, poor stamina, decreased lean body mass, increased mortality from vascular disease	Serum insulin-like growth factor (IGF-1), insulin tolerance test (ITT)	Growth hormone
Adrenocorticotropin hormone (ACTH), cortisol	Hypotension (and orthostasis), hyponatremia, weakness, confusion, fever, abdominal pain, nausea/vomiting, weight loss	Serum cortisol and ACTH (morning), ACTH stimulation test, ITT, Glucagon test	Steroids (hydrocortisone, prednisone, dexamethasone)
Thyroid-stimulating hormone (TSH)	Cognitive dysfunction, fatigue, depressive symptoms, weight gain	Serum free T4, TSH	Synthetic T4
Luteinizing hormone (LH), follicle-stimulating hormone (FSH), testosterone, estradiol	Sexual dysfunction, decreased bone mass	Serum FSH, LH, testosterone (in men), estradiol (in women)	Gonadal hormone

Diagnosis

Signs and symptoms of neuroendocrine abnormalities include cognitive dysfunction (eg, deficits in memory, attention, processing speed, executive function), depressive symptoms, hypernatremia or hyponatremia, hypotension, seizure, fatigue, and hypoglycemia (**Table 5** for anterior pituitary deficiency). It is noted that many of these symptoms mimic neurologic deficits commonly seen after brain injury. Therefore, clinicians should stay vigilant on neuroendocrine dysfunction and not assume that all deficits are caused by "brain injury" itself. Posterior pituitary deficiency usually causes sodium/water imbalance. Clinicians need to be familiar with differential diagnosis of syndrome of inappropriate antidiuretic hormone (SIADH), cerebral salt wasting (CSW), diabetes insipidus (DI); relevant information could be found online or in other textbooks.

Treatment

Treatment for most anterior pituitary deficiencies consists of replacement of the deficient hormone as listed in **Table 5**. For sodium dysregulation related to posterior pituitary deficiency, treatment mainly consists of addressing fluid status. DI and CSW are usually hypovolemic and could be life-threatening if not managed promptly. They both require fluid replacement; however, it is not effective in central DI if vasopressin or antidiuretic hormone (ADH) is not supplemented. SIADH is usually euvolemic or hypervolemic, requiring fluid restriction and salt tabs.

INFECTION
Background

Recognizing and treating infections, especially sepsis, are of utmost importance as they may compromise a patient's level of consciousness and significantly correlated with mortality.[52,53] Infections, especially pneumonia and urinary tract infections (UTIs), are one of the most frequent complications in patients with DoC.[1,2,4] Other types of infections (eg, osteomyelitis, *Clostridium Difficile* infection, infections associated with intravenous lines or surgical implants) also occur frequently, which are treatable and are important premises for functional recovery.

Diagnosis

Diagnosing infection is straightforward; however, it can be challenging in DoC due to communication deficits as well as frequent abnormalities in vital signs (eg, hyperthermia, tachycardia, hypertension, tachypnea) and laboratory results (eg, leukocytosis) caused by other complications (eg, PSH, seizures). Despite the abovementioned abnormalities, patients with DoC commonly exhibit declines in the arousal level, loss of their previously achieved behavioral capacity; sometimes, PSH and seizure-like activities are the initial signs of an infection.

Treatment

To err on the side of caution, it is imperative to consider and treat possible infection in the event of medical and neurologic decline. Empirical use of broad-spectrum antibiotics with subsequent de-escalation as the investigation proceeds is reasonable. Internists and infectious disease specialists are valuable resources to collaborate with in the medical management for patients with DoC. General preventative measures (eg, strict oral care, early Foley removal, targeted use of antibiotics) are often helpful and easy to institute but commonly overlooked.

DISCLOSURE

The authors have nothing to disclosure.

REFERENCES

1. Whyte J, Nordenbo AM, Kalmar K, et al. Medical complications during inpatient rehabilitation among patients with traumatic disorders of consciousness. Arch Phys Med Rehabil 2013;94(10):1877–83.
2. Ganesh S, Guernon A, Chalcraft L, et al. Medical comorbidities in disorders of consciousness patients and their association with functional outcomes. Arch Phys Med Rehabil 2013;94(10):1899–907.
3. Lucca LF, Lofaro D, Leto E, et al. The impact of medical complications in predicting the rehabilitation outcome of patients with disorders of consciousness after severe traumatic brain injury. Front Hum Neurosci 2020;14:570544.
4. Zhang B, Huang K, Karri J, et al. Many faces of the hidden souls: medical and neurological complications and comorbidities in disorders of consciousness. Brain Sci 2021;11(5):608.
5. Rabinstein AA. Paroxysmal sympathetic hyperactivity in the neurological intensive care unit. Neurol Res 2007;29(7):680–2.
6. Alofisan TO, Algarni YA, Alharfi IM, et al. Paroxysmal sympathetic hyperactivity after severe traumatic brain injury in children: prevalence, risk factors, and outcome. Pediatr Crit Care Med J Soc Crit Care Med World Fed Pediatr Intensive Crit Care Soc 2019;20(3):252–8.
7. Baguley IJ, Perkes IE, Fernandez-Ortega JF, et al. Paroxysmal sympathetic hyperactivity after acquired brain injury: consensus on conceptual definition, nomenclature, and diagnostic criteria. J Neurotrauma 2014;31(17):1515–20.
8. Perkes I, Baguley IJ, Nott MT, et al. A review of paroxysmal sympathetic hyperactivity after acquired brain injury. Ann Neurol 2010;68(2):126–35.
9. Rabinstein AA. Autonomic Hyperactivity. Contin Minneap Minn 2020;26(1):138–53.
10. Ripley DL, Driver S, Stork R, et al. Pharmacologic management of the patient with traumatic brain injury. In: Eapen BC, Cifu DX, editors. Rehabilitation after traumatic brain injury. St. Louis, MO: Elsevier; 2019. p. 133–63.
11. Pucks-Faes E, Hitzenberger G, Matzak H, et al. Intrathecal baclofen in paroxysmal sympathetic hyperactivity: Impact on oral treatment. Brain Behav 2018;8(11):e01124.
12. Rekate HL. A contemporary definition and classification of hydrocephalus. Semin Pediatr Neurol 2009;16(1):9–15.
13. Williams MA, Relkin NR. Diagnosis and management of idiopathic normal-pressure hydrocephalus. Neurol Clin Pract 2013;3(5):375–85.
14. Daou B, Klinge P, Tjoumakaris S, et al. Revisiting secondary normal pressure hydrocephalus: does it exist? A review. Neurosurg Focus 2016;41(3):E6.
15. Kim M, Park SW, Lee JY, et al. Differences in brain morphology between hydrocephalus ex vacuo and idiopathic normal pressure hydrocephalus. Psychiatry Investig 2021;18(7):628–35.
16. Arnts H, van Erp WS, Sanz LRD, et al. The dilemma of hydrocephalus in prolonged disorders of consciousness. J Neurotrauma 2020;37(20):2150–6.
17. Williams MA, Malm J. Diagnosis and treatment of idiopathic normal pressure hydrocephalus. Contin Minneap Minn 2016;22(2 Dementia):579–99.

18. Marmarou A, Bergsneider M, Klinge P, et al. The value of supplemental prognostic tests for the preoperative assessment of idiopathic normal-pressure hydrocephalus. Neurosurgery 2005;57(3 Suppl):S17–28 ; discussion ii-v.
19. Kowalski RG, Weintraub AH, Rubin BA, et al. Impact of timing of ventriculoperitoneal shunt placement on outcome in posttraumatic hydrocephalus. J Neurosurg 2018;23:1–12.
20. Weintraub AH, Gerber DJ, Kowalski RG. Posttraumatic hydrocephalus as a confounding influence on brain injury rehabilitation: incidence, clinical characteristics, and outcomes. Arch Phys Med Rehabil 2017;98(2):312–9.
21. Martens G, Laureys S, Thibaut A. Spasticity management in disorders of consciousness. Brain Sci 2017;7(12):162.
22. Zhang B, Karri J, O'Brien K, et al. Spasticity management in persons with disorders of consciousness. Pharm Manag PM R 2021;13(7):657–65.
23. Cruse D, Chennu S, Chatelle C, et al. Bedside detection of awareness in the vegetative state: a cohort study. Lancet Lond Engl 2011;378(9809):2088–94.
24. Zhang B, Darji N, Francisco GE, et al. The Time course of onset and peak effects of phenol neurolysis. Am J Phys Med Rehabil 2021;100(3):266–70.
25. Al-Khodairy AT, Wicky G, Nicolo D, et al. Influence of intrathecal baclofen on the level of consciousness and mental functions after extremely severe traumatic brain injury: brief report. Brain Inj 2015;29(4):527–32.
26. Halbmayer LM, Kofler M, Hitzenberger G, et al. On the recovery of disorders of consciousness under intrathecal baclofen administration for severe spasticity-An observational study. Brain Behav 2022;12(5):e2566.
27. Sarà M, Pistoia F, Mura E, et al. Intrathecal baclofen in patients with persistent vegetative state: 2 hypotheses. Arch Phys Med Rehabil 2009;90(7):1245–9.
28. Stevens RD, Dowdy DW, Michaels RK, et al. Neuromuscular dysfunction acquired in critical illness: a systematic review. Intensive Care Med 2007;33(11):1876–91.
29. Latronico N, Fenzi F, Recupero D, et al. Critical illness myopathy and neuropathy. Lancet Lond Engl 1996;347(9015):1579–82.
30. Jarrett SR, Mogelof JS. Critical illness neuropathy: diagnosis and management. Arch Phys Med Rehabil 1995;76(7):688–91.
31. Zhou C, Wu L, Ni F, et al. Critical illness polyneuropathy and myopathy: a systematic review. Neural Regen Res 2014;9(1):101–10.
32. Venkatesan A, Frucht S. Movement disorders after resuscitation from cardiac arrest. Neurol Clin 2006;24(1):123–32.
33. Moon D. Disorders of movement due to acquired and traumatic brain injury. Curr Phys Med Rehabil Rep 2022;10(4):311–23.
34. Unal A, Bulbul F, Alpak G, et al. Effective treatment of catatonia by combination of benzodiazepine and electroconvulsive therapy. J ECT 2013;29(3):206–9.
35. Van Deun B, Van Den Noortgate N, Van Bladel A, et al. Managing paratonia in persons with dementia: short-term effects of supporting cushions and harmonic techniques. J Am Med Dir Assoc 2019;20(12):1521–8.
36. Ganguly J, Kulshreshtha D, Almotiri M, et al. Muscle tone physiology and abnormalities. Toxins 2021;13(4):282.
37. Scheibe F, Neumann WJ, Lange C, et al. Movement disorders after hypoxic brain injury following cardiac arrest in adults. Eur J Neurol 2020;27(10):1937–47.
38. Seder DB, Sunde K, Rubertsson S, et al. Neurologic outcomes and postresuscitation care of patients with myoclonus following cardiac arrest. Crit Care Med 2015;43(5):965–72.

39. Zhang B, O'Brien K, Won W, et al. A Retrospective analysis on clinical practice-based approaches using zolpidem and lorazepam in disorders of consciousness. Brain Sci 2021;11(6):726.

40. Lejeune N, Zasler N, Formisano R, et al. Epilepsy in prolonged disorders of consciousness: a systematic review. Brain Inj 2021;35(12–13):1485–95.

41. Briand MM, Lejeune N, Zasler N, et al. Management of epileptic seizures in disorders of consciousness: an international survey. Front Neurol 2021;12:799579.

42. Hantus S. Monitoring for seizures in the intensive care unit. Handb Clin Neurol 2019;161:103–7.

43. Benbadis SR, Chen S, Melo M. What's shaking in the ICU? The differential diagnosis of seizures in the intensive care setting. Epilepsia 2010;51(11):2338–40.

44. Fisher RS. Serum prolactin in seizure diagnosis. Neurol Clin Pract 2016;6(2):100–1.

45. Fierain A, Gaspard N, Lejeune N, et al. Beware of nonconvulsive seizures in prolonged disorders of consciousness: Long-term EEG monitoring is the key. Clin Neurophysiol Off J Int Fed Clin Neurophysiol 2022;136:228–34.

46. Angeleri F, Majkowski J, Cacchiò G, et al. Posttraumatic epilepsy risk factors: one-year prospective study after head injury. Epilepsia 1999;40(9):1222–30.

47. Lamar CD, Hurley RA, Rowland JA, et al. Post-traumatic epilepsy: review of risks, pathophysiology, and potential biomarkers. J Neuropsychiatry Clin Neurosci 2014;26(2):iv–113.

48. Agrawal A, Timothy J, Pandit L, et al. Post-traumatic epilepsy: an overview. Clin Neurol Neurosurg 2006;108(5):433–9.

49. Estraneo A, Loreto V, Masotta O, et al. Do medical complications impact long-term outcomes in prolonged disorders of consciousness? Arch Phys Med Rehabil 2018;99(12):2523–31.e3.

50. Molaie AM, Maguire J. Neuroendocrine abnormalities following traumatic brain injury: an important contributor to neuropsychiatric sequelae. Front Endocrinol 2018;9:176.

51. Tudor RM, Thompson CJ. Posterior pituitary dysfunction following traumatic brain injury: review. Pituitary 2019;22(3):296–304.

52. Romaniello C, Bertoletti E, Matera N, et al. Morfeo Study II: clinical course and complications in patients with long-term disorders of consciousness. Am J Med Sci 2016;351(6):563–9.

53. Ventura T, Harrison-Felix C, Carlson N, et al. Mortality after discharge from acute care hospitalization with traumatic brain injury: a population-based study. Arch Phys Med Rehabil 2010;91(1):20–9.

Strategy and Philosophy for Treating Pain and Sleep in Disorders of Consciousness

Amanda Appel, MD, MPH[a,b,c,1], Eric Spier, MD[d,*]

KEYWORDS

• Brain injury • Disorders of consciousness • Pain • Sleep • Coma

KEY POINTS

• Despite the rapid evolution of brain injury medicine, there is still a lot that needs to be learned for providers to fully understand the complex neural networks involved in consciousness and how they are affected in disorders of consciousness.

• Most patients with DOC have disordered sleep and the return of normal sleep architecture is essential to the emergence of consciousness and the healing brain.

• In the treatment of pain and sleep in DOC, clinicians have the responsibility to learn and understand the pathophysiology at play in DOC and use the tools available for individualized treatment that evolves with the patient's emergent consciousness.

Disorders of sleep and pain are central concerns in the care of people with disordered consciousness. In routine practice, these issues are thought of as purely clinical phenomena. Although not mistaken, we believe that embedding issues of sleep and pain into a larger context may help clinicians better conceptualize the issues involved and, possibly, enhance bedside assessment and treatment. Specifically, we believe that viewing pain and sleep through the prism of the process of the recovery of consciousness, especially in terms of the emergence of "self," may shed light on how these issues present in patients with disorders of consciousness (DOC).

Comments made by families and clinicians illustrate conventional assumptions about the relationship between "self" and consciousness (eg, "I wonder if he is still 'in there'?" or "When will she wake up"?). The implicit assumption behind these comments is that, in DOC, a patient's "self" is intact but simply dormant, and that the recovery of consciousness simply involves a patient's self "waking-up," analogous to

[a] Department of Pediatric Rehabilitation Medicine, Children's Hospital Colorado, Aurora, CO, USA; [b] Department of Pediatrics, Children's Hospital Colorado, Aurora, CO, USA; [c] Department of Physical Medicine and Rehabilitation, University of Colorado Anschutz School of Medicine, Aurora, CO, USA; [d] Craig Hospital
[1] Present address: 1016 Cook Street, Denver, CO 80206.
* Corresponding author.
E-mail address: erictspier@gmail.com

Phys Med Rehabil Clin N Am 35 (2024) 145–154
https://doi.org/10.1016/j.pmr.2023.06.022
1047-9651/24/© 2023 Elsevier Inc. All rights reserved.

the process of awakening each morning after sleep. Although a reasonable assumption, recent discoveries in neuroscience have suggested that the self is the product of a series of discrete neurologic processes,[1] processes that may come back "on-line" in a gradual and piecemeal fashion during the recovery of consciousness.

In this new paradigm, the self is seen as a construct; an emergent property of mind as more and more networks are recruited and connected, whether during evolution, development, or recovery of consciousness. Although knowledge is still nascent, the neural networks that underpin our states of mind and emergent consciousness, such as the default mode, the salience, and executive networks are better understood. Much work is also being done to understand the connectome, or the systems of neuronal interconnections, that are responsible for the properties of selfhood associated with recovery from brain injury. Protocols used to identify covert consciousness, such as the Coma Recovery Scale-Revised, functional MRI, electroencephalography (EEG), and the "ABCD" model, show promise in screening and classifying patients with DOC.[2] Knowledge of areas of the brain and their neuroanatomic correlates is also becoming more nuanced and specific allowing providers to be symptom specific in neuropharmacologic treatment and targeted with therapeutic approaches. In addition, there are tools to define how sleep progresses, and for identifying pain and nociception in patients with DOC. The transition from a coma to a level of consciousness that allows an individual to exert some agency in their environment is defined by a spectrum of emergent awareness.

Damasio[3] describes different levels of awareness that are correlated with the Rancho Los Amigos Scale (RLAS). Whereas the RLAS describes the emerging patient with primarily diffuse axonal injury in descriptive terms, Damasio explains what may be happening anatomically in the healing brain to describe the emerging self/ego. Early in recovery the patient emerging from an unresponsive wakeful syndrome (UWS) to a minimally conscious state (MCS) has an emerging ability to follow basic commands and possibly primitive responses to pain but lacks the interconnections (return of connectome function) to normalize sleep architecture, experience pain, or form memories because this does not become evident until later in recovery. These concepts of emerging self, as defined by a protoself, a core-self, and an autobiographical-self, map well onto what is observed in the recovery of patients with DOC and can therefore be helpful in understanding and teaching about emerging consciousness for treatment planning. This starts in part with Damasio's idea of the protoself. The protoself describes an emergent consciousness capable of feeling states and requires little cortical function. Like a patient emerging from anesthesia there is a basic feeling state but no self to experience it; a bit like the George Berkeley inspired thought experiment of a tree falling in the forest with no witness.

Once a patient emerges to a more confused and automatic state (RLAS III-VI) or into a posttraumatic amnesia (PTA) and/or confusional state they can also be described as possessing a core-self. The beginnings of suffering and pain emerge with the core-self. There is some awareness of self, but without short-term declarative memory. This lack of awareness is protective and although pain and sleep are more easily treated in these emerging patients, they often still do not have the same sadness, or sense of loss and anger associated with patients with an autobiographical-self who have emerged from PTA. Patients with a core-self may become more tactile defensive, motor restless, and even have proactive interference, all elements pathognomonic for patients at this level of recovery. What all these symptoms have in common is elements of a cogent sense-of-self that is still fragmented and without a dimensional connection to time and spatial awareness. Once a patient emerges from PTA, the capacity for planning and participation in care is facilitated by emergent agency in what is called the autobiographical-self. The autobiographical-self is the merger of the proto-self and core-self in time and place. The feeling states associated with the protoself and the sensory maps of sight, sound, and tactile or physical embodiment of the core-self placed in the context of time and space is the autobiographical-self. When this final property of self is met the patient can regain the ability to navigate of their own care.

Patients with DOC are best reflected in Damasio's idea of protoself, which he describes as "an integrated collection of separate neural patterns that map, moment by moment, the most stable aspects of the organism's physical structure."[3] Anatomic structures that he posits may contribute to the protoself are those required for basic interoceptive integration. Such structures include the nucleus tractus solitarius, the parabrachial nucleus, the periaqueductal gray, the area postrema, the hypothalamus, and the deep layers of the superior colliculus. All these structures are present in the posterior aspect of the brainstem and when injured can result in a coma. At the level of the cortex, it includes the insular cortex and anterior cingulate cortex. The basic feeling states and the nuclei needed for arousal lack the higher cortical machinery needed for emotions but are sufficient to create the protoself. Thus, the awareness and arousal needed to interpret feeling states into emotions, such as hunger, fear, or pain, are lacking. At this level of consciousness treatment of nociception can be geared to minimizing autonomic symptoms and treatment of sleep can focus on preparing a person for normal sleep architecture by clustering daytime arousal and fatigue at night. It is the job of the clinician to discover the emergent consciousness and help families and treatment teams navigate care. With increasing awareness, memory, and attention the navigation of care is placed incrementally onto the patient. As recovery progresses and greater complexity of self/ego returns with memory, metacognition, and attention, then complex emotions of the autobiographical-self (ambivalence, contempt, guilt, shame, and others) emerge. The increasing awareness in turn necessitates more complex strategies of neuropsychological care on the odyssey of recovery.

EVALUATING AND TREATING SLEEP IN DISORDERS OF CONSCIOUSNESS

Sleep itself is a state of altered consciousness that is naturally recurring in healthy individuals, and quality and quantity of sleep can affect memory, attention, mood, executive function, and many other processes integral to life. Sleep deprivation has been associated with significant cognitive dysfunction (eg, deficits in attention, memory, executive function).[4] The mechanistic link between cognition and sleep is not fully understood, but it has been proposed that the increase in convective exchange between cerebral spinal fluid and interstitial fluid during quality sleep aids in the clearance of neuronal waste. A complex architecture of events must unfold overnight for the brain to store memories, recover, and prepare for the following day. It is the breakdown of this architecture that results in dysregulated sleep, which can have significant ramifications to the function of a recovering brain. It is the clinician's responsibility to assist patients with DOC on their journey to recovery, and sleep architecture is key in the progression from proto to core to autobiographical-self.

The science surrounding sleep in DOC has increased steadily over recent years, and studies estimate that 66% to 84% of individuals with brain injury have disordered sleep.[5] Disordered sleep consists of lack of normal sleep architecture, need for increased duration of sleep, and increased mean sleep latency.[6] Considering most patients with DOC experience disordered sleep, it is crucial that we explore methods to better evaluate sleep; learn the natural progression of sleep architecture through emerging consciousness; and develop strategies that allow one to augment, not hinder, the progression toward typical sleep-wake cycles and its normal architecture. There are many unique methods that have been developed to try to evaluate not only the quantity but quality of a patient's sleep, such as polysomnography, EEG, actigraphy, and patient report. Of note, patients with brain injury are unreliable when it comes to self-report and significantly underestimate the amount of excessive daytime sleepiness and need for sleep.[6]

Historically it was thought that the presence of periods of eyes open and closed represented sleep-wake cycles. However, it is now known that periods of eyes open and closed do not correlate with preserved electrophysiological sleep architecture.[7] Furthermore, evidence suggests that quality and quantity of sleep spindles correlates with changes in metabolism and network structure[8] and can possibly be used for outcome prediction in patients with DOC.[7] Given that improvement in sleep efficiency is correlated with emergence from PTA,[9] a strategy for treating a patient's sleep at this stage becomes even more important.

In the hospital setting there are many factors that can negatively or positively affect the quality of a patient's sleep, such as environmental factors, comorbid sleep disorders, and pharmacologic intervention. Although it often goes overlooked, sleep hygiene is one of the most critical, basic, and feasible nonpharmacologic interventions that can significantly improve sleep quality and quantity.[10] Common sleep hygiene interventions include minimizing interruptions at night, keeping light and sound down in a patient's room in the evenings, maintaining light greater than 100 lux during the day, minimizing napping or maintaining naps at or less than 30 minutes during the day, and keeping patients out of bed as much as possible during the day. In addition to sleep hygiene, it is important to adequately treat sleep disorders that often co-occur with brain injuries considering obstructive and central sleep apnea are more prevalent in this population.[5] After exhausting nonpharmacologic interventions providers should consider pharmacologic interventions that aid in sleep without obliterating normal sleep architecture. When considering pharmacologic intervention, less is more and pharmacy should facilitate natural recovery, meaning augmenting slow wave sleep (trazodone),[11] facilitating diurnal rhythms (melatonin/hypocretin),[12] or addressing rumination associated with sleep onset (selective serotonin reuptake inhibitors/ketamine). By taking advantage of physiological fluctuations in neurotransmitters native to normalized sleep architecture the clinician can avoid less nuanced dosing of sedating benzodiazepines and antipsychotics where possible because these have deleterious effects on slow wave sleep. This basic principle helps to facilitate normal recovery and not be a barrier to it. Suvorexant/lemborexant/daridorexant are some of the agents now available to inhibit hypocretin/orexin in an attempt to mimic physiologic fluctuations.[12] Melatonin is usually supplemented using a nutraceutical despite the availability of ramelteon, a Food and Drug Administration–approved alternative to melatonin, which induces sleep with a 1 and 2 receptor agonist.[13] Ramelteon may also help with slow wave sleep like trazodone and quetiapine.[11,14] Another common approach is to help patients cluster sleep at night and maintain arousal during the day using appropriately timed stimulants.[15] This approach is especially effective in patients with hypersomnolence. For patients with sleep dysregulation that is more difficult to manage using typical pharmacologic approaches, more-sedating medications are often used. However, when using more-sedating medications, care should be taken to minimize the effect on normal sleep architecture and therefore memory, alertness, and executive function. One approach is to start with less potent γ-aminobutyric acid–positive allosteric modulators or nonbenzodiazepine hypnotics. In patients for which sleep onset is the primary target of treatment, suggestions are short-acting nonbenzodiazepine sedatives, such as zaleplon, zopiclone, zolpidem, or alternatively eszopiclone, which is more sedating and long-acting. A combination of sleep medications is often required, and a one-size-fits-all approach is dangerous and deleterious in such a varied and diverse patient population. Providers should strive to individualize treatment based on each patient's unique sleep dysfunction, arousal, mood, and behaviors while also ensuring that the patient's medication list is constantly reviewed for medications that can have a negative effect on sleep.

EVALUATING AND TREATING PAIN IN DISORDERS OF CONSCIOUSNESS

Although normal sleep is critical to healing, effective pain management is equally as important. Intrinsic to the human condition is the want to reduce pain and suffering for those we love and care for. At the forefront of the minds of family and caregivers of patients with DOC is whether they are in pain, and if it is adequately treated. This is even more complicated in patients with DOC because of the many possible pain generators including central pain, traumatic comorbidities (fractures, soft tissue injury, solid organ injury), myofascial pain, neuropathic pain, spasticity, dystonia, contractures, infection, changes in ICP, heterotopic ossification, and skin breakdown. Adequately treating pain in this population is vital not only to minimize suffering, but also to eliminate barriers to participation in therapies and recovery. However, to adequately treat pain, one must first be able to establish that the patient is in fact experiencing pain. When discussing the notion of distress caused by pain it is important to distinguish the difference between nociception and pain. Nociception is the process of encoding and processing noxious stimuli or tissue damage, and pain is the suffering associated with higher level processing of that nociceptive input. The International Association for the Study of Pain defines pain as an "unpleasant sensory and emotional experience associated with actual or potential tissue damage or described in terms of such damage."[16] Therefore, one cannot experience pain without extensive cortico-cortical, thalamocortical, and thalamostriatal interconnectivity, or emergence of a self/ego to experience it. The core-self and autobiographical-self reflect a mental state where feeling states in a body are mapped into an experiencing being capable of reflecting on or experiencing said unpleasant sensations. Stated differently it is the experiencing self that is necessary for nociception to become pain.

Historically it was thought that patients with DOC were unable to experience pain. However, this has been refuted in patients with MCS, and is now being questioned in some patients with UWS because studies have found evidence of pain processing in small subsets of patients with UWS.[17,18] It is arguable that the patients with UWS who show evidence of higher cortical processing of pain are misclassified using the CRS-R and are better classified as MCS or having cognitive motor dissociation. Patients with true UWS therefore theoretically should have no conscious perception of pain despite having the ability to have reflexive responses to nociception. Patients with MCS, however, have started to emerge and connect the complex, higher level cortical pathways to be able to consciously perceive pain. This has been shown in multiple imaging studies that exhibit activity of the entire "pain matrix," and more specifically regions that are thought to be involved in the cognitive and affective responses to pain in patients with DOC.[17,19–21] However, because of the possibility of misdiagnosis of patients with DOC, patients with UWS are often treated with the assumption that they may have capacity to perceive pain to minimize suffering.[18] In fact, pain is a sine qua non of the transition from the autonomic response in the vessel to the experience of the conscious individual with the ability not only to perceive but comprehend and remember the experience. Before the emergence of consciousness, it is possible that the physical body or vessel is experiencing nociceptive inputs, and the body has autonomic and reflexive responses to those nociceptive inputs despite being unable to consciously perceive them as pain. This can often be a difficult concept for families to accept, and a way to objectively describe the difference between nociception and pain helps to shape a treatment strategy that is empowering for the family and treatment team and simultaneously reduce ambiguous suffering.

Considering that patients with DOC are unable to consistently and accurately communicate their experience of pain with caregivers, there are many different pain scales that have been developed to evaluate nociception and pain ranging from scales that were developed for nonverbal children to scales that were developed specifically for the brain-injured population (**Table 1**).[22-28] Different tools are used based on the strengths, preferences, and biases in various setting of care. Most of these scales focus on the detection of nociception using behavioral and physiologic ques, which may not accurately identify the subjective experience of pain. Because nociception tends to be a prerequisite for pain, then identifying and treating it can prevent the suffering associated with pain albeit at the potential expense of emergent consciousness. The Nociception Coma Scale-Revised (NCS-R)[23] is a scale that has been validated for use in the intensive care unit, neurosurgery/neurology units, rehabilitation centers, and nursing homes for this population. Despite it being a scale developed to evaluate nociception, there is a correlation between NCS-R scores and brain metabolism in the anterior cingulate cortex suggesting it could be tapping into some cortical pain processing.[29] This is because the anterior cingulate cortex has been shown to be involved with executive frontal network processing. The Brain Injury Nociception Assessment Measure has been developed to provide a measure of nociceptive pain using behavioral and physiological items in patients with DOC who do not have a level of consciousness that allows them to have cortically mediated responses to pain, which are in turn required to achieve the highest scores on the NCS-R.[30] There are many other pain scales that are used in patients with DOC that have not been validated for use in the population. Pain scales that look at physiological responses to nociceptive input, such as increased heart rate, diaphoresis, or other autonomic signs, can help to avoid chronic use of pain medications or around-the-clock strategies but can alternatively result in the overuse of pain medications. Using these measures can also be problematic in that changes in autonomic signs are indicators of other problems, such as infection or paroxysmal autonomic hyperactivity not related to nociception or pain. Additionally, providers must differentiate motor restlessness and akathisia as being caused by nociception versus other causes. As such the physiologic capture

Table 1	
Tools commonly used for assessment of pain in disorders of consciousness	
Tool	**Patient Population**
Nociceptive Coma Scale (NCS, NCS- R, and NCS-R-PS)	Adults with disorders of consciousness/brain injury[23]
Brain Injury Nociception Assessment Measure (BINAM)	Adults with disorders of consciousness/brain injury[30]
Face, Legs, Activity, Cry, and Consolability (FLACC and rFLACC)	Nonverbal pediatric patients[28]
Behavioral Pain Scale (BPS)	Critically ill and sedated adults[25]
Checklist of Nonverbal Pain Indicators (CNPI)	Cognitively impaired adults[26]
Critical Care Pain Observation Tool (CPOT)	Nonverbal critically ill adults[27]

of these tools can include more than just nociception and the clinician must remain vigilant to the evolving needs of care.

Other techniques have been used to evaluate pain include EEG[31] and advanced imaging,[19–21] but these are not always realistic in practice and do not provide real-time feedback on pain for an adequate treatment response. Additionally, when evaluating pain in a patient with DOC it is important to evaluate all the adjuncts to pain including subcortical responses to noxious stimuli. For example, although a patient with UWS may not be able to consciously experience pain, the reflexive response to nociceptive stimuli may cause a plethora of additional symptoms that is problematic for recovery including increased tone, elevated ICP, adverse neuroendocrine responses, and so forth.[32] Treating reflexive nociceptive responses in these patients and the sequalae of pain is important to make progress in neurologic recovery. Regardless of the tools used they should be considered in the wider context of emergent consciousness and best practices for care of the vessel for whom one expects that self/ego to reemerge.

Once the presence or absence of pain is established, the clinician must determine the best treatment course. Similar to treating sleep dysfunction in patients with DOC, when considering pharmacologic intervention for pain most providers operate using the guiding principle that one should use as little as possible and tend toward medications that are less likely to impair cognitive recovery or memory. Generally, one of the more difficult tasks for the provider is determining the cause of the pain when there is often an overabundance of possible pain generators. Adequately identifying the cause of the pain allows providers to first attempt to treat pain with nonpharmacologic treatment strategies that may optimize patient recovery without hindering patient alertness, awareness, memory, and overall cognitive function. If nonpharmacologic interventions are deemed inadequate for appropriate pain control, there are many pharmacologic options to consider. When starting pharmacologic pain intervention, many physicians subscribe to the "start low and go slow" mentality, which is ideal for optimizing patient cognition but may lead to longer periods of patient suffering by prolonging subtherapeutic treatment. As such, treatment aggressiveness and pace should be in proportion to the clinical need. In addition, although some may prefer a hierarchical approach to pain management, it is often best to consider a more nuanced and patient-centered approach that capitalizes on the intricacies of the pharmacotherapeutics available. In the absence of contraindications, nonsedating medications, such as nonsteroidal anti-inflammatory drugs and acetaminophen, and topical medications (eg, diclofenac gel, lidocaine gel or patches, capsaicin cream) are helpful in providing baseline pain control without affecting cognitive recovery. GABAergic medications, such as gabapentin and pregabalin, are important and often overlooked options for pain control in patients with DOC. They not only aid in the treatment of neuropathic pain, which is common in this population, but they also act as antiepileptics, can decrease spasticity, and aid in treatment of anxiety.[33] However, care must be taken because they are sedating. Antidepressants are useful in the treatment of neuropathic pain and tricyclic antidepressants are considered in patients who may benefit from the added effects on sleep. Many antiepileptic drugs can also be used in the treatment of pain and can aid in treatment of posttraumatic headaches or migraines.[34] Opioids and benzodiazepines can also be used in the treatment of pain but should be used with caution because of the detrimental effects on arousal and cognition. Although often overlooked, more directed interventions are extremely beneficial for patients and may aid in the avoidance of systemic sedating medications. For example, an intrathecal baclofen pump or local chemodenervation for a patient with spasticity can significantly decrease the amount of systemic sedating medication required. Finally, it is vital that clinicians continuously evaluate the patient's medications list and wean medications as soon as appropriate and possible. Patients emerging from DOC have a rapidly evolving clinical picture, and their pharmacotherapeutics should constantly be reevaluated to ensure optimization of cognition, alertness, and participation in therapies.

SUMMARY

Despite the rising number of people with DOC and a collective scientific knowledge base that is rapidly evolving, there is still a significant amount of work to do in the classification and understanding of the complex neural networks or connectomes at play in DOC. Clinicians caring for patients with DOC have a responsibility to strive to understand the anatomy of sleep and pain in the emerging patient, use the tools available to best assess and treat using a patient-centered approach, and continuously reevaluate patients because of the constantly evolving nature of emergence. Normalization of sleep architecture is vital for consciousness to evolve and reinforces the importance of appropriate clinical assessment. Similarly, pain can lead to unnecessary suffering and the available information suggests the capacity for patients diagnosed with MCS and in some cases UWS to experience pain and should be treated as such.[22] Although more research is needed to empower better treatment in the future it is worth noting how much progress has been made in the short history of brain injury medicine as a specialty. The emergent properties of the self and ego are now understood in terms of the neural networks or connectomes and key cortical zones of convergence. Medications and treatment strategies are now symptom specific and can be targeted for a brain injury population. Validated tools now exist for evaluation of emergent consciousness, pain, and sleep. This is a foundation of knowledge to build on to be sure, but a solid foundation for future progress.

DISCLOSURE

Nothing to disclose.

REFERENCES

1. Damasio A. Making minds conscious. Pantheon Books; 2021.
2. Curley WH, Bodien YG, Zhou DW, et al. Electrophysiological correlates of thalamocortical function in acute severe traumatic brain injury. Cortex 2022;152: 136–52.
3. Damasio A. Self comes to mind: constructing the conscious brain. Vintage Books a Division of Random House, Inc.; 2010.
4. Durmer JS, Dinges DF. Neurocognitive consequences of sleep deprivation. Semin Neurol 2005;25(1):117–29.
5. Nakase-Richardson R, Sherer M, Barnett SD, et al. Prospective evaluation of the nature, course, and impact of acute sleep abnormality after traumatic brain injury. Arch Phys Med Rehabil 2013;94(5):875–82.
6. Imbach LL, Büchele F, Valko PO, et al. Sleep-wake disorders persist 18 months after traumatic brain injury but remain underrecognized. Neurology 2016; 86(21):1945–9.
7. Cologan V, Drouot X, Parapatics S, et al. Sleep in the unresponsive wakefulness syndrome and minimally conscious state. J Neurotrauma 2013;30(5):339–46.
8. Thengone DJ, Voss HU, Fridman EA, et al. Local changes in network structure contribute to late communication recovery after severe brain injury. Sci Transl Med 2016;8(368):368re5.

9. Makley MJ, Johnson-Greene L, Tarwater PM, et al. Return of memory and sleep efficiency following moderate to severe closed head injury. Neurorehabil Neural Repair 2009;23(4):320–6.

10. Makley MJ, Gerber D, Newman JK, et al. Optimized sleep after brain injury (OSABI): a pilot study of a sleep hygiene intervention for individuals with moderate to severe traumatic brain injury. Neurorehabilitation Neural Repair 2020;34(2):111–21.

11. Wichniak A, Wierzbicka AE, Jarema M. Treatment of insomnia: effect of trazodone and hypnotics on sleep. Psychiatr Pol 2021;55(4):743–55. Leczenie bezsenności – wpływ trazodonu i leków nasennych na sen.

12. Baumann CR, Bassetti CL. Hypocretins (orexins) and sleep-wake disorders. Lancet Neurol 2005;4(10):673–82.

13. Liu J, Clough SJ, Hutchinson AJ, et al. MT1 and MT2 melatonin receptors: a therapeutic perspective. Annu Rev Pharmacol Toxicol 2016;56:361–83.

14. Cohrs S, Rodenbeck A, Guan Z, et al. Sleep-promoting properties of quetiapine in healthy subjects. Psychopharmacology (Berl) 2004;174(3):421–9.

15. Trotti LM, Arnulf I. Idiopathic hypersomnia and other hypersomnia syndromes. Neurotherapeutics 2021;18(1):20–31.

16. Raja SN, Carr DB, Cohen M, et al. The revised International Association for the Study of Pain definition of pain: concepts, challenges, and compromises. Pain 2020;161(9):1976–82.

17. Chatelle C, Thibaut A, Whyte J, et al. Pain issues in disorders of consciousness. Brain Inj 2014;28(9):1202–8.

18. Schnakers C, Chatelle C, Demertzi A, et al. What about pain in disorders of consciousness? AAPS J 2012;14(3):437–44.

19. Laureys S, Faymonville ME, Peigneux P, et al. Cortical processing of noxious somatosensory stimuli in the persistent vegetative state. Neuroimage 2002;17(2):732–41.

20. Boly M, Faymonville ME, Schnakers C, et al. Perception of pain in the minimally conscious state with PET activation: an observational study. Lancet Neurol 2008;7(11):1013–20.

21. Kassubek J, Juengling FD, Els T, et al. Activation of a residual cortical network during painful stimulation in long-term postanoxic vegetative state: a 15O-H2O PET study. J Neurol Sci 2003;212(1–2):85–91.

22. Schnakers C, Chatelle C, Majerus S, et al. Assessment and detection of pain in noncommunicative severely brain-injured patients. Expert Rev Neurother 2010;10(11):1725–31.

23. Chatelle C, Majerus S, Whyte J, et al. A sensitive scale to assess nociceptive pain in patients with disorders of consciousness. J Neurol Neurosurg Psychiatr 2012;83(12):1233–7.

24. Schnakers C, Zasler ND. Pain assessment and management in disorders of consciousness. Curr Opin Neurol 2007;20(6):620–6.

25. Dehghani H, Tavangar H, Ghandehari A. Validity and reliability of behavioral pain scale in patients with low level of consciousness due to head trauma hospitalized in intensive care unit. Arch Trauma Res 2014;3(1):e18608.

26. Feldt KS. The checklist of nonverbal pain indicators (CNPI). Pain Manag Nurs 2000;1(1):13–21.

27. Boitor M, Fiola JL, Gélinas C. Validation of the critical-care pain observation tool and vital signs in relation to the sensory and affective components of pain during mediastinal tube removal in postoperative cardiac surgery intensive care unit adults. J Cardiovasc Nurs 2016;31(5):425–32.

28. Malviya S, Voepel-Lewis T, Burke C, et al. The revised FLACC observational pain tool: improved reliability and validity for pain assessment in children with cognitive impairment. Paediatr Anaesth 2006;16(3):258–65.

29. Chatelle C, Thibaut A, Bruno MA, et al. Nociception coma scale-revised scores correlate with metabolism in the anterior cingulate cortex. Neurorehabilitation Neural Repair 2014;28(2):149–52.

30. Whyte J, Poulsen I, Ni P, et al. Development of a measure of nociception for patients with severe brain injury. Clin J Pain 2020;36(4):281–8.

31. Haenggi M, Ypparila-Wolters H, Bieri C, et al. Entropy and bispectral index for assessment of sedation, analgesia and the effects of unpleasant stimuli in critically ill patients: an observational study. Crit Care 2008;12(5):R119.

32. Zasler ND, Formisano R, Aloisi M. Pain in persons with disorders of consciousness. Brain Sci 2022;12(3). https://doi.org/10.3390/brainsci12030300.

33. Stahl SM. Anticonvulsants as anxiolytics, part 2: pregabalin and gabapentin as alpha(2)delta ligands at voltage-gated calcium channels. J Clin Psychiatry 2004;65(4):460–1.

34. Langdon R, Taraman S. Posttraumatic headache. Pediatr Ann 2018;47(2):e61–8.

Pharmacology in Treatment of Patients with Disorders of Consciousness

Michael H. Marino, MD[a,b,*]

KEYWORDS

- Disorders of consciousness • Traumatic brain injury • Amantadine • Bromocriptine
- Levodopa • Apomorphine • Modafinil • Methylphenidate

KEY POINTS

- High-level evidence exists for the use of amantadine to promote recovery from traumatic disorders of consciousness between 4 and 16 weeks after injury.
- Zolpidem is effective at improving the level of consciousness in a small percentage of patients with disorders of consciousness.
- No distinguishing clinical features have been identified to accurately predict zolpidem responders versus nonresponders.
- Zolpidem and intrathecal baclofen likely increase responsiveness via the mesocircuit pathway.
- There is a large body of literature supporting the use of dopaminergic medications to improve alertness and responsiveness in patients with disorders of consciousness.
- It can be worthwhile to initiate treatment with medications such as dopaminergics, methylphenidate, and modafinil if patients are monitored closely for therapeutic response.

INTRODUCTION

Disorders of consciousness (DOC) are severe acquired brain injuries leading to alterations of arousal, awareness, and responsiveness. Traditionally, DOC comprised three distinct states: coma (or comatose state), vegetative state/unresponsive wakefulness syndrome (VS/UWS), and the minimally conscious state (MCS). The MCS can be further divided into MCS "plus" (MCS+) or MCS "minus" (MCS−) based on the presence or absence of language abilities. There is a movement within the field that proposes to include the PTCS as the fourth state of DOC.[1] As research on DOC has progressed, the nomenclature of the different states of DOC may have changed, but our desire to understand the pathophysiology of injury and the neural systems

[a] Moss Rehab, 60 Township Line Road, Elkins Park, PA 19027, USA; [b] Remed Residential Brain Injury Center
* 60 Township Line Road, Elkins Park, PA 19027.
E-mail address: marino01@einstein.edu

Phys Med Rehabil Clin N Am 35 (2024) 155–165
https://doi.org/10.1016/j.pmr.2023.06.023
1047-9651/24/© 2023 Elsevier Inc. All rights reserved.

underlying consciousness has not abated. While we still do not have full understanding of how the brain manifests consciousness, research has elucidated the key neurotransmitters involved in many brain functions. For most clinicians, utilizing a neurotransmitter-based approach remains the most practical method of directing pharmacologic intervention for DOC. This article will explore pharmacologic treatments, organized by the neurotransmitter systems they mediate, and how they apply to our current behavior-based classification of DOC (ie, phenotypes). As research into DOC progresses, identification of patients by endotypes will be possible. An endotype considers clinically observable behaviors and structural imaging but also has the ability to incorporate data from advanced nonbehavioral diagnostics yielding information including, but not limited to, the functional status of brain structures and networks, loss of functional connectivity, and injury at the cellular and even molecular level. More targeted and specific therapies, including pharmacologic interventions, may be possible by identifying patient endotypes.[2]

MONOAMINES INCLUDING DOPAMINE
Amantadine

Dopaminergic medicines are among the most studied medicines in DOC. Dopaminergic medicines studied as treatments for DOC include amantadine, bromocriptine, apomorphine, and levodopa (commonly combined with carbidopa). Amantadine initially came to market in the 1960s as an antiviral agent used to treat and prevent influenza type A. Its dopaminergic properties later led to its use as an antiparkinsonian agent.[3] More recently, amantadine has been prescribed as an agent to treat cognitive and behavioral changes related to traumatic brain injury (TBI). Amantadine research in brain injury continued to expand into the 1980s and through today. There are several properties of amantadine that make it a popular choice for research and clinical use in patients with acquired brain injuries. Amantadine has both presynaptic and postsynaptic mechanisms. Presynaptic actions include increase in the release of dopamine and also the delay of re-uptake which leads to an increase in dopamine concentration in the synaptic space. In the postsynaptic space, amantadine is purported to increase the number of dopamine receptors. In addition, it works as an N-methyl-D-aspartate (NMDA) glutamate receptor antagonist which may play a role in neurologic protection by decreasing the effects of excitotoxicity.[3,4] Dopaminergic medications including bromocriptine and amantadine have been purported to improve a wide variety of neurocognitive functions including wakefulness/arousal, fatigue, behavioral initiation, attention, processing time, and recovery of speech.[5,6] Amantadine dosage ranges from 50 mg to 400 mg per day in two divided doses. Steady state of drug concentrations is achieved within 4 days, and a clinical effect has been noted within days to weeks of amantadine initiation.[3,7] The half-life of amantadine is approximately 16 hours in healthy adults.[8] Although generally considered well-tolerated, there are potential side effects which include insomnia, nausea and vomiting, livedo reticularis, orthostatic hypotension, dizziness, edema, ataxia, and possibly seizures.[3]

Important early work using amantadine for patients with severe TBI was done by Meythaler and colleagues in 2002.[9] Thirty-five patients with acute severe TBI (initial Glasgow Coma Scale [GCS] < 10) were enrolled. Group 1 received 200 mg of amantadine daily for 6 weeks, followed by placebo for another 6 weeks. Group 2 received placebo for 6 weeks, then amantadine for another 6 weeks. All patients were enrolled within 6 weeks of injury. There was a consistent trend toward more rapid cognitive and functional improvement when the patients were given amantadine, regardless of when it was administered with the first 3 months after injury.[9]

Research on amantadine's role in DOC continued in a 2012 study by Giacino and colleagues in patients with DOC.[10] This was a multicentered, randomized controlled trial of 184 patients admitted to acute inpatient rehabilitation hospitals who were in a vegetative or MCS between 4 and 16 weeks after injury. Patients were randomized to an amantadine group or the placebo group for 4 weeks, followed by a 2-week washout and observation period. Dosing started at 100 mg twice daily, with an increase to 150 mg at week 3. Dosage was further increased to 200 mg twice daily at week 4 if the was insufficent clinical improvement. Insufficient clinical improvement was defined by a Disability Rating Scale (DRS) score that had not yet increased by 2 points from baseline. They found the rate of recovery was significantly faster, as measured by DRS score, in the amantadine group than that in the placebo group. They did not find any increased risk of adverse events (including seizures) in the treatment group.[10] Based on the results of this single, well-designed, randomized controlled trial, amantadine administration is considered standard of care for traumatic DOC patients within 4 and 16 weeks of injury.

The timing of administration of amantadine is important as conflicting evidence exists for its role in the acute setting. Notably, a recent study comparing the use of modafinil and the use of amantadine to standard of care in acute traumatic disorder of consciousness revealed no improvement in recovery of consciousness for either drug at the time of hospital discharge. In this study, the median starting time for each medicine was 8 days after injury. The standard of care treatment group had improved GCS scores and shorter hospital length of stay than the amantadine group.[11] Ghalaonovi and colleagues conducted a randomized controlled trial in which they administered amantadine 100 mg twice daily to severe TBI patients (GCS < 9) within the first week after injury.[12] Amantadine was continued for 6 weeks and then stopped. While there was improvement in GCS score within the first week of medication administration, there were no differences between the amantadine group and placebo group at 6-month follow-up as measured by Mini-Mental Status Exam, Glasgow Outcome Scale, DRS, and Karnofsky Performance Scale.[12]

No strong body of literature exists to guide the use of amantadine for nontraumatic DOC. There are some case reports that suggest its efficacy in improving level of consciousness and functional abilities in both the acute and chronic phases of nontraumatic DOC.[13,14] A particularly compelling and well-designed case report was performed by Estraneo and colleagues in 2015.[15] They described a 57-year-old female with non-TBI due to intracranial hypertension from third ventricular colloid cyst, who was in an MCS+ for greater than 1 year on Coma Recovery Scale-Revised (CRS-R). Baseline electroencephalogram (EEG) recordings revealed background theta activity with occasional low-frequency posterior alpha activity. Amantadine was initiated in an on-off fashion over the course of 36 weeks with doses ranging from 50 mg twice daily to 100 mg twice daily. At 50 mg twice daily dosing, CRS-R scores increased within 3 days. At 100 mg twice daily dosing, the patient was able to communicate and demonstrate functional object use consistent with emergence from MCS. With discontinuation of the medication, her condition returned to baseline. EEG findings paralleled the clinical observations with increased alpha activity recorded during periods of amantadine administration.[15]

The use of advanced neuroimaging techniques is shedding light on how pharmacologic interventions like amantadine work in DOC patients. Chen and colleagues published a case report of a 52-year-old man in a VS/UWS following TBI.[16] He underwent baseline functional MRI (fMRI) examination with passive and active protocols. The passive protocols involved listening to familiar and unfamiliar voices. The active protocol involved the command to imagine playing tennis. The patient then underwent

3 months of rehabilitation and 4 weeks of amantadine treatment starting at 100 mg twice daily with gradual uptitration to a goal dose of 200 mg twice daily. Repeat fMRI was performed after 3 months and showed increased areas of activation in the passive and active conditions. Clinically, the patient was able to demonstrate signs of MCS following amantadine treatment.[16]

Bromocriptine

Bromocriptine is another dopaminergic medicine with a long history of use for TBI. Its mechanism of action is thought to be related to decreasing dopamine turnover rate in the striatum and stimulation of central dopaminergic systems by direct activation of dopaminergic receptors. However, studies have also suggested that the system for dopamine synthesis must be intact for the drug to be effective.[17] It is rapidly absorbed and reaches peak plasma concentration in 30 to 150 minutes and remains effective for up to 4 hours.[7] In 2002, Passler and Riggs published a retrospective review of 5 patients with traumatic DOC in VS/UWS admitted in acute inpatient rehabilitation.[5] They were treated with bromocriptine starting at 1.25 mg twice daily with uptitration to 2.5 mg twice daily. Bromocriptine was continued for 2 to 6 months. As a control, the patients were compared to a cohort of TBI patients in vegetative state (TBI-VS) who did not receive bromocriptine. After 12 months, the patients treated with bromocriptine had an average DRS score of 4.4 (moderate disability) compared with the TBI-VS DRS average score of 19 (extremely severe disability). In fact, the group treated with bromocriptine showed greater recovery than a cohort of TBI patients who were already in MCS at the time of the study, but were not treated with bromocriptine (DRS 8.2 at 12 months).[5] This study suggested that bromocriptine could alter the long-term recovery of traumatic DOC patients, but further study is required.

Apomorphine

Apomorphine is another dopaminergic drug that has been studied in DOC. It is considered a potent direct agonist of dopamine at D1 and D2 receptors and can be administered via a continuous subcutaneous infusion through an external pump.[7,18,19] Fridman published a case study of a 25-year-old male who sustained a severe closed TBI and was in the MCS for more than 100 days. He was treated with a subcutaneous infusion of apomorphine for 179 days, while concurrently receiving rehabilitation. Rapid improvement was seen, with improved command following within days of starting the apomorphine infusion. Gains in physical function and cognition measured on the Coma Near Coma Scale (CNCS) and DRS were reversed when the pump was turned off.[19] Fridman followed this up in 2010 with prospective open-labelled clinical feasibility trial of subcutaneous apomorphine for chronic traumatic DOC between 1 and 4 months after injury. The 8 study patients were also receiving inpatient rehabilitation. Two were in VS, 6 in MCS, but none were responding to commands. Improvements in CNCS were seen in all patients. All patients responded to command after administration of apomorphine (4 patients within 10 days, and 4 within 62 days). All patients who completed the study showed long-term improvements on DRS after 1 year. Four patients were independent in walking, and 2 regained full independence.[18]

Levodopa

Administration of levodopa is considered dopamine replacement therapy as it is an amino acid that serves as a precursor molecule for dopamine. Levodopa is almost always combined with carbidopa or benserazide to improve the tolerance of levodopa, increase the serum concentration of levodopa, and increase the proportion available to cross the blood-brain barrier. Levodopa/carbidopa reaches peak serum concentration between 30 and 120 minutes.[7] It has not been studied extensively in DOC outside of case series and case reports. In 2003, Matsuda and colleagues reported a case series of 3 patients who sustained TBI and were in VS/UWS for more than 1 month.[20] All displayed parkinsonian features and had MRI findings indicative of injuries involving the substantia nigra or ventral tegmental area. The patients were treated with carbidopa/benserazide 100 mg/25 mg twice daily, levodopa 450 mg daily (later converted to levodopa/benserazide 100 mg/25 mg three times per day), and levodopa/carbidopa 100 mg/10 mg three times per day, respectively. All showed improvements in level of consciousness with progression from VS/UWS to MCS+, with 2 patients emerging from MCS.[20] In 2018, Bancalari and colleagues published a case study in which levodopa/carbidopa 100 mg/25 mg three times daily was used to treat a nontraumatic DOC patient after neurologic recovery had stalled.[21] Within 4 days of administration, improvements were seen in eye opening and motor movements, and within 8 days, she produced her first verbalizations. Her communication skills regressed after the discontinuation of levodopa/carbidopa and recovered when it was restarted. Notably, this patient showed no signs of parkinsonism on examination.[21]

Methylphenidate

Methylphenidate is a centrally acting stimulant medication that exerts its effects on monoamines. It works by blocking reuptake of norepinephrine and dopamine, thereby increasing their availability in the extraneural space.[22] The impact of elevated levels of monoamines is purported to effect a wide range of cognitive functions from improved frontal attention function to improved arousal via increased activity in the brain stem.[23,24] While many formulations are available, including long acting, the immediate-acting formulation is most likely to be used in patients with DOC because it can be given via a feeding tube for patients with dysphagia. Immediate-release methylphenidate is rapidly absorbed and reaches peak plasma concentration in approximately 2 hours, with a half-life extending to 3.5 hours.[22,25] Despite its widespread use in the field of brain injury, there is a paucity of evidence supporting its role in DOC. One notable attempt was a meta-analysis of n-of-1 studies by Martin and Whyte in 2007.[24] All subjects were from a single center and were treated with methylphenidate in a repeated crossover trial of symmetric design to control for the impact of spontaneous recovery over time. Seventeen patients were analyzed. The population consisted of traumatic and nontraumatic injuries with a mean age of 30 years, and time since injury was subacute to chronic. They demonstrated no significant effect of methylphenidate on response rate to commands or on accuracy of following a command.[24] Methylphenidate's quick onset and short half-life make it conducive to n-of-1 trials in which it can be administered in an on-off protocol (ie, A-B-A-B) in order to control for the effects of time and natural recovery.[24]

Modafinil

Modafinil is a centrally acting stimulant medication with an uncertain mechanism of action. It promotes wakefulness, which may be mediated by increased extracellular levels of monoamines, including norepinephrine and dopamine.[26] Research on the role of modafinil in DOC is limited. However, in 2017, Dhamapurkar and colleagues published a retrospective pilot study of 24 patients with prolonged DOC of traumatic and nontraumatic origin.[27] Modafinil was started at 100 mg daily and uptitrated to 300 mg daily as tolerated. Eleven of 12 traumatic DOC patients showed improvements in Western Head Injury Matrix Scale scores while on modafinil. Six of 12 nontraumatic DOC patients showed improvements in Western Head Injury Matrix Scale scores, while 4 showed no improvement, and 2 showed worsening scores from baseline. In terms of improved level of consciousness, 50% of the traumatic and nontraumatic DOC patients demonstrated an improved level of consciousness while treated with modafinil. While this was an uncontrolled pilot study, the apparent discrepancy of response in traumatic versus nontraumatic patients is noteworthy.[27]

GABA
Baclofen

Medications that affect the inhibitory gamma-aminobutyric acid (GABA) neurotransmitter system, specifically intrathecal baclofen (ITB) and zolpidem, have shown promising improvements in wakefulness and consciousness in some patients with DOC. Promoting consciousness by potentiating the inhibitory GABA system was initially believed to be a paradoxic effect, but it can be explained by the mesocircuit theory **(Fig. 1)**. In this hypothesis, GABAergic inhibition of the globus pallidus interna facilitates increased excitatory output from the central thalamus. Essentially, these medications inhibit a structure that is inhibiting the thalamus.[28] In 2009, Sara and colleagues published a case series of 5 DOC patients treated with ITB. All patients were in the VS, 6 to 10 months following a traumatic or nontraumatic injury. They were selected for ITB based on their spasticity. Over the course of 6 months of treatment with ITB, all showed improvement that ranged from increased alertness to full recovery of consciousness on CRS-R. Natural recovery could have certainly played a role for some of the patients in this series. However, natural recovery is less likely for nontraumatic DOC patients after 6 months, further implicating the effect of ITB

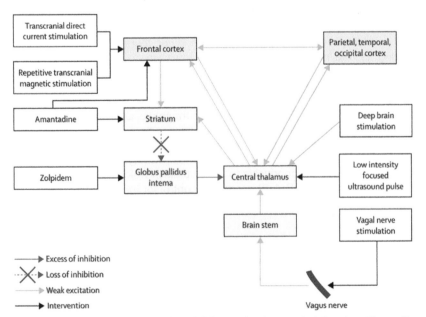

Fig. 1. The mesocircuit frontoparietal model for mechanisms underlying the effects of interventions in severe brain injuries. (Reprinted with permission from Elsevier. The Lancet Neurology, 2019, 18 (6), 600-614.)

in their improved clinical condition.[29] A logical question to ask regarding the role of ITB in DOC is if these patients had severe motor restrictions due to spasticity that essentially prevented them from demonstrating consciousness by moving their limbs to command. In other words, were these patients conscious/minimally conscious before but lacked sufficient observable motor output? To answer this question, Halbmayer and colleagues published a retrospective chart analysis of DOC patients treated with ITB. In their sample of 26 patients of traumatic and nontraumatic etiology, improvements were noted in CRS scores, level of consciousness, and spasticity as measured by Modified Ashworth Scale (MAS). However, a careful sub-analysis showed that improvements in CRS scores did not correspond to improved MAS scores. This indicates that the reduction of spasticity itself is insufficient in improving consciousness.[30]

Zolpidem

The wakefulness effects of zolpidem were discovered spuriously in 2000 when it was given to a young South African male patient in a nontraumatic chronic VS (greater than 3 years after injury) to treat his restlessness. Within 15 minutes after zolpidem was administered, he became more alert and was able to demonstrate some behaviors consistent with emergence from MCS.[31] This report spurred great interest in zolpidem, a short-acting nonbenzodiazepine hypnotic medication that potentiates GABA. Zolpidem has a rapid onset within 15 to 30 minutes, as demonstrated in the aforementioned case report, reaching maximum effect at 1 hour, with a 2- to 3-hour duration of clinical effect.[32] Multiple case reports of zolpidem "responders" (ie, increased movement, social interaction, command following, communication attempts, functional object use) have been published.[33–36] Notably, Clauss and Nel reported on 3 chronic DOC patients in VS who were zolpidem responders.[33] In their case series, the medication efficacy did not decrease with regular daily administration over a period of 3 to 6 years.[33] The most common dosage in published case reports is 10 mg, but dosages of 20 mg to 30 mg have been used.[37,38]

The largest controlled trials of zolpidem in DOC were conducted by Whyte in 2009 and 2014. The 2009 trial was a double-blind, placebo-controlled, crossover design involving 15 DOC patients in VS or MCS. Only 1 of 15 (6.7%) patients was a responder, and there was no identifiable trend toward improvement in the nonresponders. This led to the conclusion that zolpidem produces a bimodal rather than a graded response.[35] The 2014 trial was a placebo-controlled, double-blind, single-dose, crossover study involving 84 chronic DOC patients in VS or MCS. Approximately 5% (4 out of 84 patients) were responders.

Lorazepam

Although infrequently used currently, benzodiazepines may also enhance arousal and initiation. One case report discussed a DOC patient receiving 1 mg of lorazepam with significant improvement in cognition, language, and mobility[39,40]; the benefit was attributed to its therapeutic effect on an underlying catatonia. Recently, a retrospective study based on practice in a DOC rehabilitation program reported a 14.0% (6/43) overall positive rate to lorazepam, compared to 6.3% (5/79) to zolpidem, which was similar to the previous reports.[41] Among lorazepam responders, the positive response rate in TBI-related DOC was 6.9% (2/29), and in anoxic brain injury–related DOC, it was 28.6% (4/14).[41] One hypothesis for the efficacy of benzodiazepines in these patients is that they may have had underlying catatonia partially contributing to their clinical presentation.[41] The use of lorazepam is well documented in the diagnosis and treatment of catatonia.[42]

Utilization of Paradoxic Stimulating Responses to GABAergic Agents in Disorders of Consciousness

Currently, no demographic or clinical features are predictive of responders or nonresponders to zolpidem or lorazepam.[36,41] However, when these medications are effective, they can have a significant, even life-changing, impact on an individual's function and trajectory of recovery.[43] Since both zolpidem and lorazepam are relatively safe and inexpensive, and considering the very limited treatment options currently available for this population, performing trials with zolpidem and/or lorazepam for all patients with DOC seems reasonable.[35,41] It should be noted that one trial with an equivocal or negative response does not denote that a patient will not benefit from future trials. Periodically repeating the trials (eg, every 30–150 days) needs to be considered to re-evaluate a patient's response as neural recovery is a dynamic process and continues to evolve over time. Trials with these medications should also be considered in patients who may have emerged (eMCS); if they respond, these patients can also show an improvement in their arousal and initiation.

DISCUSSION

Despite the lack of high-level evidence to guide the clinician, pharmacologic treatment of DOC remains a vital part of providing care for the DOC population. However, several questions remain regarding the role of pharmacologic treatment. For example, if administered at the right timeframe after injury, can a medication lead to a better long-term outcome, or does it just temporarily enhance cognitive ability with no effect on the maximum level of improvement? How should a clinician choose a medication when there is no high level of evidence supporting its use? Ultimately, clinicians must use the existing evidence for pharmacologic treatment in conjunction with basic principles of brain injury medicine. Basic principles of brain injury medicine include such concepts as minimizing sedating medications, restoring normal sleep-wake cycle, monitoring for medication interactions, and identifying underlying medical conditions that may interfere with demonstration of consciousness. When possible, obtaining baseline objective data with frequent monitoring of medication response will help to guide pharmacologic treatment. Hopefully, our ability to treat DOC patients effectively will only be enhanced by ongoing research in nonbehavioral assessments of DOC and identification of patient endotypes.

DISCLOSURE

The author has nothing to disclose.

REFERENCES

1. Sherer M, Katz D, Bodien Y, et al. Post-traumatic Confusional State: A Case Definition and Diagnostic Criteria. Arch Phys Med Rehabil 2020;101(11):2041–50. https://doi.org/10.1016/j.apmr.2020.06.021.

2. Kondziella D, Menon D, Helbok R, et al. A Precision Medicine Framework for Classifying Patients with Disorders of Consciousness: Advanced Classification of Consciousness Endotypes (ACCESS). Neurocrit Care 2021;35(Suppl 1): 27–36. https://doi.org/10.1007/s12028-021-01246-9.

3. Zafonte R, Lexell J, Cullen N. Possible Applications for Dopaminergic Agents Following Traumatic Brain Injury: Part 2: Update on Pharmacology. J Head Trauama Rehabil 2001;16(1):112–6.

4. Danysz W, Dekundy A, Scheschonka A, et al. Amantadine: reappraisal of the timeless diamond—target updates and novel therapeutic potentials. J Neural Transm 2021;128(2):127–69.
5. Passler MA, Riggs RV. Positive outcomes in traumatic brain injury-vegetative state: patients treated with bromocriptine. Arch Phys Med Rehabil 2001;82(3):311–5.
6. Powell JH, al-Adawi S, Morgan J, et al. Motivational deficits after brain injury: effects of bromocriptine in 11 patients. J Neurol Neurosurg Psychiatry 1996;60(4):416–21.
7. Deleu D, Northway M, Hanssens Y. Clinical Pharmacokiinetic and Pharmacodynami Properties of Drugs Used in the Treatment of Parkinson's Disease. Clin Pharmacokinet 2002;41(4):261–309.
8. Hayden FG, Minocha A, Spyker DA, et al. Comparative Single-Dose Pharmacokinetics of Amantadine Hydrochloride and Rimantadine Hydrochloride in Young and Healthy Adults. Antimicrob Agents Chemother 1985;28(2):216–21.
9. Meythaler JM, Brunner RC, Johnson A, et al. Amantadine to improve neurorecovery in traumatic brain injury-associated diffuse axonal injury: A pilot double-blind randomized trial. J Head Trauma Rehabil 2002;17(4):300–13.
10. Giacino Joseph T, Whyte J, Bagiella E, et al. Placebo-Controlled Trial of Amantadine for Severe Traumatic Brain Injury. N Engl J Med 2012;366:819–26.
11. Hintze TDP, Small CE, Montgomery J, et al. Comparison of amantadine, modafinil, and standard of care in the acute treatment of disorders of consciousness after severe traumatic brain injury. Clin Neuropharmacol 2022;45(1):1–6.
12. Ghalaenovi H, Fattahi A, Koohpayehzadeh J, et al. The effects of amantadine on traumatic brain injury outcome: a double-blind, randomized, controlled, clinical trial. Brain Inj 2018;32(8):1050–5. https://doi.org/10.1080/02699052.2018.1476733.
13. Avecillas-Chasín JM, Barcia JA. Effect of amantadine in minimally conscious state of non-traumatic etiology. Acta Neurochir 2014;156(7):1375–7.
14. Lehnerer SM, Scheibe F, Buchert R, et al. Awakening with amantadine from a persistent vegetative state after subarachnoid haemorrhage. BMJ Case Rep 2017;2017. https://doi.org/10.1136/bcr-2017-220305.
15. Estraneo A, Pascarella A, Moretta P, et al. Clinical and electroencephalographic on-off effect of amantadine in chronic non-traumatic minimally conscious state. J Neurol 2015;262(6):1584–6.
16. Chen X, Tang C, Zhou H, et al. Effect of amantadine on vegetative state after traumatic brain injury: a functional magnetic resonance imaging study. J Int Med Res 2019;47(2):1015–24.
17. Trabucchi M, Spano PF, Tonon GC, et al. Effects of Bromocriptine on Central Dopaminergic Receptors. Life Science 1976;19225–35.
18. Fridman EA, Kimchansky B, Bonetta M, et al. Continuous subcutaneous apomorphine for severe disorders of consciousness after traumatic brain injury. Brain Inj 2010;24(4):636–41. https://doi.org/10.3109/02699051003610433.
19. Fridman EA, Calvar J, Bonetto M, et al. Fast awakening from minimally conscious state with apomorphine. Brain Inj 2009;23(2):172–7. https://doi.org/10.1080/02699050802649662.
20. Matsuda W, Matsumura A, Komatsu Y, et al. awakenings from persistent vegetative state: report of three cases with parkinsonism and brain stem lesions on MRI. J Neurol Neurosurg Psychiatry 2003;741571–3.

21. Bancalari E, Rabinstein A, Machiavello F, et al. Accelerated emergence from a nontraumatic minimally conscious state with levodopa/carbidopa. Neurol Clin Pract 2018;8(6):541–2.

22. IBM Micromedex® DRUGDEX® (electronic version). (Methylphenidate Hydrochloride) Internet. IBM Watson Health/EBSCO Information Services, Greenwood Village, Colorado, Cambridge, Massachusetts, USA. Available at: https://www. dynamed.com. Accessed May 8, 2023.

23. Whyte J, Vaccaro M, Grieb-Neff P, et al. Effects of methylphenidate on attention deficits after traumatic brain injury: a multidimensional, randomized, controlled trial. Am J Phys Med Rehabil 2004;83(6):401–20. https://doi.org/10.1097/01. phm.0000128789.75375.d3.

24. Martin RT, Whyte J. The effects of methylphenidate on command following and yes/no communication in persons with severe disorders of consciousness: a meta-analysis of n-of-1 studies. Am J Phys Med Rehabil 2007;86(8):613–20.

25. Wargin W, Patrick K, Kilts C, et al. Pharmacokinetics of Methyiphenidate in Man, Rat and Monkey. The Journal of Pharmacology and Experimental Therapeutics 1983;226(2):382–6.

26. Schwartz J. Modafi nil in the treatment of excessive sleepiness. Drug Des Dev Ther 2008;271–85.

27. Dhamapurkar SK, Wilson BA, Rose A, et al. Does Modafinil improve the level of consciousness for people with a prolonged disorder of consciousness?: a retrospective pilot study. Disabil Rehabil 2017;39(26):2633–9.

28. Thibaut A, Schiff N, Giacino J, et al. Therapeutic interventions in patients with prolonged disorders of consciousness. Lancet Neurol 2019;18(6):600–14.

29. Sarà M, Pistoia F, Mura E, et al. Intrathecal baclofen in patients with persistent vegetative state: 2 hypotheses. Arch Phys Med Rehabil 2009;90(7):1245–9.

30. Halbmayer L-M, Kofler M, Hitzenberger G, et al. On the recovery of disorders of consciousness under intrathecal baclofen administration for severe spasticity-An observational study. Brain Behav 2022;12(5):e2566. https://doi.org/10.1002/brb3. 2566.

31. Clauss RP, Giildenpfennig WM, Nel HW, et al. Extraordinary Arousal from Semi-Comatose State on Zolpidem. S Afr Med J 2000;90(1):68–72.

32. Clauss R. Disorders of Consciousness and Pharmaceuticals that act on Oxygen Based Amino Acid and Monoamine Neurotransmitter Pathways of the Brain. Curr Pharmaceut Des 2014;20(26):4140–53.

33. Clauss R, Nel W. Drug induces arousal from the permanent vegetative state. NeuroRehabilitation 2006;2123–8.

34. Shames JL, Ring H. Transient reversal of anoxic brain injury-related minimally conscious state after zolpidem administration: a case report. Arch Phys Med Rehabil 2008;89(2):386–8.

35. Whyte J, Myers R. Incidence of clinically significant responses to zolpidem among patients with disorders of consciousness: a preliminary placebo controlled trial. Am J Phys Med Rehabil 2009;88(5):410–8.

36. Whyte J, Rosenbaum R, Katz D, et al. Zolpidem and restoration of consciousness. Am J Phys Med Rehabil 2014;93(2):101–13. https://doi.org/10.1097/PHM. 0000000000000069.

37. Bomalaski MN, Claflin ES, Townsend W, et al. Zolpidem for the Treatment of Neurologic Disorders: A Systematic Review. JAMA Neurol 2017;74(9):1130–9.

38. Calabro RS, Arico I, De Salvo S, et al. Transient awakening from vegetative state: Is high-dose zolpidem more effective? Psychiatr Clin Neurosci 2014;69(2):122–3.

39. Luz J, Jang EJ. Poster 354 lorazepam trial for a patient with a disorder of consciousness: A case report. PM&R 2014;6:S309.

40. Mancuso CE, Tanzi MG, Gabay M. Paradoxical reactions to benzodiazepines: literature review and treatment options. Pharmacotherapy 2004;24(9):1177–85.

41. Zhang B, O'Brien K, Won W, et al. A Retrospective Analysis on Clinical Practice-Based Approaches Using Zolpidem and Lorazepam in Disorders of Consciousness. Brain Sci 2021;11(6):726.

42. Sienaert P, Dhossche DM, Vancampfort D, et al. A clinical review of the treatment of catatonia. Front Psychiatry 2014;5:181.

43. Interlandi, J. A Drug that Wakes the Near Dead. The New York Times Magazine. 1 December 2011. Available at: https://www.nytimes.com/2011/12/04/magazine/can-ambien-wake-minimally-conscious.html.

Prognostication and Trajectories of Recovery in Disorders of Consciousness

Mary E. Russell, DO, MS[a],*, Cindy B. Ivanhoe, MD[b],
Eboni A. Reed, MD[c]

KEYWORDS

- Prognostication • Disorders of consciousness (DoC) • Outcomes • Rehabilitation
- Minimally conscious • Trajectories of recovery
- Withdrawal of life-sustaining treatment (WoLST)

KEY POINTS

- Reviewing the natural history of prognostication in disorders of consciousness (DoC).
- Discussing withdrawal of life-sustaining treatment in patients with DoC.
- Highlighting the current guidelines for prognostication in DoC.
- Summarizing the considerations, limitations, and future goals of predictions trajectories of recovery in DoC.

BACKGROUND

Natural History of Recovery in Disorders of Consciousness

Historically one of the most difficult aspects of managing patients with disorders of consciousness (DoC) has been predicting outcomes, that is, prognostication. When discussing possible trajectories in DoC, common outcomes are improvement of disability, emerging consciousness, and death. Outcomes can be influenced by a variety of factors such as the mechanism of injury, duration of coma, and level of consciousness. For many decades, and still to date, there are many uncertainties surrounding recovery in patients with DoC. There is a paucity of large research studies that report long-term functional outcomes (**Fig. 1**).[1,2]

Withdrawal of Life-Sustaining Treatment

With the current gaps in scientific evidence regarding the natural history of recovery in DoC, many providers may feel limited in their ability to discuss prognosis. Traditionally,

[a] Physical Medicine and Rehabilitation Department, UT McGovern School of Medicine, TIRR Memorial Hermann-The Woodlands, Houston, TX 77030, USA; [b] Physical Medicine and Rehabilitation Department, UT McGovern School of Medicine, TIRR Memorial Hermann, Houston, TX 77030, USA; [c] Physical Medicine and Rehabilitation Department, Baylor College of Medicine, Houston, TX 77030, USA
* Corresponding author. TIRR Memorial Hermann, 1333 Moursund, Houston, TX 77030.
E-mail address: mary.e.russell@uth.tmc.edu

Phys Med Rehabil Clin N Am 35 (2024) 167–173
https://doi.org/10.1016/j.pmr.2023.09.001

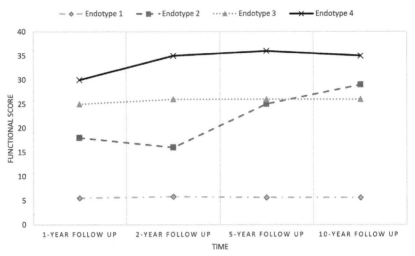

Fig. 1. At the 2-year follow-up, endotype 2 seems markedly different from endotype 3 and seems to have declined from the 1-year follow-up. However, by the 5-year follow-up, endotype 2 progresses past endotype 3. At the present time, variables for identifying markers to assign a patient to a particular endotype are lacking. In addition, the common trajectories and meaningful markers (*y* axis) are not adequately identified

goals of care conversations take place very early and often result in overestimation or underestimation of recovery. The mortality in DoC is estimated to be around 32% yet 70% of death in DoC is due to withdrawal of life-sustaining treatment (WoLST).[3] These striking numbers lead to many clinical, ethical, and moral questions. The most pressing question is what drives withdrawal from life-sustaining treatment. There are several possible answers to this question.

1. Lack of knowledge about prognosis among health-care providers. Limited scientific evidence of good recovery may lead to more frequent conversations recommending life support withdrawal. Implicit bias and limitations to prognostication so shortly after injury may be confounding the clinical picture in these individuals. Providers tend to provide overly pessimistic prognoses, which may negatively influence WoLST decisions.[4,5]
2. Lack of access to further care after acute hospitalization. Patients limited by financial constraints, including insurance denials, may be limited in rehabilitation options that can lead to poorer outcomes. When forced to make early decisions, families may choose to withdraw life-sustaining treatment rather than be limited in care options after severe brain injury.
3. Advance directives expressing wishes for withdrawal of life support in the event of coma, vegetative state, or minimally conscious state. Often patients have preexpressed wishes and underestimate the potential quality of life after severe brain injuries.

Late recovery and functional independence are possible with many patients with severe brain injury and should be considered a potential outcome. Anecdotally and data shown in the Traumatic Brain Injury Model Systems have demonstrated this.[6] Despite this, early WoLST remains a major contributor to acute care deaths and unfortunately outcome data on these individuals is not available, although a good outcome may still be a potential outcome.[3]

Current Methods to Assess Prognosis

Clinical guidelines from the American Congress of Rehabilitation Medicine and the American Academy of Neurology (ACRM/AAN) were developed in 2018 to help guide prognostication in persons with DoC.[7,8]

Key takeaways from the latest ACRM/AAN guidelines with regard to prognostication:

- One should wait 28 days postinjury before making a universally poor prognosis.
- For patients in posttraumatic vegatative state/unresponsive wakefulness state (VS/UWS): Clinicians should perform the following for prognostication of 1-year recovery of consciousness.
  - MRI at 6 to 8 weeks to evaluate for corpus callosum, dorsolateral upper brainstem, or corona radiata lesions.
  - Single-photon emission computed tomography (SPECT) scan 1 to 2 months.
  - Disability Rating Scale, P300, and/or electroencephalogram (EEG) at 2 to 3 months postinjury.
  - Blood oxygen level-dependent functional MRI 1 to 60 months postinjury in response to a familiar voice speaking the patient's name.
- For nontraumatic/anoxic VS/UWS prognostication for recovery of consciousness at 24 months.
  - Coma recovery scale-revised (CRS-R)
  - Somatosensory evoked potentials (SEPs)
- Permanent VS/UWS is antiquated given the ability of persons to recover consciousness post 3 months in non traumatic brain injury (NTBI)/anoxia and post 12 months in traumatic brain injury (TBI). Chronic UWS/VS followed by the amount of time should be given instead, for example, chronic traumatic VS/UWS for 6 months.
- Counseling recommendations:
  - Traumatic UWS/VS: The ability to emerge to minimally conscious state (MCS) within 5 months of injury provides a more favorable outcome.
  - Nontraumatic UWS/VS: associated with poorer outcomes; however, individual outcomes vary and prognosis is not universally poor.
- Prognostic study findings in traumatic VS/UWS:
  - Favorable
    - Normal SPECT scan 1 to 2 months postinjury
    - Disability rating scale (DRS) less than 26 2 to 3 months postinjury
    - Detectable p300 2 to 3 months postinjury
    - Reactive EEG at 2 to 3 months postinjury
    - Higher level activation of the auditory association cortex using blood oxygen level-dependent fMRI in response to a familiar voice speaking patient's name
  - Unfavorable
    - Corpus callosal lesion on MRI 6 to 8 weeks postinjury
    - Dorsolateral upper brainstem injury on MRI 6 to 8 weeks postinjury
    - Corona radiata injury on MRI 6 to 8 weeks postinjury
- Prognostic study findings in nontraumatic/anoxic VS/UWS suggest the likelihood of recovery consciousness within 24 months postinjury.
  - CRS-R of 6 or greater 1 month or longer after injury
  - Somatosensory evoked potentials present (bilateral median nerve stimulation)

Katz and colleagues in 2009 looked at DoC in both TBI and non-TBI populations who were admitted to a specialized acute inpatient rehabilitation facility up to 4 years postinjury and found the following[8]:

- Seventy-two percent emerged from MCS
- Fifty-eight percent emerged from confusional state/posttraumatic amnesia (CS/PTA)
- The duration of MCS is a strong predictor of the duration of CS/PTA.
- One year follow-up:
  - ○ Nearly 50% achieved daytime independence at home
  - ○ Twenty-two percent returned to work/school within 2 years
  - ○ Seventeen percent at or near preinjury levels.
- Best predictors of DRS outcomes:
  - ○ Discharge functional independence measure (FIM)
  - ○ Age
- DRS scores continued to improve 2 to 3 years postinjury.

These individuals can often have varying arousal and multiple medications and treatments that may additionally affect arousal. Before making a diagnosis of DoC, sedating medications should be weaned as able.

Accuracy on current best available predictive tools and models yields 70% to 80% positive predictive value. Considerable errors in prognostication can abound. Additionally, approximately 40% of clinical assessments on the level of consciousness are misdiagnosed.[9]

DISCUSSION

Prognosis is defined as the likely course of a disease or ailment. Many considerations affect the course of the patient with DoC. From the above discussion, it is clear that there are limitations to prognostication about the future of persons with DoC. This comes not only from conflicting data in the research but also from education and biases that are hard to change.

Behavioral evaluation is a mainstay of the clinical evaluation of the patient with DoC. Behavioral observations may be limited by the many physical and cognitive deficits these individuals exhibit.[10] This may include deficits of vision, tone, language, effects of sedating medications, disrupted sleep–wake cycles, and so forth. Pain is also a powerful confounder that can limit consistent participation in clinical evaluations. Potentially positive predictive behaviors in the patient with DoC may go unobserved, depending on when they occur or if they extinguish quickly. Variability in clinical presentation may be coupled with the variability of clinical expertise across rehabilitation programs.

Variability in Clinical Assessment

Biases can affect the interpretation of subtle interactions, in both positive and negative directions. Clinicians with the best of intentions, may overinterpret or underinterpret what they see. Clinically, the same is true of family members, who may gauge consciousness by a clinical presentation that is not considered valid by clinicians. Furthermore, clinicians may get caught up in a momentary finding or become focused on a small improvement and express to a family member that their loved one is doing well. Although this may be true, it is important to be sensitive to the interpretation of the family. There are differences in interpretation of what is an acceptable outcome and who gets to decide. The expectations of the loved ones might be for return to their former life. Although, in contrast, the expectation of the clinician may be nothing more than the patient is able to tolerate therapy better each day. Families will make decisions not only based on what they are told by a rehabilitation professional but also by their understanding of what their loved one would want, how the message is delivered, and the many factors that constitute their lives, and their new reality.

Access to assorted medical settings may also affect expectations and outcomes based on the variable quality of care and attitudes in the acute care setting. Various acute neurosurgical settings and rehabilitation settings can offer different levels of expertise and medical expectations. There are differences in the level of advocacy for a patient among health-care providers. Quality of life for many persons with acquired brain injury will be interpreted by those around them, whose own quality of life may also be affected in the short term and long term.

Limitations in Access to Care

Many states have a law or policy that allows health-care facilities to withdraw care when care is deemed "futile." Who assesses the patient and when has a bearing on the information given to families. Consideration of the influence of short-term interventions on long-term outcomes can be missed by payor sources. Initial costs of care and pressures of health-care coverage are invariable factors, whether acknowledged or not, in the decisions about withdrawal of care, length of stay in rehabilitation, chosen equipment, and approach to care given. Not everyone who has the potential for more improvement will gain access to the interventions that may permit more.

If a patient with DoC receives rehabilitation care, there are still many limitations and factors that influence outcomes such as personal and family finances. For example, if a patient's partner/spouse needs to leave employment in order to provide care or supervision, then we must ask, are there financial considerations to extending health insurance for and how long? This comes with additional emotional and social costs.

Insurance constraints and peer-to-peer reviews can affect outcomes. Although some medical reviewers will understand the point of rehabilitation for patients with DoC, many believe that if a patient will be referred to a nursing home anyway, then inpatient rehabilitation does not make sense. It becomes incumbent on the treating physician to make sense of inpatient rehabilitation interventions. Whether their ultimate home will be in a nursing home or home, their care needs can be favorably affected by inpatient rehabilitation. Although a patient with DoC may remain with disabilities, they have the potential to be healthier with fewer comorbidities and a better quality of life. The patient may even eventually be able to live with family, or with less supervision.

Cost-effectiveness frameworks are likely to provoke serious limitations in drawing direct comparisons of health utility across diverse clinical populations.[11–13] We may aspire to a more inclusive health-care system where all patients, regardless of their condition, have equal opportunity to receive a certain standard of medical treatment, such that the cost of rare or expensive diseases is seen as a societal rather than an individual burden and where the well-being and opportunities of one population cannot necessarily be traded off for that of another. This is not to say that cost-effectiveness has no place in DoC medicine; it could be an important guiding principle for deciding between treatments that are otherwise equally effective and safe, and help to guide research and development of more cost-effective options for managing and treating DoC, which ought to remain an important research priority. Determining what constitutes equal access to treatment across clinical populations may pose further challenges but considering more inclusive principles places the health-care system at less risk of disadvantaging those who already have the misfortune of having a medical condition such as DoC with an evolving, uncertain science where cost-effective treatments are not yet available.

SUMMARY

Acquired brain injury, especially severe brain injury, is a chronic medical condition. There is a trove of information on acute care management and large-scale studies; however, there is a gap in research studies on prognostication and trajectory analysis in postacute care and long-term outcomes. Major challenges to obtaining this data include a lack of large-scale data sources outside of those that have participated in acute inpatient rehabilitation, early WoLST, varied recovery trajectories, and inequalities in access to care.

Furthermore, there is a paradox between the current state of medicine and the needs of the special population with DoC. Health-care systems are often focused on meeting metrics and quality indicators, such as decreased length of stay and morbidity/mortality, and oftentimes, reimbursement and financial health of the institution are tied to these metrics. Guidelines for the care of persons with severe brain injury require time, resources, and knowledge of the population and the outcomes possible. In summation, the paucity of national guidelines/recommendations suggests an international need for standardization of admission criteria (which may in part be driven by resource availability and monetary allocation), clinical and instrumental diagnostic tools and prognostic protocols that should be developed, endorsed, and disseminated.

Finally, but remarkably important, there are also implicit biases and differing perspectives on what constitutes meaningful recovery and quality of life.[1] This raises a question that is difficult to answer, especially early after injury. What is quality of life? Is recovery of consciousness enough of a goal? Emerging from a DoC state is not a linear event. Patients do not emerge predictively and delayed emergence is neither uncommon nor does it indicate a poor outcome from a traumatic brain injury. As health-care professionals, evidence-based prognostic expectations need to be considered but we also must consider the interplay of personal histories, family dynamics, injury severity, acceptance of disability, health-care coverage, and societal socioeconomics.

CLINICS CARE POINTS

- There are very few research studies that report long-term functional outcomes.
- There are also major considerations that affect prognosis including mechanism of injury, duration of coma, advance directives, access to quality rehabilitation, family support, personal finances, and socioeconomic status.
- Late recovery and functional independence are possible with many patients with severe brain injury and should be considered a potential outcome.
- Early WoLST remains a major contributor to acute care deaths, approximately 70%.
- Clinical guidelines from the American Congress of Rehabilitation Medicine and the American Academy of Neurology were developed in 2018 to help guide prognostication in persons with DoC.
- Accuracy on current best available predictive tools and models yields 70% to 80% positive predictive value; approximately 40% of clinical assessments on level of consciousness are misdiagnosed.
- There are implicit biases and differing perspectives on what constitutes meaningful recovery and quality of life.

DISCLOSURE

The authors have nothing to disclose.

REFERENCES

1. Hammond FM, Katta-Charles S, Russell MB, et al. Research Needs for Prognostic Modeling and Trajectory Analysis in Patients with Disorders of Consciousness. Neurocrit Care 2021;35(Suppl 1):55–67.
2. Schnakers C, Vanhaudenhuyse A, Giacino J, et al. Diagnostic accuracy of the vegetative and minimally conscious state: clinical consensus versus standardized neurobehavioral assessment. BMC Neurol 2009;9:35.
3. Turgeon AF, Lauzier F, Burns KE, et al. Determination of neurologic prognosis and clinical decision making in adult patients with severe traumatic brain injury: a survey of Canadian intensivists, neurosurgeons, and neurologists. Crit Care Med 2013;41(4):1086–93.
4. Hammond FM, Giacino JT, Nakase Richardson R, et al. Disorders of Consciousness due to Traumatic Brain Injury: Functional Status Ten Years Post-Injury. J Neurotrauma 2019;36(7):1136–46.
5. Izzy S, Compton R, Carandang R, et al. Self-fulfilling prophecies through withdrawal of care: do they exist in traumatic brain injury, too? Neurocrit Care 2013;19(3):347–63.
6. Nakase-Richardson R, Whyte J, Giacino JT, et al. Longitudinal outcome of patients with disordered consciousness in the NIDRR TBI Model Systems Programs. J Neurotrauma 2012;29(1):59–65.
7. Giacino JT, Katz DI, Schiff ND, et al. Practice guideline update recommendations summary: Disorders of consciousness: Report of the Guideline Development, Dissemination, and Implementation Subcommittee of the American Academy of Neurology; the American Congress of Rehabilitation Medicine; and the National Institute on Disability. Neurology 2018;91(10):450–60.
8. Katz DI, Polyak M, Coughlan D, et al. Natural history of recovery from brain injury after prolonged disorders of consciousness: outcome of patients admitted to inpatient rehabilitation with 1-4 year follow-up. Prog Brain Res 2009;177:73–88.
9. O'Donnell JC, Browne KD, Kilbaugh TJ, et al. Challenges and demand for modeling disorders of consciousness following traumatic brain injury. Neurosci Biobehav Rev 2019;98:336–46.
10. Giacino JT, Sherer M, Christoforou A, et al. Behavioral Recovery and Early Decision Making in Patients with Prolonged Disturbance in Consciousness after Traumatic Brain Injury. J Neurotrauma 2020;37(2):357–65.
11. Peterson AB, Thomas KE. Incidence of Nonfatal Traumatic Brain Injury–Related Hospitalizations — United States, 2018. MMWR. Morbidity and Mortality Weekly Report 2021;70(48):1664–8.
12. Geurts M, Macleod MR, van Thiel GJ, et al. End-of-life decisions in patients with severe acute brain injury. Lancet Neurol 2014;13(5):515–24.
13. Formisano R, Giustini M, Aloisi M, et al. An International survey on diagnostic and prognostic protocols in patients with disorder of consciousness. Brain Inj 2019; 33(8):974–84.

Emergence from Disorders of Consciousness

Optimizing Self-Agency Through Communication

Brooke Murtaugh, OTD, OTR/L, CBIST, BT-C[a],*,
Susan Fager, PhD, CCC-SLP[b], Tabatha Sorenson, OTD, OTR/L, ATP[c]

KEYWORDS

- Consciousness disorders • Brain injury • Communication disorders
- Assistive devices

KEY POINTS

- Language and communication impairments are inherent to the disorders of consciousness (DoC) population.
- Functional communication is a key behavioral feature of recovery of consciousness.
- Language and communication deficits should be considered during behavioral assessment to mitigate errors and decrease risk of misdiagnosis.
- Utilization of assistive technology and augmentative communication devices can support early intentional and functional communication in patients with DoC.
- Providing avenues for communication is key for patients with severe brain injury to support self-agency.

INTRODUCTION

Communication is recognized as an important marker of the return of consciousness in patients with a disorder of consciousness (DoC).[1-3] However, it also has intrinsic value, providing an avenue for the expression of thoughts and desires, the exercise of autonomy, the conveying of our identity and individuality, and the creation of emotional connection to others. Indeed, families caring for loved ones experiencing DoC identify communication as one of the most important capacities that they hope their loved one will regain.[4] Not only communication allows family members to

[a] Department of Rehabilitation Programs, Madonna Rehabilitation Hospitals, 5401 South Street, Lincoln, NE 68506, USA; [b] Research Institute, Madonna Rehabilitation Hospitals, 5401 South Street, Lincoln, NE 68506, USA; [c] Department of Occupational Therapy, Madonna Rehabilitation Hospitals, 5401 South Street, Lincoln, NE 68506, USA
* Corresponding author.
E-mail address: bmurtaugh@madonna.org

Phys Med Rehabil Clin N Am 35 (2024) 175–191
https://doi.org/10.1016/j.pmr.2023.07.002
1047-9651/24/© 2023 Elsevier Inc. All rights reserved.

know that their loved ones are conscious it also reestablishes the personal identity of the patient for the family. Absence of reciprocal communication can lead to feelings of loss of the emotional and psychological personhood of the patient, even though their "body" is still present.[5]

The emergence of communication is also important for clinicians caring for patients with a DoC. One key behavioral feature for the identification of the minimally conscious state (MCS) and emergence from MCS (eMCS) is communication.[6] In recent years, MCS has been further stratified into MCS minus (−) and MCS plus (+) based on the presence of linguistically mediated behaviors such as following commands or communication.[3] Return of communication has implications for prognosis. Martens and colleagues[6] identified a linear relationship between recovery and 6 key behaviors including intelligible speech and reliable yes/no communication. For each behavior recovered, the Disability Rating Score improved by 2 points.

The purpose of this article is to provide an overview of communication and language in the context of recovery after DoC. Authors will review DoC standardized assessments that include evaluation of communication and various confounds related to severe brain injury that can mask a patient's ability to communicate. In addition, rehabilitation interventions to promote functional communication as a patient emerges from DoC will be highlighted, including compensatory strategies, assistive technology, and emerging neurotechnologies.

NEUROANATOMY OF LANGUAGE

Injury to the brain can result in language and communication deficits. Neurological injury can not only affect speech production and structures involved in speech creation but also affect the anatomical and physiological substrates for language formulation and comprehension. Acoustic processing of verbal and nonverbal sounds is achieved in the bilateral auditory cortex and adjacent superior temporal cortex. Processing the phonetics of language involve the previously mentioned structures as well as the bilateral posterior superior temporal gyri and superior and temporal sulci. Speech production ability is housed in the superior temporal lobe and frontal lobe (especially Broca's area) but it also includes subcortical structures such as the thalamus, putamen, and pallidum. The cerebellum also plays a key role in speech production and oral motor coordination.[7] Thus, functional language and communication relies on multiple cortical and subcortical structures and anatomical and physiological integration between those structures. Damage or dysfunction of these areas due to acquired brain injury can result in various language disorders[8–10] (**Fig. 1**).

BEDSIDE ASSESSMENT OF COMMUNICATION

Emergence of communication after severe brain injury is a key behavioral sign that a patient is progressing toward consciousness and a main avenue for consciousness to be identified by others. It is important to recognize that the initial recovery of communication behaviors can be simplistic, nonverbal, and inconsistent. Clinicians should observe for behaviors such as head nodding, thumbs up/down, and mouthing words. Qualitative bedside observation should be supplemented by the use of standardized neurobehavioral assessments.[11] Most, if not all, of these DoC assessment tools evaluate communication abilities.[12–14] An assessment tool that has been endorsed as reliable, valid, and sensitive in differentiating among coma, UWS, MCS, and eMCS is the Coma Recovery Scale-Revised (CRS-R).[12,15,16] The CRS-R has a communication subscale to assess a patient's ability to initiate communication as well as to evaluate the accuracy and consistency of that communication.[12] A top score of 2 within the

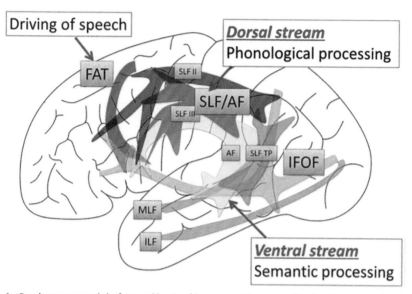

Fig. 1. *Dual stream model of neural basis of language.* The neural basis of language has been evolving to a more complex model with involvement of many cortical areas and white matter tracts than the classic model simply consisting of the Broca and Wernicke centers and the arcuate fasciculus (AF) connecting the above two. Adding to the dual stream model, there is another system inside the frontal lobe for "driving of speech." Recently named the frontal aslant tract (FAT) is associated with initiation and spontaneity of speech. The dorsal stream is associated with phonological processing via the superior longitudinal fasciculus (SLF) as a major trunk of the network. The SLF/AF consists of several subcomponents in 2 layers, the SLF II, the SLF III, and the SLF temporo-parietal (SLF TP) in the superficial layer and the classic AF in the deep layer. The ventral stream is associated with semantic processing. It is assumed that the network consists of intratemporal network, such as the middle longitudinal fasciculus (MLF) and the inferior longitudinal fasciculus (ILF) and the inferior fronto-occipital fasciculus (IFOF) as an interlobe network. (*From:* Fujii M, Maesawa S, Ishiai S, Iwami K, Futamura M, Saito K. Neural Basis of Language: An Overview of An Evolving Model. Neurol Med Chir (Tokyo). 2016;56(7):379-386. https://doi.org/10.2176/nmc.ra.2016-0014. Open Access.)

subscale denotes eMCS.[12] In 2020, the CRS-R underwent revisions to include "Test Completion Codes" that allow scorers to identify any barriers or errors that could influence the total score of the evaluation[17] (**Figs. 2** and **3**). It is recommended that neurobehavioral assessments be completed multiple times during a few weeks to compensate for the expected inconsistency of patient performance.[18,19]

THE ROLE OF IMAGING

During the last 2 decades, multiple studies have reported that specialized imaging studies can detect language and communication abilities in patients with DoC who lack overt signs of responsiveness at bedside.[20–24] This condition has been labeled cognitive motor dissociation (CMD). The first studies by Schiff,[25] Owens and colleauges[26,27] used functional magnetic resonance imaging (fMRI) to observe patients' brain activation when provided meaningful auditory and linguistic stimuli and motor figure commands. They found that some behaviorally unresponsive patients with DoC were able to activate the language-processing centers of their brains, thus suggesting that they were conscious, especially those patients that were able to willfully

JFK COMA RECOVERY SCALE ©2004										
Record Form										
This form should only be used in association with the "CRS-R ADMINISTRATION AND SCORING GUIDELINES" which provide instructions for standardized administration of the scale.										
Patient:		Diagnosis:								
Date of onset:		Date of Admission:								
Date										
Assessment		1		2		3		4		5
AUDITORY FUNCTION SCALE	#	TCC	#	TCC	#	TCC	#	TCC	#	TCC
4 – Consistent Movement to Command[b]										
3 – Reproducible Movement to Command[b]										
2 – Localization to Sound										
1 – Auditory Startle										
0 – None										
VISUAL FUNCTION SCALE	#	TCC	#	TCC	#	TCC	#	TCC	#	TCC
5 – Object Recognition[b]										
4 – Object localization: Reaching[a]										
3 – Visual Pursuit[a]										
2 – Fixation[a]										
1 – Visual Startle										
0 – None										
MOTOR FUNCTION SCALE	#	TCC	#	TCC	#	TCC	#	TCC	#	TCC
6 – Functional Object Use[c]										
5 – Automatic Motor Response[a]										
4 – Object Manipulation[a]										
3 – Localisation to Noxious Stimulation[a]										
2 – Flexion Withdrawal										
1 – Abnormal Posturing										
0 – None										
OROMOTOR/VERBAL FUNCTION SCALE	#	TCC	#	TCC	#	TCC	#	TCC	#	TCC
3 – Intelligible Verbalization[b]										
2 – Vocalization/Oral Movement										
1 – Oral Reflexive Movement										
0 – None										
COMMUNICATION SCALE	#	TCC	#	TCC	#	TCC	#	TCC	#	TCC
2 – Functional: Accurate[c]										
1 – Non-functional: Intentional[b]										
0 – None										
AROUSAL SCALE	#	TCC	#	TCC	#	TCC	#	TCC	#	TCC
3 – Attention										
2 – Eye Opening w/o Stimulation										
1 – Eye Opening with Stimulation										
0 – Unarousable										
TOTAL SCORE										

Updated 2020

Fig. 2. *CRS-R Score Sheet.* [a]Denotes minimally conscious state minus (MCS−). [b]Denotes minimally conscious status plus (MCS+). [c]Denotes emergence from eMCS. TCC test completion code. (*From*: Kalmar K, Giacino J. The JFK coma recovery scale-revised. Neuropsychological Rehabilitation. 2005;15(3–4):454- 460. https://doi.org/10.1080/09602010443000425.)

modulate their brain activity to command. Additional studies have confirmed these findings.[28,29] Consequently, it is now recommended that fMRI or specific electrophysiological examinations be used to attempt to identify covert signs of consciousness[18,30] when the results of serial bedside assessments are consistently ambiguous or negative (**Figs. 4** and **5**).

CONFOUNDS IN ASSESSMENT

Complicating the accuracy of consciousness assessments is the high incidence of comorbid conditions and deficits that can "mask" a patient's true level of consciousness.

Test Completion Codes (TCC)

A TCC should be assigned to each CSR-R subscale to indicate the validity of the subscale score.

Test Completion Codes	
1	test completed in full - results valid
Test attempted, not completed due to:	
2.1	impaired sensory function (cortical or peripheral)
2.2	aphasia
2.3	physical injury (e.g., fracture, brachial plexus, hemiparesis)
2.4	primary language barrier
2.5	illness/medical instability
2.6	examiner error
2.7	logistical reasons
2.8	other (specify):
Test not attempted due to:	
3.1	impaired sensory function (cortical or peripheral)
3.2	aphasia
3.3	physical injury (e.g., fracture, brachial plexus, hemiparesis)
3.4	primary language barrier
3.5	illness/medical instability
3.6	examiner error
3.7	logistical reasons
3.8	other (specify):

Fig. 3. CRS-R Test Completion Codes to be applied to subscale scores. (*Adapted from*: Kalmar K, Giacino J. The JFK coma recovery scale-revised. Neuropsychological Rehabilitation. 2005;15(3–4):454-460. https://doi.org/10.1080/09602010443000425. *Update by:* Yelena Bodien, PhD, Camille Chatelle, PhD, Joseph Giacino, Ph.D. (2020).)

These confounds can include medical complications, sensory and motor deficits, and language impairments.[31,32] Multiple language confounds can limit the patient's ability to demonstrate intentional and functional communication after severe brain injury. For example, patients with DoC can have concomitant aphasia (expressive and/or receptive), which can interfere with the patient's ability to understand commands and/or produce language.[33] Oral motor apraxia may also be present; this is a condition characterized by a lack of coordination of eccentric breathing, vocal cord control, and coordination of tongue and mouth movements to produce intelligible speech.

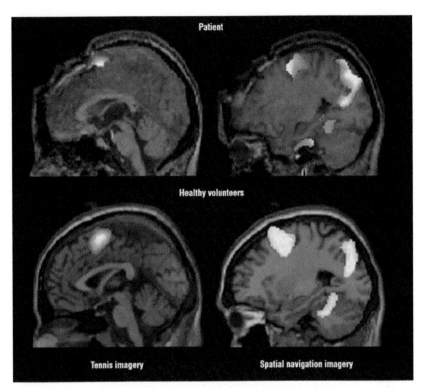

Fig. 4. Functional MRI imaging during mental imagery comparison. (Top) DoC patient and (Bottom) healthy volunteers. (*From*: Owen AM, Coleman MR, Boly M, Davis MH, Laureys S, Pickard JD. Using Functional Magnetic Resonance Imaging to Detect Covert Awareness in the Vegetative State. Arch Neurol. 2007;64(8):1098. https://doi.org/10.1001/archneur.64. 8.1098. With permission.)

Other conditions, although not strictly disorders of language, can affect the patient's capacity to communicate. For example, aphonia due to paralysis of the vocal cords can interfere with the ability to vocalize. Akinetic mutism is a neurological disorder that presents as a drive state disorder in which initiation is severely compromised, impairing the ability to engage in goal-directed behaviors including communication[34] (**Table 1**). The patient is fully conscious but lacks the motivation to engage in communication.

Potential confounds to assessment should be identified and addressed. Understanding the neuroanatomical location of the patient's injury, especially because it relates to language centers at the subcortical and cortical levels, can provide insights into potential communication barriers. Successful identification and skilled interventions to alleviate these communication and language confounds will improve the accuracy, reliability, and validity of assessments of consciousness.[18,19]

PATTERNS OF RECOVERY

Predicting recovery of natural speech with DoC can be challenging. However, there are predictable patterns of recovery for communication as a patient's level of consciousness improves. A recent prospective study by Martens and colleagues[6] evaluated patients using the CRS-R while in an inpatient rehabilitation program during an 8-

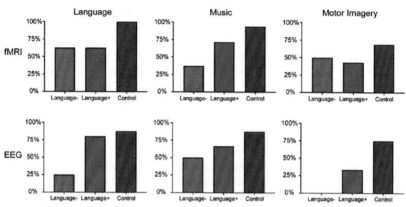

Fig. 5. *Percentage of functional MRI and EEG responders in patients and healthy subjects when presented with language, music, and motor imagery stimulus.* Results for patients without behavioral evidence of language function (Language–; ie, CRS-R/CAP-based behavioral diagnosis indicates coma, vegetative state, or MCS) are represented as red bars. Results for patients with behavioral evidence of language function (Language +; ie, CRS-R/CAP-based behavioral diagnosis indicates MCS + or posttraumatic confusional state) are represented as blue bars. Results for healthy subjects (Control) are represented as purple bars. (*From*: Edlow BL, Chatelle C, Spencer CA, et al. Early detection of consciousness in patients with acute severe traumatic. Brain. 2017 Sep 1;140(9):2399-2414. https://doi.org/10.1093/brain/awx176.)

Table 1	
Potential confounds masking consciousness within disorders of consciousness	
Medical	• Seizures
	• Intracranial complications (hydrocephalus, hygroma, and so forth)
	• Illness/infection (ie, pneumonia, UTI)
	• Pharmacological side effects (ie, sedating medications)
	• Sleep disorders
	• Paroxysmal autonomic hyperactivity
	• Neuro-endocrine disorders
Sensory/motor	• Spasticity
	• Contractures
	• Movement disorders
	• Fractures
	• Pain
	• Vision deficits
	• Hearing deficits
	• Concomitant spinal cord injury
	• CMD
	• Peripheral neuropathies/myopathies
	• Ideomotor/ideational apraxia
Language	• Aphasia (receptive/expressive)
	• Oral motor apraxia
	• Dysarthria
	• Akinetic mutism
	• Aphonia
	• Language processing disorders

week period. Martens identified varying, yet distinct, patterns of communication recovery. They found that 52% of patients recovered functional communication within 8 weeks of rehabilitation admission. They also found that most patients recovered intentional communication first, followed by improved accuracy and functionality. This occurred as early as 10 days after admission and suggests that intentional communication is a building block to functional communication.[6] These findings can provide clinicians and families with potential predictive signals for the return and recovery of communication.

THE ROLE OF REHABILITATION

Specialized interdisciplinary rehabilitation is recommended for individuals in DoC.[18,19,35] Interdisciplinary rehabilitation should comprise of specialists in communication and cognition including speech language pathologists, neuropsychologists, and occupational therapists. These disciplines are trained to assess; identify' and treat cognitive, language, and communication deficits after neurological injury. They also have the knowledge to implement assistive and augmentative communication techniques and technologies to improve a patient's ability to interact verbally and nonverbally.

Access to these specialties after severe brain injury is imperative to ensure accurate DoC assessment, address identified confounds, and implement effective rehabilitation strategies. Unfortunately, many patients in DoC are not referred to or, if referred, lack the means to access expert DoC postacute care.[36] These limitations can leave patients, who may have naturally recovered consciousness but continue to live with communication barriers, unable to meaningfully interact with caregivers, thereby depriving them of their autonomy and ability to participate in decision-making.[4]

THE USE OF AUGMENTATIVE AND ALTERNATIVE COMMUNICATION IN EARLY RECOVERY

Augmentative and alternative communication (AAC) plays an important role in communication assessment and intervention at all levels of DoC recovery.[37,38] Low/light-tech AAC strategies are often the first methods of communication explored by rehabilitation teams. Early in recovery, the team may use readily available familiar objects and technology (eg, iPads/tablets with apps that make use of lights and/or sound, personally relevant photos and messages, and so forth) to elicit general attention and response to a request.[39] The team focuses on shaping these early behaviors into a functional response (eg, following a command/request, indicating a choice, communicating yes/no). As the consistency and reliability of these response modalities increase, low-tech AAC methods can be used including eye gaze, partner-dependent scanning, and use of communication boards.[37,40] The exact type of strategy, access methods, and message representations used will vary based on the patient's physical, cognitive, and visual capabilities.

The use of switches can be introduced early to shape response modalities into communication. Successful use of switch technology to access single message devices and control basic environmental options (eg, fans, music, lights, TV, recordings of family voices) is well documented for patients who have been described as persistently minimally conscious.[41,42] Depending on the specific physical capabilities of the patient, a wide range of switches are available to capture physical movement (eg, light touch, proximity, grasp, button, sensor, and electromyography switches).

AUGMENTATIVE AND ALTERNATIVE COMMUNICATION STRATEGIES AND TECHNOLOGY TO SUPPORT LONG-TERM COMMUNICATION NEEDS

As patients recover and responses become more consistent, access to speech-generating devices (SGDs) and computers to support communication may be explored. A wide range of alternative access methods exist for those with persistent severe physical impairments including switch-activated scanning, eye tracking, and head tracking. Finding a direct means of alternative access (ie, eye tracking or head tracking) is preferable to switch-activated scanning due to the cognitive and physical requirements required to successfully use switch-scanning (eg, attention, vigilance, timing, motor planning, and execution).

Eye-tracking alternative access uses an infrared light source to produce a reflection on the user's pupil that translates eye movement into cursor control on a computer or item selection on an SGD.[43] Use of eye tracking research technology to identify visual-cognitive processing capabilities of individuals with brain injury is well documented. However, there is a paucity of literature on the use of this technology as an alternative access method in the DoC population. Clinical anecdotal evidence suggests that this may be due to challenges associated with diminished attention and impaired oculomotor control[44] that can be present throughout recovery. Modifications such as decreasing the number and increasing the size of communication targets may facilitate the functional use of this technology. Head-tracking technology uses an infrared light source that is picked up by a reflective dot affixed to the user's forehead or cap. This technology requires extensive head movement abilities to move a cursor across the screen and to recalibrate during use.[40,44]

If physical impairments preclude the use of eye or head-tracking technology, head-mounted laser pointers can be used as a hybrid low/high-tech AAC solution. Laser pointers have been documented to be useful in cases of individuals with locked-in syndrome and can provide an early method of direct alternative access for some.[37] When direct methods are unsuccessful, the team may use switch-activated scanning methods with a capability switch that matches a patient's physical abilities. Activation of the switch causes communication software on an SGD to be scanned often by rows and columns for the user to make selections. As mentioned earlier, this method can be difficult due to the attention, timing, and vigilance required to compose messages. Some useful adaptations include limiting the number of messages to be scanned, using 2-switch scanning when physical abilities permit, and implementing auditory cues to facilitate the use of this technology for those with significant vision issues.[45]

In addition to alternative access solutions, how messages are represented require ongoing evaluation and modification to accommodate any concomitant cognitive, language, and visual processing issues that may be present. Early in recovery, the attention required to use alternative methods to spell messages may limit their use. Expression is best supported through displays that include full messages, photographs and/or icons. Visual-cognitive processing literature suggests that using icons only (versus text only or icon + text) displays,[46] contextualized (versus decontextualized) photographic content,[47] and photographic Figure (versus icon-based) grid displays[48] may result in improved use of communication interfaces. When individuals are able to use spelling-based message construction, overlearned and familiar keyboard layouts (eg, Traditional keyboard on a computer or laptop with QWERTY in the top left part of the letters of the standard keyboard [QWERTY]) can optimize access compared with other layouts such as alphabetic[49] (**Table 2**).

Table 2
Levels of augmentative and alternative communication communication for individuals with brain injury, specific goal targets, and description of strategies and technologies that can be used to support communication at the different levels

Levels of AAC Communication	Goals	Strategies/Technology
Early in recovery	• Attention • Following commands • Identifying consistent/reliable response modalities	• Use of personally relevant photos/objects • Familiar mobile technologies (tablet/iPad) to display personally relevant content or apps with visual interest for attention, tracking • Specific eye gaze or other physical response to personally relevant content
Emerging communication	• Shaping response modalities into communicative responses	• Low-tech AAC strategies such as eye gaze cards/boards, communication boards • Yes/no response modes (head nods, thumbs up/down, eye gaze, eye blinks, other physical movements) • Switch-activated radio, fan, lights with latch-timer • Switch-adapted call-light • Single message communication devices • Laser pointer to low tech communication boards • Introduction to head tracking/eye tracking or switch-scanning access to speech generating devices as appropriate with simplified displays of personally relevant communication content
Supporting long-term communication	• Support long-term communication needs	• Iterative expansion of use of speech-generating device technology • Spelling to communicate messages • Navigating and accessing messages within complex communication displays • Adjusting amount and complexity of communication content to increase successful use • Accommodating visual processing/visual motor issues using customized communication displays and auditory cues

NEW AND EMERGING COMMUNICATION TECHNOLOGIES FOR DISORDERS OF CONSCIOUSNESS

There are emerging technologies that demonstrate potential to support communication for patients with DoC. In one approach, patients used eye tracking to target a gross location on a communication interface on a computer. Then patients used switch scanning of a few items to make a specific selection. This combined approach mitigated the challenges often experienced by individuals with severe brain injury by (1) decreasing the high level of resolution required to use eye tracking so that patients with eye motor impairments could be successful and (2) decreasing the number of targets that were required to be scanned to make a selection, thereby decreasing the attention and vigilance required.[44]

Brain computer interface (BCI) is another emerging technology that has the potential to support consciousness assessment and communication with survivors of severe brain injury.[50,51] However, the use of BCI as a communication tool has primarily focused on individuals with locked-in syndrome due to brainstem strokes or late-stage amyotrophic lateral sclerosis.[52–56] BCI uses EEG electrodes on the head to measure neuronal activity and provide real-time feedback.[52,53] Initial studies concluded that BCI was safe, feasible and effective in identifying consciousness in patients with DoC who were unable to produce an observable response during bedside assessment.[50,51] Expanding on past studies, BCI is being tested as an avenue for "cerebral communication" through brain wave interfacing with the computer and computing language externally.[50,57] It is noted however that currently BCI is used predominantly in research settings and is not easily accessible for patients to use clinically. The hope is, by demonstrating its efficacy in DoC, BCI will be available for future clinical application. BCI might not only improve the identification of consciousness but also provide a communication strategy that has a great potential to enhance a patient's ability to engage with others, externalize their needs, and promote self-determination (**Fig. 6**).

EMERGING CONSCIOUSNESS, COMMUNICATION, AND THE FAMILY

Families describe the return of communication as an important milestone in recovery from severe brain injury.[58] Involving families in the process of assessment of consciousness allows them to better understand the potential barriers to communication. Furthermore, families may be able to identify patient attempts at purposeful communication before the clinical team. Evidence has supported that patients demonstrate increased consistency of arousal and response when their family is interacting with them versus medical or rehabilitation professionals.[58,59] As verbal or nonverbal communication avenues begin to emerge, it is imperative to educate caregivers on how to effectively engage with their loved one. This includes (1) training on use of AAC, (2) educating them about the increased time required for auditory processing and response, and (3) phrasing questions for binary choice. Families may not recognize that the patient will not immediately regain premorbid language and communication abilities and will require adaptive strategies because they continue to recover linguistic and cognitive skills. Involving families in the process of developing communication strategies can assist them in reestablishing relationships and participation in familial roles. Caregivers that can effectively communicate with their loved ones, in order to meet their wants and needs, are better prepared to care for them in a home setting. Family competence and comfort in using adaptive communication strategies can decrease overall burden of care and promote a patient's autonomy and self-agency.

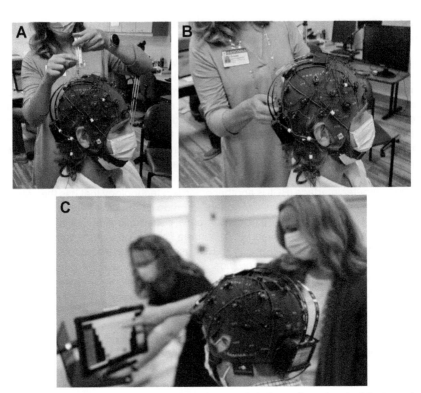

Fig. 6. BCI technology. (*A* and *B*): EEG-Based BCI cap and electrodes example. (*C*): Example of patient utilizing EEG-Based BCI with computer feedback.

COMMUNICATION, SELF-AGENCY, AND ETHICAL CONSIDERATIONS

The recovery of communication is imperative for a patient to reestablish their sense of self, autonomy, and decision-making capacity (DMC). Frequently, however, the communication established is limited and inconsistent, especially early in recovery. The partial recovery of communication raises several ethical issues, especially regarding the extent to which a patient is able to participate in decisions about their care. The ability to communicate in and of itself does not imply the ability to make informed decisions.[57,60,61] Although emerging technologies show promise as a way of augmenting the patient's communication capacity, especially because it relates to decision-making, several questions remain. The interpretation of brain activity through fMRI, EEG, or BCI has yet to be widely applied and accepted clinically as evidence of consciousness and capacity. Thus, there remain questions about whether these neurotechnologies can be a valid means to confirm a patient's DMC. This is a result of the lack of empirical evidence regarding the use of these new technologies to identify additional aspects of cognition—such as memory and comprehension of complex information—that are required for self-determination.[23,50,57] Finally, questions arise as to how best to incorporate the "voice" and wishes of the patient who has only partial DMC. Rather than simply shifting all of the decision-making authority back to the legally recognized surrogate in these situations, a better approach might be for the surrogate to try to incorporate whatever the patient is able to communicate into the process of coming to a decision. Such an approach is the most likely to preserve and enhance a patient's self-agency and even civil rights.[4,62,63]

SUMMARY

Families and professionals identify the recovery and augmentation of communication as an overriding goal in the care of patients in DoC. Knowledge of subcortical and cortical neuroanatomical substrates of language and communication is required for clinicians to suspect potential language deficits that may be present after severe brain injury. The importance of accurate neurobehavioral assessment as well as the identification and alleviation of confounds to consciousness and communication were emphasized. Rehabilitation specialists hold the expertise to implement compensatory and adaptive communication strategies for patients in DoC. Therefore, it is crucial that brain injury professionals advocate for access to specialized rehabilitation. Finally, current and future technologies hold the promise to expand available options for patients to communicate early and effectively. Promoting communication after severe brain injury will facilitate an individual's autonomy, self-advocacy, and participation in meaningful relationships with family and community.

CLINICS CARE POINTS

- Recovery of functional communication is a key behavioral feature of emergence from disorders of consciousness.
- Clinical care teams should identify and address confounds that can negatively influence the assessment of DoC and potentially lead to diagnostic inaccuracy.
- Interdisciplinary rehabilitation can promote communication through use of AAC and technology.
- Clinical teams should engage families in the DoC assessment and rehabilitation interventions related to optimizing communication and communication techniques to decrease caregiver burden and promote patient autonomy.

DISCLOSURE

Authors BM & TS do not have any commercial, financial or nonfinancial conflicts of interest or disclosures related to the content included within this article. Author SF discloses contents of this article were partially developed under a grant to the Rehabilitation Engineering Research Center on Augmentative and Alternative Communication (RERC on AAC) from the U.S. Department of Human Services, United States, National Institute on Disability, Independent Living, and Rehabilitation Research, United States (NIDILRR grant #90E5017 & #90REGE0014). Contents do not necessarily represent the policy of the funding agency, endorsement by the federal government should not be assumed.

REFERENCES

1. Giacino J, Katz DI, Schiff ND, et al. Assessment and rehabilitative management of individuals with disorders of consciousness. In: Zasler ND, Katz DI, Zafonte RD, et al, editors. *Brain injury medicine: principles and practice*. third. New York, NY: Demos Medical Publishing; 2022. p. 447–61.

2. Giacino J, Ashwal S, Childs N, et al. The minimally conscious state: definition and diagnostic criteria. Neurology 2002;58(3):349–53.
3. Bruno MA, Vanhaudenhuyse A, Thibaut A, et al. From unresponsive wakefulness to minimally conscious PLUS and functional locked-in syndromes: recent advances in our understanding of disorders of consciousness. J Neurol 2011; 258(7):1373–84.
4. Fins JJ. Rights come to mind: brain injury, ethics, and the struggle for consciousness. New York, NY: Cambridge University Press; 2015.
5. Zaksh Y, Yehene E, Elyashiv M, et al. Partially dead, partially separated: establishing the mechanism between ambiguous loss and grief reaction among caregivers of patients with prolonged disorders of consciousness. Clin Rehabil 2019; 33(2):345–56.
6. Martens G, Bodien Y, Thomas A, et al. Temporal profile of recovery of communication in patients with disorders of consciousness after severe brain injury. Arch Phys Med Rehabil 2020;101(7):1260–4.
7. Majerus S, Bruno MA, Schnakers C, et al. The problem of aphasia in the assessment of consciousness in brain-damaged patients. Prog Brain Res 2009;177: 49–61. Elsevier.
8. Van Lancker Sidtis D, Sidtis JJ. Cortical-subcortical production of formulaic language: a review of linguistic, brain disorder, and functional imaging studies leading to a production model. Brain Cognit 2018;126:53–64.
9. Nasios G, Dardiotis E, Messinis L. From broca and wernicke to the neuromodulation era: insights of brain language networks for neurorehabilitation. Behav Neurol 2019;2019:1–10.
10. Fujii M, Maesawa S, Ishiai S, et al. Neural basis of language: an overview of an evolving model. Neurol Med -Chir 2016;56(7):379–86.
11. Whyte J, DiPasquale MC, Vaccaro M. Assessment of command-following in minimally conscious brain injured patients. Arch Phys Med Rehabil 1999;80(6): 653–60.
12. Kalmar K, Giacino J. The JFK coma recovery scale—revised. Neuropsychol Rehabil 2005;15(3–4):454–60.
13. Pape TLB, Mallinson T, Guernon A. Psychometric properties of the disorders of consciousness scale. Arch Phys Med Rehabil 2014;95(9):1672–84.
14. Chatelle C, Schnakers C, Bruno MA, et al. La sensory modality assessment and rehabilitation technique (SMART) : une échelle comportementale d'évaluation et de revalidation pour des états altérés de conscience. Rev Neurol 2010;166(8–9): 675–82.
15. Seel RT, Sherer M, Whyte J, et al. Assessment scales for disorders of consciousness: evidence-based recommendations for clinical practice and research. Arch Phys Med Rehabil 2010;91(12):1795–813.
16. Bodien YG, Carlowicz CA, Chatelle C, et al. Sensitivity and specificity of the coma recovery scale–revised total score in detection of conscious awareness. Arch Phys Med Rehabil 2016;97(3):490–2.e1.
17. Giacino JT, Bodien Y, Chatelle C. Coma Recovery Scale Revised. Published online 2020. Available at: https://www.sralab.org/sites/default/files/downloads/2021-12/CRS-R_Manual20201210%5B2%5D.pdf. Accessed March 10, 2023.
18. Giacino JJT, Katz DI, Schiff ND, et al. Practice guideline update recommendations summary: disorders of consciousness. Arch Phys Med Rehabil 2018; 99(9):1699–709.
19. Giacino JJT, Whyte J, Nakase-Richardson R, et al. Minimum competency recommendations for programs that provide rehabilitation services for persons with

disorders of consciousness: a position statement of the american congress of rehabilitation medicine and the national institute on disability, independent living and rehabilitation research traumatic brain injury model systems. Arch Phys Med Rehabil 2020;101(6):1072–89.

20. Schnakers C, Bauer C, Formisano R, et al. What names for covert awareness? A systematic review. Front Hum Neurosci 2022;16:971315.

21. Kondziella D, Stevens RD. Classifying disorders of consciousness: past, present, and future. Semin Neurol 2022;42(03):239–48.

22. Kondziella D, Friberg CK, Frokjaer VG, et al. Preserved consciousness in vegetative and minimal conscious states: systematic review and meta-analysis. J Neurol Neurosurg Psychiatr 2016;87(5):485–92.

23. Sanz LRD, Thibaut A, Edlow BL, et al. Update on neuroimaging in disorders of consciousness. Curr Opin Neurol 2021;34(4):488–96.

24. Gosseries O, Pistoia F, Charland-Verville V, et al. The role of neuroimaging techniques in establishing diagnosis, prognosis and therapy in disorders of consciousness. TONIJ 2016;10(1):52–68.

25. Schiff ND, Rodriguez-Moreno D, Kamal A, et al. fMRI reveals large-scale network activation in minimally conscious patients. Neurology 2005;64(3):514–23.

26. Owen AM, Coleman MR, Boly M, et al. Detecting awareness in the vegetative state. Science 2006;313(5792):1402.

27. Owen AM, Coleman MR, Boly M, et al. Using functional magnetic resonance imaging to detect covert awareness in the vegetative state. Arch Neurol 2007;64(8):1098.

28. Edlow BL, Chatelle C, Spencer CA, et al. Early detection of consciousness in patients with acute severe traumatic brain injury. Brain 2017;140(9):2399–414.

29. Claassen J, Doyle K, Matory A, et al. Detection of brain activation in unresponsive patients with acute brain injury. N Engl J Med 2019;380(26):2497–505.

30. Kondziella D, Bender A, Diserens K, et al. European academy of neurology guideline on the diagnosis of coma and other disorders of consciousness. Eur J Neurol 2020;27(5):741–56.

31. Bodien YG, Katz DI, Schiff ND, et al. Behavioral assessment of patients with disorders of consciousness. Semin Neurol 2022;42(03):249–58.

32. Ganesh S, Guernon A, Chalcraft L, et al. Medical comorbidities in disorders of consciousness patients and their association with functional outcomes. Arch Phys Med Rehabil 2013;94(10):1899–907.e3.

33. Schnakers C, Bessou H, Rubi-Fessen I, et al. Impact of aphasia on consciousness assessment: a cross-sectional study. Neurorehabil Neural Repair 2015;29(1):41–7.

34. Arnts H, van Erp WS, Lavrijsen JCM, et al. On the pathophysiology and treatment of akinetic mutism. Neurosci Biobehav Rev 2020;112:270–8.

35. Seel RT, Douglas J, Dennison AC, et al. Specialized early treatment for persons with disorders of consciousness: program components and outcomes. Arch Phys Med Rehabil 2013;94(10):1908–23.

36. Giacino J, Bodien YG, Zuckerman D, et al. Empiricism and rights justify the allocation of health care resources to persons with disorders of consciousness. AJOB Neuroscience 2021;12(2–3):169–71.

37. Fager S, Doyle M, Karantounis R. Traumatic brain injury. In: Beukelman DR, Garrett KL, Yorkston KM, editors. Augmentative communication strategies for adults with acute or chronic medical conditions. Baltimore, MD: Paul H. Brooks Publishing Co.; 2007. p. 131–62.

38. Fager Susan, Karantounis R. AAC assessment and intervention. In: Hux KK, editor. Assistive survivors of traumatic brain injury. 3rd ed. Autsin, TX: Pro-Ed Inc; 2022. p. 264–86.

39. Lancioni GE, Singh NN, O'Reilly MF, et al. Mainstream technology to support basic communication and leisure in people with neurological disorders, motor impairment and lack of speech. Brain Inj 2020;34(7):921–7.

40. Fager S, Beukelman DR. Individuals with traumatic brain injury. In: Beukelman DR, Light J, editors. Augmentative & Alternative communication: supporting children and adults with complex communication needs. 5th ed. Baltimore, MD: Paul H. Brooks Publishing Co.; 2020. p. 637–46.

41. Lancioni GE, Singh NN, O'Reilly MF, et al. Promoting adaptive behavior in persons with acquired brain injury, extensive motor and communication disabilities, and consciousness disorders. Res Dev Disabil 2012;33(6):1964–74.

42. Lancioni GE, Singh NN, O'Reilly MF, et al. Occupation and communication programs for post-coma persons with or without consciousness disorders who show extensive motor impairment and lack of speech. Res Dev Disabil 2014; 35(5):1110–8.

43. Hammoud R. Passive eye monitoring: algorithms, applications, and experiments. Heidelberg, Germany: Springer-Verlag; 2008.

44. Fager S, Gormley J, Sorenson T. Access to AAC for individuals with acquired conditions: challenges and solutions in early recovery. In: Ogletree B, editor. Augmentative and alternative communication challenges and solutions. San Diego, CA: Plural Publishing Inc.; 2021. p. 199–228.

45. Fager S, Spellman C. Augmentative and alternative communication intervention in children with traumatic brain injury and spinal cord injury. J Pediatr Rehabil Med 2010;3(4):269–77.

46. Brown J, Thiessen A, Beukelman D, et al. Noun representation in AAC grid displays: visual attention patterns of people with traumatic brain injury. Augment Altern Commun 2015;31(1):15–26.

47. Thiessen A, Brown J, Beukelman D, et al. Effect of message type on the visual attention of adults with traumatic brain injury. Am J Speech Lang Pathol 2017; 26(2):428–42.

48. Brown J, Thiessen A, Freeland T, et al. Visual processing patterns of adults with traumatic brain injury when viewing Figure-based grids and visual scenes. Augment Altern Commun 2019;35(3):229–39.

49. Gormley J, Koch Fager S. Personalization of patient–provider communication across the life span. Top Lang Disord 2021;41(3):249–68.

50. Ortner R, Allison BZ, Pichler G, et al. Assessment and communication for people with disorders of consciousness. JoVE 2017;(126):53639. https://doi.org/10.3791/53639.

51. Wang F, He Y, Qu J, et al. Enhancing clinical communication assessments using an audiovisual BCI for patients with disorders of consciousness. J Neural Eng 2017;14(4):046024.

52. Sellers EW, Vaughan TM, Wolpaw JR. A brain-computer interface for long-term independent home use. Amyotroph Lateral Scler 2010;11(5):449–55.

53. Oken BS, Orhan U, Roark B, et al. Brain–computer interface with language model–electroencephalography fusion for locked-in syndrome. Neurorehabil Neural Repair 2014;28(4):387–94.

54. Vaughan TM. Brain-computer interfaces for people with amyotrophic lateral sclerosis. Handb Clin Neurol 2020;168:33–8. Elsevier.

55. Akcakaya M, Peters B, Moghadamfalahi M, et al. Noninvasive brain-computer interfaces for augmentative and alternative communication. IEEE Rev Biomed Eng 2014;7:31–49.
56. Peters B, Bedrick S, Dudy S, et al. SSVEP BCI and eye tracking use by individuals with late-stage ALS and visual impairments. Front Hum Neurosci 2020;14: 595890.
57. Farisco M, Laureys S, Evers K. Externalization of consciousness. Scientific possibilities and clinical implications. In: Lee G, Illes J, Ohl F, editors. *Ethical issues in behavioral neuroscience*. Vol 19. Current topics in behavioral neurosciences. Heidelberg, Germany: Springer Berlin Heidelberg; 2014. p. 205–22. https://doi. org/10.1007/7854_2014_338.
58. Moretta P, Trojano L, Masotta O, et al. Family caregivers' opinions about interaction with the environment in consciousness disorders. Rehabil Psychol 2017; 62(2):208–13.
59. Formisano R, Contrada M, Iosa M, et al. Coma recovery scale-revised with and without the emotional stimulation of caregivers. Can J Neurol Sci 2019;46(5): 607–9.
60. Tamburrini G, Mattia D. Disorders of consciousness and communication. Ethical motivations and communication-enabling attributes of consciousness. Funct Neurol 2011;4:51–4.
61. Evers K. Neurotechnological assessment of consciousness disorders: five ethical imperatives. Dialogues Clin Neurosci 2016;18(2):155–62.
62. Fins JJ, Bernat JL. Ethical, palliative, and policy considerations in disorders of consciousness. Neurology 2018;91(10):471–5.
63. Fins JJ, Wright MS. Rights language and disorders of consciousness: a call for advocacy. Brain Inj 2018;32(5):670–4.

Education, Training, and Support Across the Continuum of Recovery for Caregivers of Persons with Disorders of Consciousness

Amy Shapiro-Rosenbaum, PhD[a,b,c,*], Michelle P. Jaffe, PhD[a,c,d,1]

KEYWORDS

- Consciousness • Disorders • Family • Caregiver • Burden • Education • Support
- Training

KEY POINTS

- Caregivers of persons with disorders of consciousness (DoC) experience high levels of perceived burden.
- Level of perceived burden has been shown to have an adverse impact on caregiver emotional, psychosocial, and financial well-being and engenders greater expressed need for information and support.
- DoC caregivers' information and support needs are diverse and evolve over time.
- Providing individually tailored education, training, and support may help ease caregiver burden and increase the likelihood of community discharge, thereby potentially translating to reduced long-term costs of care for this population.

INTRODUCTION

Given the crucial role that caregivers play in the overall functioning of persons with disorders of consciousness (DoC), recognizing factors that influence their perceived level of burden and targeting interventions that address their needs are critical. DoC caregivers often experience stress related to the uncertainty of their loved one's condition and the weight of feeling responsible for making informed decisions on their

[a] Department of Brain Injury Rehabilitation, Park Terrace Care Center, Queens, NY, USA; [b] TBI Model System, Icahn School of Medicine at Mount Sinai, New York, NY, USA; [c] BrainMatters Neuropsychological Services, PLLC, Plainview, NY, USA; [d] North Shore University Hospital, Northwell Health, Kings Point, NY, USA
[1] Present address: c/o Park Terrace Care Center, 59-20 Van Doren Street, Rego Park, NY 11368.
* Corresponding author. c/o Park Terrace Care Center, 59-20 Van Doren Street, Rego Park, NY 11368.
E-mail address: ashapi1@hotmail.com

Phys Med Rehabil Clin N Am 35 (2024) 193–208
https://doi.org/10.1016/j.pmr.2023.06.015
1047-9651/24/© 2023 Elsevier Inc. All rights reserved.

pmr.theclinics.com

behalf. On the whole, they report high levels of burden and low levels of quality of life.[1] To maintain consistency with how the term has been used in the literature, for the purposes of this article, the term caregiver includes family members, partners, friends, and any other persons who feel responsible for providing formal or informal care in terms of time dedicated to the person with DoC. Most commonly, this is a middle-aged woman who is either the spouse/partner or parent of the person with DoC.[2–6]

There are many factors that encompass perceived caregiver burden, some specific to personal characteristics of the caregiver (eg, their individual coping style, resilience), some to situational (eg, health condition of the person with DoC, daily hours of caregiving), and some to environmental (eg, place of domicile, financial resources, availability of social supports). Collectively, these variables have a multifaceted impact on the overall well-being of caregivers, adversely affecting social and interpersonal relationships, physical health, and psychological and financial well-being.[1,3,6–8] For example, caregivers report lower levels of social support[1] and high levels of anxiety and depression, with higher levels of anxiety being associated with negative mental health outcomes in both men and women.[2–4,6] The number of daily hours of caregiving has also been shown to significantly impact the level of perceived burden,[1] in part due to repercussions on financial stability. Among caregivers of persons with DoC that live in institutional settings, as many as one in three have to temporarily or permanently resign from their job as a result of the time demands required to care for their loved one.[2,3,5,6]

Given the psychosocial, emotional, and financial impact on caregivers, it is not surprising that higher levels of perceived burden are associated with a greater expressed need for information and support across all phases of recovery.[1,6] Despite abundant research highlighting the negative impact of caregiver burden, caregiver needs are an often-overlooked aspect of DoC care management. This article provides an overview of current knowledge about the needs of DoC caregivers, identifies targets for caregiver education, training, and support central to each level of care, and offers practical guidance to optimize communication efforts between DoC care providers and caregivers across the continuum of recovery.

RESEARCH

Ensuring effective communication between providers and caregivers is essential to help mitigate the level of perceived burden and, in turn, reduce the strain felt by health care professionals who are often targets of caregiver expressed stress. To that end, the type of information and support, stage of recovery, and method of conveying information must all be considered, as the nature, amount, and timing of information may either serve to alleviate or exacerbate caregiver perceived burden.

Studies of DoC caregiver expressed needs collectively distinguish among the following three categories of support needs:[1–3,5,6,9,10]

- Instrumental needs—hands-on training and help accessing resources
- Informational needs—understanding the person with DoCs health condition, what to expect throughout the course of recovery, and how to be involved in making decisions affecting their loved one's care
- Emotional and social support needs—resources to help alleviate caregiver burden

Needs can be further categorized based on whether the information and support centers on practical versus sensitive issues. *Practical* matters include hands-on training, information about tests the person with DoC may undergo, medications and current treatments, and assistance finding appropriate placements and accessing resources. *Sensitive* issues include information related to prognosis, decisions regarding withdrawal of care, and discussions related to long-term disability and care needs.

Designed for caregivers of stroke survivors, the Timing it Right (TIR) model provides a useful framework for conceptualizing how the nature and type of support needs may change over time.[11] The model highlights the importance of timing the provision of education, training and support based on individual caregiver needs and readiness, both of which can be expected to change throughout the continuum of their loved one's recovery, and even within any given stage. Of note, the TIR model delineates caregiver needs based on the patient's transition across three stages from (1) intensive care to (2) the ward/hospital unit, where the focus is on medical stabilization and preparation for discharge to (3) discharge home.[11] Unlike what is typical in stroke recovery, persons with DoC are rarely discharged home straight from the hospital. In DoC, there is great diversity in the care pathways taken and thus among the experiences of individual caregivers (**Fig. 1**), making it difficult to adopt a uniform framework based on the stage of recovery for this population. To adapt the TIR model for DoC caregivers, herein we consider caregiver needs in terms of three general phases of recovery: (1) intensive care and acute hospitalization; (2) inpatient rehabilitation (eg, hospital-based, skilled nursing facility); and (3) transition to a less intensive care setting (ie, for long-term care) or a more intensive care setting (ie, for inpatient rehabilitation), irrespective of time post-injury.

According to the TIR model, although caregivers collectively seek out practical information and instrumental guidance early on and throughout the continuum of care, there is more variability with respect to timing regarding individual caregiver readiness to receive sensitive information. Caregivers often need time before they are prepared to consider more diverse and complex issues such as those related to

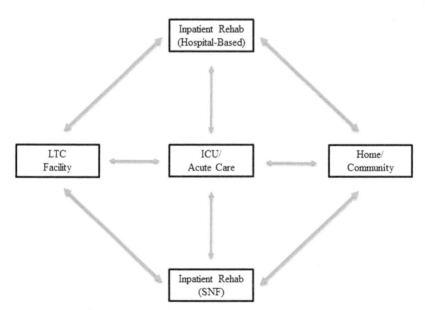

Fig. 1. Transition of care pathways for persons with disorders of consciousness. ICU, intensive care unit; LTC, long-term care; SNF, skilled nursing facility.

long-term recovery or decisions related therein.[11] In addition, there may be discrepancy between what information caregivers want or are able to hear and what physicians and other health care professionals perceive their needs to be.[12] Consequently, a more individualized approach is required when it comes to discussing sensitive issues, one that prioritizes topics considered essential for developing a plan of care, while taking into consideration caregiver receptiveness and the amount of information they can process at any given time. **Fig. 2** provides an overview of caregiver needs and how they change over time.

GUIDELINES

Both DoC practice guidelines[13] and minimal competency recommendations for programs that provide rehabilitation to persons with DoC[14] reinforce the importance of having a mechanism in place to identify and address support needs based on the specific patient and DoC caregiver (**Boxes 1** and **2**). The minimal competency recommendations state that programs should have procedures in place to determine how individualized education and training will be delivered (eg, who will provide it, when, and how). Only individuals with an appropriate level of training, expertise, and experience in a given topic area should provide information relative to that topic, especially with respect to sensitive issues such as diagnosis, prognosis, and withdrawal of care.[14] Finally, as shown in **Boxes 1** and **2**, at a minimum, educational efforts should include information about the diagnosis, prognosis, and care needs of the person with DoC, as well as guidance and assistance with medical decision-making, short- and long-term care planning, and accessing resources.[13,14]

CONSIDERATIONS FOR ADDRESSING CAREGIVER NEEDS ACROSS THE CONTINUUM OF RECOVERY
Intensive Care Unit and Acute Hospitalization

Early post-injury caregivers want practical information to, at a minimum, help them better understand the events surrounding their loved one's intensive care unit (ICU) admission, including information on their condition, and what to expect throughout the course of their hospital stay.[15] Caregivers for individuals in the ICU also express needs for ready access to care team members and to receive repeated, clear, easily

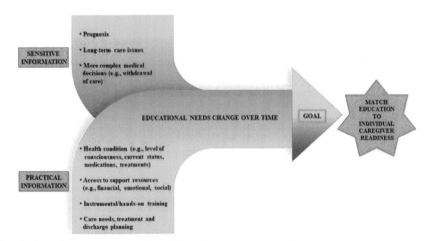

Fig. 2. Caregiver support needs and how they change over time.

Box 1
Practice guidelines for disorders of consciousness caregiver communication across the continuum of recovery

Guidelines for communicating prognosis
- Clinicians must avoid statements suggesting a universally poor prognosis when discussing prognosis with caregivers of patients with a DoC of 28 days or less (Level A)[a]
- Clinicians should counsel caregivers that outcomes are more favorable when MCS is diagnosed within 5 months of a traumatic injury, whereas a diagnosis of VS/UWS due to nontraumatic etiology is associated with poorer outcomes. However, it should also be communicated that individual outcomes vary and prognosis is not universally poor (Level B)[b]
- Caregivers of children with prolonged DoC (>28 days) should be counseled that the natural history and prognosis is not well-defined in this population and there are no current evaluations established to improve prognostic accuracy (Level B)

Guidelines to assist family caregivers with decision-making
- For persons with prolonged DoC, clinicians must identify patient and caregiver preferences early on and throughout all phases of recovery to help guide the decision-making process (Level A)
- Caregivers should be counseled regarding the uncertainty surrounding the degree of pain and suffering experienced by patients with DoC (Level B)
- Given caregivers are often in distress and vulnerable, counseling should be provided about the limitations of existing evidence on treatment effectiveness and the potential risks related to interventions that lack evidentiary support
- When discussing non-validated treatments with caregivers, evidence-based information about the potential benefits and risks should be presented as well as the level of uncertainty associated with any particular treatment(s) being considered
- Caregivers should be counseled that it is often impossible to discern whether improvements observed early on in recovery are related to a specific intervention versus spontaneous recovery (Level B)
- Caregivers should be counseled that there are no established therapies for children with a prolonged DoC (Level B)

Guidelines regarding support and resources for long-term care planning
- In patients with a prolonged DoC with a likelihood of severe long-term disability, clinicians must counsel caregivers to seek assistance in establishing goals of care and completing state-specific forms regarding medical decision-making, applying for disability benefits, and starting estate, caregiver, and long-term care planning (Level A)
- For patients in chronic VS/UWS (ie, 3 months after non-TBI and 12 months after TBI), prognostic counseling should emphasize the likelihood of permanent severe disability and the need for long-term assistive care (Level B)

[a]Level A is the strongest recommendation level and is denoted by use of the helping verb must.[b]Level B corresponds to the helping verb should. Such recommendations are still associated with confidence in the rationale and a favorable benefit–risk profile.*Abbreviations:* DoC, disorder of consciousness; MCS, minimally conscious state; TBI, traumatic brain injury; UWS, unresponsive wakefulness syndrome; VS, vegetative state.

Giacino JT, Katz DI, Schiff ND, Whyte J, Ashman EJ, Ashwal S, Barbano R, Hammond FM, Laureys S, Ling GSF, Nakase-Richardson R, Seel RT, Yablon S, Getchius TSD, Gronseth GS, Armstrong MJ. Practice guideline update recommendations summary: Disorders of consciousness: Report of the Guideline Development, Dissemination, and Implementation Subcommittee of the American Academy of Neurology; the American Congress of Rehabilitation Medicine; and the National Institute on Disability, Independent Living, and Rehabilitation Research. Neurology. 2018 Sep 4;91(10):450-460.

---

understandable communication throughout the hospital stay.[1,3,4,15] However, many ICU caregivers may not know what questions to ask or what information they need to know.[15] Therefore, it is important to offer guidance to caregivers about the kinds of information and resources available to them.

Box 2
Minimal competency recommendations for programs providing rehabilitation to persons with disorder of consciousness: caregiver education, training, and support

Recommendation regarding communication of diagnosis and prognosis
- Clinical information provided regarding diagnosis and prognosis (eg, diagnostic features, prognostic indicators) should be communicated using language that is easy to understand and include an explanation about the limits of certainty based on the current state of the evidence

Recommendations regarding caregiver education, training, and access to resources
- Programs should have procedures in place to identify caregiver needs
- Programs should have procedures in place to provide individualized education and training to caregivers. Topics to cover include:
  ○ Level of consciousness
  ○ Prognosis
  ○ Care needs
  ○ Estimated length of stay
  ○ Resources to address common emotional, legal, financial, and social support needs
  ○ Information on appropriate disposition sites
- Procedures for accessing community-based services for those who require more intensive services should be available on-site. This includes but is not limited to:
  ○ Registries listing mental health providers
  ○ Attorneys specializing in legal rights for persons with disability
  ○ Financial consultants

Recommendations regarding transition of care
- Programs should have procedures in place for ensuring that information necessary to support continuity of care is communicated to professional and lay caregivers. At a minimum, transfer of care should include information about:
  ○ Current level of consciousness
  ○ Overall level of functioning
  ○ Prognosis
  ○ Ongoing comorbid medical conditions and current treatments
  ○ Equipment needs
  ○ Caregiver educational needs
  ○ Recommendations for follow-up appointments with appropriate specialists

Abbreviation: DoC, disorder of consciousness.

Giacino JT, Whyte J, Nakase-Richardson R, Katz DI, Arciniegas DB, Blum S, Day K, Greenwald BD, Hammond FM, Pape TB, Rosenbaum A, Seel RT, Weintraub A, Yablon S, Zafonte RD, Zasler N. Minimum Competency Recommendations for Programs That Provide Rehabilitation Services for Persons With Disorders of Consciousness: A Position Statement of the American Congress of Rehabilitation Medicine and the National Institute on Disability, Independent Living and Rehabilitation Research Traumatic Brain Injury Model Systems. Arch Phys Med Rehabil. 2020 Jun;101(6):1072-1089.

With respect to discussing sensitive topics early on when caregivers can become overwhelmed easily, more information is not necessarily better. For instance, when communicating about prognosis, even if caregivers express wanting to know whether their loved one will recover, emotionally, not everyone is able to hear and process this information, especially when they are told the outcome looks grim. More often, caregivers are looking to hear messages that reinforce feelings of hope and optimism, rather than those that focus on harsh realities. Although ICU professionals may feel responsible for providing definitive information to caregivers regarding their loved one's prognosis, research shows that except in cases of brain death, it is not possible to make accurate predictions regarding long-term recovery so early post-injury.

Considering that it can take months before a desired level of prognostic confidence can be achieved, the nature and timing of these conversations can and should be tailored based on individual caregiver readiness.[13] To that end, early discussions regarding prognosis should aim to strike a balance between hope and realism by presenting information within the context of the patient's injury, stage of recovery, and always couched by some level of uncertainty.[14]

As the person with DoC achieves medical stability and is approaching completion of their ICU stay, discharge planning becomes a key focus. Caregivers are often left on their own to research and find an appropriate placement for their loved one's next level of care. There is a need to make information and resources more readily available to guide them through this process. Social-emotional interventions should also be incorporated to address the physical and mental health effects of caregiving, in light of research suggesting the level of burden and its impact on mental health is greatest early post-injury.[1,5]

Importantly, at this stage, care team goals are primarily focused on medical stabilization, survival, and addressing complications. Once medically stable, patients are often quickly moved off the unit or are discharged from the hospital. In this setting, the critical care team typically does not have ample time to provide repeated face-to-face education, though this is encouraged if possible. Strategies to address this issue include supplementing educational efforts with pamphlets, videos, or other materials that can be reviewed on their own, and referring caregivers to trustworthy websites and/or brain injury organizations where more information can be found about the topics being discussed.

Although instrumental needs such as hands-on training are less of a focus at this early stage, caregivers do express a desire to be actively involved in patient care.[3] Teaching sensory stimulation techniques such as how to safely massage or perform passive range of motion exercises may help reduce the risk of secondary complications due to lack of mobility (eg, foot drop, contractures, blood clots) while also countering the shock and distress experienced by caregivers by providing some semblance of control over the situation. A comprehensive list of specific topics to address at this level of care is presented in **Box 3**.

Inpatient Rehabilitation

According to the practice guidelines, medically stable persons with DoC should be referred to settings staffed by multidisciplinary rehabilitation teams with specialized training in DoC care. Beyond attempting to maximize functional recovery, specialized rehabilitation should focus on ongoing diagnostic assessment, medical monitoring, and care management, as well as outcome monitoring and prognostication.[13] Per the minimal competency recommendations, rehabilitation goals should be individualized, cross-disciplinary, and centered on enhancing health, self-care, mobility, communication, and active participation.[14]

On admission to inpatient rehabilitation, efforts should be made to identify caregiver needs including determining:

- Their baseline understanding of DoC
- What information/education topics they are interested in (or would benefit from) learning more about
- How much information they want and/or can handle
- Their interest and ability to participate with their loved one's daily care
- What aspects of hands-on care they are interested in (or would benefit from) training in

---

Box 3
Educational needs during intensive care unit and acute hospitalization

Informational needs
Practical
- Information about the patient's condition, medications, and current health status
- Information about tests and procedures
- Plan for preventing secondary complications due to impaired mobility (eg, bed sores, contractures, pneumonia, blood clots)
  - Explanations of complications as they develop (eg, seizures)
- Treatment plan and current treatment interventions
- Information related to the patient's personal care, hygiene, and comfort including but not limited to:
  - Tracheostomy management and daily care
  - Nutrition and peg tube
  - Assessment and management of pain
  - Strategies being used to promote daytime arousal and sleep at night
- As patients progress toward preparation for hospital discharge:
  - Information on progress made
  - Information on discharge plan and options to consider
  - Information on treatments and/or medications needed to support/ensure ongoing recovery

Sensitive
- Prognosis and long-term recovery potential
- Discussions regarding more complex medical decisions including but not limited to:
  - Withdrawal of care
  - Palliative care
  - Identifying decision-making surrogates
  - Need to pursue guardianship
  - Dealing with ethical issues that may arise during the course of care
- Discussions about long-term care planning

Instrumental needs
- Hands-on training (eg, range of motion, turning and positioning protocols if not contraindicated)

Support needs
- Access to resources for:
  - Finding an appropriate placement for the next level of care (eg, identifying and exploring discharge options, criteria for admission for rehabilitation)
  - Financial planning and assistance
- Information regarding federal, state, local, and private resources including but not limited to:
  - Mental health provider registries
  - Attorneys specializing in legal rights for persons with disability
  - Financial consultants
- Guidance regarding transition of care needs
- Normalization of caregivers' emotional response
- Strategies for caregiver wellness, coping and self-care

Abbreviation: ICU, intensive care unit.

- What their goals are and what outcomes they view as important
- What types of supports (legal, financial, social/emotional) are needed.

Caregivers should be viewed as an integral part of the rehabilitation team; they should be actively involved in all aspects of care planning and goal setting. However, caregivers often tend to think in terms of big picture goals and may need help breaking down larger expectations into smaller, measurable steps. For example, caregivers often identify ambulation or independent toileting as a goal for their loved one. They may need education to understand the smaller key milestones that reflect more realistic and tangible progress in persons with DoC such as sitting balance, upright tolerance, command following, and the ability to actively participate with tasks. Several studies show that even among persons with prolonged post-traumatic DoC who are unable to follow commands at the time of inpatient rehabilitation admission, many will have good functional outcomes as measured by eventually achieving at least partial independence. Nevertheless, it can take years for a person with DoC to achieve some level of functional independence in self-care, mobility, and cognition.[16–18] Caregivers should be prepared to expect a protracted recovery curve, as the rate of progress is notoriously slow in this population.

With respect to instrumental needs, providing hands-on training in how to actively participate with daily care tasks can impart a sense of control and empowerment while facilitating the caregivers' ability to interact with their loved one in a meaningful and productive way.[12] Caregivers can be trained to participate with daily activities through learning how to:

- Perform stretching, turning, and positioning
- Safely transfer the person with DoC in and out of bed
- Perform oral hygiene and tracheostomy care
- Accurately interpret behavioral responses
- Monitor for changes in function

Seel and colleagues incorporated comprehensive individualized education, training, and support for caregivers as one of the key components of a specialized treatment program for persons with DoC. Methods included a combination of didactic and hands-on training, staff modeling of techniques, training the trainer, and information provided via case conferences with families. In this study, on completion of rehabilitation, even persons who remained in a DoC were more than twice as likely to be discharged home with family versus remaining institutionalized in a long-term care facility.[19] This shows the potential benefit at a programmatic level of equipping caregivers with the knowledge and skills necessary to promote a sense of confidence and commitment to remain actively involved in their loved ones' care.

Regardless of the planned discharge setting, during inpatient rehabilitation, caregivers are generally over the initial shock of the injury and ready to move toward accepting the reality of the situation. At this stage, they are often faced less with the uncertainty of their loved one's survival and more with the uncertainty regarding what to expect and how to prepare for their loved one's recovery over the long term. Accordingly, discussions regarding sensitive issues such as prognosis and long-term care planning are more appropriate to address during this phase of recovery. Sensitive clinical information should be communicated with care and presented using simple, direct language that is easy to understand. Conversations regarding the potential for meaningful recovery should recognize the limitations of existing knowledge as well as factors that may limit prognostic certainty.[14] In persons for whom an outcome has been established and suggests a high likelihood of severe long-term disability, caregivers require counseling and guidance to establish appropriate long-term goals of care, complete medical decision-making forms (eg, orders for life-sustaining treatment), and apply for disability benefits.[13]

At this phase of care, there should also be an emphasis on emotional and social support needs, such as coping, adjustment, and stress management.[12,15] A focus should also be placed on connecting the caregiver to resources (both on site and in the community) to support long-term care planning.[13,14] Ideally, one team member

---

Box 4
Educational needs during inpatient rehabilitation

Informational needs
Practical
- Information about the patient's level of consciousness
- Information related to the patient's personal care, hygiene, and comfort (eg, tracheostomy management and daily care, nutrition and peg tube, assessment and management of pain, strategies being used to promote daytime arousal and sleep at night)
- Rehabilitation goals, treatment plan/goals of care
- Anticipated length of stay
- Information about ongoing medical conditions, medications, and current health status (including current treatments)
- Information regarding environmental modifications/strategies being used to balance periods of patient stimulation and rest

Sensitive
- Prognosis and long-term recovery potential
- Discussions regarding more complex medical decisions including but not limited to:
  o Withdrawal of care
  o Palliative care
  o Identifying decision-making surrogates
  o Need to pursue guardianship
  o Dealing with ethical issues that may arise during the course of care
- Discussions about long-term care planning

Instrumental needs
- Family training in:
  o Turning and positioning (if not contraindicated)
  o Trach care
  o Range of motion exercises
  o How to interact with their loved one
  o How to accurately interpret behavioral responses

Support needs
- Access to resources for:
  o Financial planning and assistance
  o Guardianship
- Long-term care planning
  o Identifying and exploring discharge options
  o Guidance regarding transition of care needs
  o Accessing federal, state, and local community-based support resources (eg, mental health provider registries, attorneys, financial consultants)
- Individual and/or group emotional support
- Strategies for caregiver wellness, coping, and self-care

(eg, a social worker) can serve as the primary point of contact for caregivers to direct questions to and can also provide support as well as assistance accessing resources to address their legal, financial, and emotional support needs. By serving as a liaison between caregivers and the care team, this team member can help build a relationship of trust and offer guidance in dealing with questions or issues that may arise during the course of treatment. Specific education and training topics to address with caregivers at this level of care are presented in **Box 4**.

Transitioning Care

Following the acute hospital stay, some persons with DoC may go on to inpatient rehabilitation settings; many are discharged straight to long-term care, whereas others may be preparing for discharge back to the community/home (see **Fig. 1**). Regardless of what setting they transition to and when, during this stage, there is an increased emphasis on instrumental and resource support needs including training to facilitate caregiver preparation, ensuring continuity of access to follow-up services over time, while also attending to the needs of caregivers themselves.

Owing to variability in the timeframe of recovery and the myriad care pathways that persons with DoC may follow, there is no one set time period nor track when it comes to transition of care in this population. Moreover, intensity of care needs is variable and can fluctuate over time, which influences care setting and the need for an individualized approach to caregiver support and transition of care planning. Before discharge from any given setting, caregivers should have ample time and opportunity to meet with the care team to discuss issues related to the patient's progress, transition, and discharge options. Planning discussions should be collaborative and address the goal of determining the best discharge setting based on the level of complexity of the patient's care needs, the family's interest in and ability to provide care at home, and access to appropriate long-term care options.[19] A successful transition of care at all levels requires clear communication and coordination across providers to maintain continuity of care (see **Box 2**).[14]

Transition to a More Intensive Care Setting: Inpatient Rehabilitation

Many persons with DoC regain consciousness throughout the course of their recovery and become able to participate with more active rehabilitation efforts. Regardless of time post-injury when this occurs, for these patients, transitioning care may mean shifting to a more intensive rehabilitation focus with specific treatment goals aimed at enhancing function and level of independence in mobility, self-care, communication, and participation. At this point, information to be shared with caregivers and health care professionals is largely centered around the patient's condition, medical and rehabilitation needs, and recommended interventions to support continuity of care and ongoing meaningful functional recovery. Specific education and training topics to address during inpatient rehabilitation are presented in **Box 4**.

Transition to a Less Intensive Care Setting: Long-Term Care or Community/Home

For those patients who remain in a prolonged DoC and do not demonstrate significant improvement in their functional status or abilities after an adequate period of assessment, transition to a less intensive setting may be appropriate.

Whether this transition occurs following a course of rehabilitation or a period of observation in another care setting, the focus is on how to provide adequate care for the longer term to maintain optimal long-term health and function as well as to promote increased quality of life for both the person with DoC and the caregiver. **Box 5** includes a comprehensive list of essential topics to address with family and professional caregivers when transitioning care.

During this stage of recovery, caregivers variably learn to accept their loved one's condition and prognosis, allowing for a shift, where the focus is on how to be a support. For those discharged to the community/home, even if some training was provided during the course of acute care or inpatient rehabilitation, the care plan should be revisited to ensure caregivers are trained in the skills needed to successfully manage the patient in a home environment. In this setting, there is less oversight and greater burden put on the caregiver who is responsible for providing daily care as well as needing to ensure that follow-up appointments are made and medical needs are properly managed. In some cases, particularly for those discharged home straight from an acute care setting, caregivers should understand how to identify behavioral

Box 5
Educational needs during transition of care

Informational needs
Practical
- Information about the patient's current level of consciousness and level of functioning
- Level of assistance required to ensure patient safety and address basic care needs, including but not limited to the number of people and hours of assistance needed for:
  ○ Bed mobility
  ○ Transfers
  ○ Grooming
  ○ Feeding
  ○ Bathing
  ○ Toileting
- Active comorbid medical conditions, current medications, and current treatments
- Current rehabilitative interventions and needs
- Information regarding nutrition and dietary status, such as:
  ○ Can the patient take any food or drink by mouth? If so, what consistency?
  ○ If peg fed, information about feeding (eg, timing/rate, how to administer medications through the tube, water flushes, and general peg care)
- Recommendations/referrals for follow-up testing and appointments with specialists (what, who, when, and where)
Sensitive
- Likelihood of further functional and cognitive recovery

Instrumental needs
- Evaluation of caregiver willingness/readiness/preparedness for home placement
- Evaluation of home accessibility for patient access (stairs, doorway/hallway measurements)
- Equipment and home modification needs
- Caregiver training in:
  ○ Turning and positioning
  ○ Bed mobility and transfers
  ○ How to interact with their loved one
  ○ How to accurately interpret their behavioral responses
  ○ Peg management and feeding
  ○ Wound care (if applicable)
  ○ Wheelchair mobility
  ○ How to use equipment and adaptive technologies (eg, Hoyer lifter, putting on braces, communication device)
  ○ Tracheostomy care management (if applicable)

Support needs
- Support services needs assessment
- Long-term care planning including but not limited to:
  ○ Information on appropriate options for long-term care placement
  ○ Connecting caregivers to local and state community-based agencies to assist with long-term financial planning and assistance, and accessing social and emotional support services

benchmarks that may signal late recovery and a potential to benefit from a referral for rehabilitation.

Although emotional support may have been offered onsite at earlier stages, identifying the emotional and social support service needs of caregivers at this point can facilitate more successful transition and subsequently long-term outcomes. DoC caregivers are at high risk of social isolation,[1,3] and there seems to be an inverse relation between social support and depressive symptoms.[2] In addition, some research suggests that a longer history of caregiving may be associated with more adverse mental and physical health outcomes.[9] Financial burden also remains an issue over the long term, as a result of the high level of care needed for these patients.[5]

Connecting caregivers to resources for financial planning and assistance can help alleviate the financial stress that is often experienced at this stage, while being referred to local and regional community-based agencies for social and emotional support is key to reducing social isolation and the level of perceived caregiver burden. Caregivers should be counseled about the importance of self-care and social support as requisite tools to prevent caregiver burnout and help combat the long-term negative health effects of caregiving.

DISCUSSION

This article stresses the negative impact of caregiving on the emotional, psychosocial, and financial well-being of DoC caregivers and the subsequent need for targeted interventions that address perceived level of burden. Evidence supports the practical value at both the individual and programmatic level of providing information, training, and support across the continuum of recovery, tailored to the specific needs of each patient and caregiver.

Published practice guidelines and minimum competency program recommendations outline the key topics to include in a caregiver education and training curriculum. Developing a structured curriculum requires careful consideration in light of the great diversity among caregivers in terms of type of support needs and readiness to receive such. Adopting an individualized approach that starts with an assessment of the caregiver in terms of strengths, history, composition, level of knowledge and information, skills and learning preferences, and emotional and social support needs can serve to decrease perceived level of burden, thus reducing the risk of burnout.

Caregivers typically want to be involved in their loved ones' care; as such, they should be viewed as a valuable resource and essential member of the interdisciplinary care team. Communication should be viewed as an ongoing process to ensure that they are involved in all phases of care planning, treatment, and decision-making. To streamline communication efforts, clinical care teams may consider identifying a point person to be responsible for coordinating educational efforts for each caregiver. This person may be a case manager, social worker, discharge planner, or other team member who can check in often to monitor the caregiver's changing needs over time. This care team member can also provide guidance in navigating the complexities of medical decision-making, accessing resources, and identifying appropriate discharge placement options.

Finally, providing comprehensive individualized education, hands-on training, and support services to caregivers may increase the likelihood of them remaining actively involved across the continuum of recovery, leading to higher rates of community discharge among medically stable persons with DoC. In turn, this may translate to lower post-discharge rehospitalization rates and potential long-term health care savings by reducing the number of long-term care facility placements.

FUTURE DIRECTIONS

A tool or questionnaire specifically designed to aid assessment of DoC caregiver support needs would be useful to target the development of individualized interventions aimed at optimizing the provision of support to meet their changing needs over time. There are currently efforts underway within the American Congress of Rehabilitation Medicine Brain Injury Special Interest Group DoC Task Force to create an easily accessible and centralized online library of resources to facilitate caregiver communication and education efforts. Exploring the use of other technologies (eg, app-based

---

Box 6
Clinical care points: summary of evidence-based recommendations for caregiver communication, education, and support

DO
- Conduct ongoing assessment of patient and caregiver support needs (eg, via formal assessment, semi-structured interview, or case conference)
- Plan for how *individualized* education, support, and training will be provided to the caregiver:
  ○ What information is needed and when?
  ○ Who will provide education?
  ○ In what context will education be provided (eg, via care plan meetings, family days, reading materials or videos)?
- Balance the type, amount and timing of information based on caregiver expressed needs and readiness at any given time
- At a minimum, educational efforts should include:
  ○ Information about DoC, the patient's level of consciousness and prognosis
  ○ Information about the patient's specific care needs and estimated length of stay
  ○ Guidance to help address ethical issues that may arise and assist caregivers with decision-making
  ○ Information on appropriate disposition sites
  ○ Assistance accessing support and resources for short- and long-term care planning (**Boxes 3–5**)
- Adopt a multimodal approach to education and training
  ○ Supplement verbal communication on key topics with more permanent materials (eg, pamphlets, booklets, videos, Websites) to support ongoing review
  ○ Provide opportunity for formal sit-down meetings as well as for more direct, informal interactions with team members
  ○ Include a combination of didactic and hands-on training
- When communicating about sensitive issues:
  ○ Have an expert experienced in a given topic area be responsible for providing education on that topic
  ○ Provide small amounts of information at a time
  ○ Use simple, direct language that is easy to understand
  ○ Repeat the message to aid the family in "hearing," processing, and accepting it
  ○ Keep message consistent

DON'T
- Use complex language, medical jargon, or euphemisms
- Force caregivers to give up hope
- Adopt a cookie cutter approach to education
- Make statements that suggest a universally poor prognosis for individuals who are in a DoC for 28 days or less
- Talk in definites or be overly confident—avoid overly negative statements and communicate prognosis with a level of confidence commensurate to time post-injury

---

platforms, online portals) can further aid in customizing and delivering content in a more cost-effective manner. This may additionally serve to account for efficiency of staff time, which may be a particular barrier to the implementation of practice guidelines and recommendations in the ICU and similar settings.

SUMMARY

Caregivers of persons with DoC experience high levels of perceived burden which is associated with adverse physical, emotional, psychosocial, and financial outcomes and is directly tied to expressed needs for information and support. Providing individualized education and training at each phase of recovery can enhance effective communication between providers and caregivers, helping to increase caregiver proficiency in managing their loved one's care while also helping to mitigate the challenges associated with perceived burden. This may subsequently increase the rate of community discharge among persons with DoC, potentially translating to a reduction in the long-term costs of care for this population.

CLINICS CARE POINT

- For a summary of evidence-based recommendations for caregiver communication, education, and support, see **Box 6**.

ACKNOWLEDGMENTS

The authors gratefully acknowledge Sydney McCage, MA (Department of Brain Injury Rehabilitation, Park Terrace Care Center, Rego Park, NY) for her assistance in performing the literature review, managing the references, and preparing the final article for publication and Rose Winder, CBIS (Department of Brain Injury Rehabilitation, Park Terrace Care Center, Rego Park, NY) for her assistance in designing the figures for the article.

DISCLOSURE

The authors certify that no party having a direct interest in the results of the research supporting this article has or will confer a benefit on us or on any organization with which we are associated.

REFERENCES

1. Giovannetti AM, Leonardi M, Pagani M, et al. Burden of caregivers of patient in Vegetative state and minimally conscious state. Acta Neurol Scand 2013;127(1):10–8.
2. Giovannetti AM, Covelli V, Sattin D, et al. Caregivers of patients with disorder of consciousness: burden, quality of life and social support. Acta Neurol Scand 2015;132(4):259–69.
3. Leonardi M, Giovannetti AM, Pagani M, et al. National Consortium Functioning And Disability In Vegetative And In Minimal Conscious State Patients. Burden and needs of 487 caregivers of patients in vegetative state and in minimally conscious state: results from a national study. Brain Inj 2012;26(10):1201–10.
4. Moretta P, Estraneo A, De Lucia L, et al. A study of the psychological distress in family caregivers of patients with prolonged disorders of consciousness during in-hospital rehabilitation. Clin Rehabil 2014;28(7):717–25.
5. Covelli V, Sattin D, Giovannetti AM, et al. Caregiver's burden in disorders of consciousness: a longitudinal study. Acta Neurol Scand 2016;134(5):352–9.
6. Pagani M, Giovannetti AM, Covelli V, et al. Caregiving for patients in vegetative and minimally conscious states: perceived burden as a mediator in caregivers' expression of needs and symptoms of depression and anxiety. J Clin Psychol Med Settings 2014;21(3):214–22.
7. van Heugten C, Visser-Meily A, Post M, et al. Care for carers of stroke patients: evidence-based clinical practice guidelines. J Rehabil Med 2006;38(3):153–8.
8. Chiambretto P, Rossi Ferrario S, Zotti AM. Patients in a persistent vegetative state: caregiver attitudes and reactions. Acta Neurol Scand 2001;104(6):364–8.

9. Pagani M, Giovannetti AM, Covelli V, et al. Physical and mental health, anxiety and depressive symptoms in caregivers of patients in vegetative state and minimally conscious state. Clin Psychol Psychother 2013;21(5):420–6.

10. Tooth L, McKenna K, Barnett A, et al. Caregiver burden, time spent caring and health status in the first 12 months following stroke. Brain Inj 2005;19(12):963–74.

11. Cameron JI, Naglie G, Silver FL, et al. Stroke family caregivers' support needs change across the care continuum: a qualitative study using the timing it right framework. Disabil Rehabil 2013;35(4):315–24.

12. Boegle K, Bassi M, Comanducci A, et al. Informal Caregivers of Patients with Disorders of Consciousness: a Qualitative Study of Communication Experiences and Information Needs with Physicians. Neuroethics 2022;15(3):24.

13. Giacino JT, Katz DI, Schiff ND, et al. Practice guideline update recommendations summary: Disorders of consciousness: Report of the Guideline Development, Dissemination, and Implementation Subcommittee of the American Academy of Neurology; the American Congress of Rehabilitation Medicine; and the National Institute on Disability, Independent Living, and Rehabilitation Research. Neurology 2018;91(10):450–60 [published correction appears in Neurology. 2019 Jul 16;93(3):135].

14. Giacino JT, Whyte J, Nakase-Richardson R, et al. Minimum Competency Recommendations for Programs That Provide Rehabilitation Services for Persons With Disorders of Consciousness: A Position Statement of the American Congress of Rehabilitation Medicine and the National Institute on Disability, Independent Living and Rehabilitation Research Traumatic Brain Injury Model Systems. Arch Phys Med Rehabil 2020;101(6):1072–89.

15. King J, O'Neill B, Ramsay P, et al. Identifying patients' support needs following critical illness: a scoping review of the qualitative literature. Crit Care 2019; 23(1):187.

16. Hammond FM, Giacino JT, Nakase Richardson R, et al. Disorders of Consciousness due to Traumatic Brain Injury: Functional Status Ten Years Post-Injury. J Neurotrauma 2019;36(7):1136–46.

17. Nakase-Richardson R, Whyte J, Giacino JT, et al. Longitudinal outcome of patients with disordered consciousness in the NIDRR TBI Model Systems Programs. J Neurotrauma 2012;29(1):59–65.

18. Katz DI, Polyak M, Coughlan D, et al. Natural history of recovery from brain injury after prolonged disorders of consciousness: outcome of patients admitted to inpatient rehabilitation with 1-4 year follow-up. Prog Brain Res 2009;177:73–88.

19. Seel RT, Douglas J, Dennison AC, et al. Specialized early treatment for persons with disorders of consciousness: program components and outcomes. Arch Phys Med Rehabil 2013;94(10):1908–23.

Disorders of Consciousness Rehabilitation

Ethical Dimensions and Epistemic Dilemmas

Michael J. Young, MD, MPhil

KEYWORDS

- Disorders of consciousness • Neuroethics • Coma • Minimally conscious state
- Brain injury • Covert consciousness • Unresponsive wakefulness syndrome

KEY POINTS

- Patients with disorders of consciousness (DoC) who survive to discharge following severe acute brain injury may face profoundly complex medical, ethical, and psychosocial challenges during their courses of recovery and rehabilitation.
- Capacity building efforts at local, national, and international levels are sorely needed to advance equitable and responsible approaches to identifying, supporting, and promoting recovery of consciousness in this vulnerable population.
- Awareness of the complex ethical, epistemic, and clinical challenges that arise in the course of rehabilitative management of patients with DoC can help prepare clinicians to optimally support patients and surrogates following the acute phase of injury through the continuum of recovery, adaptation, and rehabilitation.

Patients with disorders of consciousness (DoC) who survive to discharge following severe brain injury can face profoundly complex medical, ethical, and psychosocial challenges during their course of recovery and rehabilitation.[1–5] Although issues encountered in caring for persons with DoC during acute hospitalization have received substantial attention,[6–11] ethical challenges that may develop in subacute and chronic phases following transition to rehabilitation settings have been relatively underexplored. Shedding light on these distinctive dimensions, this article explores the landscape of ethical issues raised in the course of facilitating care for persons with DoC during rehabilitation and examines potential implications for patients, clinicians, family members, and society. These issues are explored through the lens of core principles of biomedical ethics, including those of autonomy, beneficence, nonmaleficence, and justice, with particular focus on equity challenges in DoC rehabilitation; barriers to access of novel neurotechnologies and interventions to aid in the detection, prediction, and recovery

Department of Neurology, Massachusetts General Hospital, Center for Neurotechnology and Neurorecovery, 101 Merrimac Street, Suite 310, Boston, MA 02114, USA
E-mail address: michael.young@mgh.harvard.edu

Phys Med Rehabil Clin N Am 35 (2024) 209–221
https://doi.org/10.1016/j.pmr.2023.06.016
1047-9651/24/© 2023 Elsevier Inc. All rights reserved.

of consciousness; and epistemic gaps in prevailing methods of DoC diagnosis and classification.

ACCESS TO NEUROREHABILITATIVE CARE

Consideration of the ethical dimensions of neurorehabilitation for persons with DoC begins, temporally, at the point of initial access. Despite the development of rehabilitative care standards for patients who experience DoC following brain injury,[12–14] and increasing recognition of the importance of multidisciplinary neurorehabilitation services to support DoC recovery and adaptation following acute hospitalization,[15–17] appropriate multidisciplinary rehabilitation may be inaccessible or unaffordable for many patients, especially among those in low-resource settings or who might be underinsured.[18–20] Racial, geographic, and socioeconomic disparities have also been described in access to rehabilitation following brain injury, with reduced odds of discharge to rehabilitation among minorities and those who are underinsured, as well as geographic factors.[21–24] Unequal access to appropriate neurorehabilitation services may generate concerning disparities in outcomes,[25,26] raising critical issues of justice.

The ethical requirements of justice requires that clinicians and health-care systems are designed and operationalized to maximize equitable distribution of resources (distributive justice) through a process that is fair (procedural justice), and in a manner that respects the dignity and rights of individuals (interactional/interpersonal justice).[27–31] Even in well-resourced settings, however, access to rehabilitation services to support recovery from adaptation to DoC may prove elusive. Patients may experience insurer coverage denials for admission to rehabilitation facilities if they do not meet prespecified standards or fail to demonstrate improvement over a circumscribed time window.[32–34] Rules and regulations governing rehabilitation access and coverage determination may not be sensitized to the unique needs of persons with DoC and could lead to suboptimal care for already marginalized patients.[35,36] Many of these ethical challenges were magnified during the coronavirus disease 2019 pandemic, where increased resource constraints forced difficult triage decisions often disadvantaging those with DoC.[37] In resource constrained settings, allocation of limited resources to patients with DoC may be disproportionately affected due to preconceived notions regarding moral status or utility; disability rights and opportunity-based frameworks challenge these tendencies and support increased advocacy efforts for patients with DoC during care transitions to support adequate provision of optimal rehabilitative resources.[38–40] Systematic efforts to facilitate access to rehabilitative care for patients with DoC are sorely needed, including policies to advance neurorehabilitation infrastructure development as a matter of ethics and equity.

ETHICS, EQUITY AND ACCESS TO DIAGNOSTIC, PROGNOSTIC AND THERAPEUTIC TECHNOLOGIES AND RESEARCH

Intertwined with the ethics of access to rehabilitative care following acute hospitalization are issues of disparities in access to diagnostic, prognostic and therapeutic tools to aid in the detection, prediction and recovery of consciousness following severe brain injury. Central among these challenges is access to advanced tools to clarify the level of awareness of patients with DoC who are behaviorally unresponsive (ie, behavioral coma or unresponsive wakefulness syndrome), among whom it has been estimated that approximately 15% to 20% may harbor covert awareness only detectable by advanced task-based neuroimaging, electrophysiologic, or other emerging examination techniques,[41–43] a finding which may importantly inform both diagnosis and prognosis.[44] Despite professional society guideline endorsement of advanced neuroimaging or electrophysiologic tools such as task-based functional magnetic resonance imaging (fMRI) or advanced electroencephalography (EEG) to detect covert consciousness among behaviorally unresponsive patients with DoC where uncertainty exists,[45–47] these tools or the expertise necessary to clinically deploy them may not be routinely available in the many centers.[8,39,43,48] Irregular distribution of knowledge surrounding optimal management of DoC, especially in nonspecialized centers, could also preclude routine provision of guideline-driven therapeutic strategies to aid in the recovery of consciousness and adaptation to brain injury.[49–51] Awareness of such tools and their importance in diagnosis and prognosis but inability to access them could generate moral distress among clinicians and surrogates facing difficult management decisions that might be meaningfully informed through clarification of a behaviorally unresponsive person's level of consciousness.[52] Strategies to harmonize and democratize access to guideline-driven diagnostic, prognostic, and therapeutic advances for DoC are thus sorely needed. Such strategies should optimally include advocacy efforts on the institutional, professional society, and healthcare policy levels to expand availability and access, as well as educational efforts to foster guideline dissemination and implementation. The advent of telemedicine and teleneurology services carries further promise to facilitate access to specialty DoC care within underserved areas,[53] which may be further facilitated through the development of hub-and-spoke model systems for DoC evaluation and management.[39] Recent research has also emphasized the importance of facilitating access to DoC clinical trials and research studies, which remains irregular especially within underserved regions.[54,55]

SUPPORTING AUTONOMY IN SETTINGS OF LIMINAL SELF-EXPRESSION AND REEMERGENT AGENCY

Among the core principles of biomedical ethics is respect for autonomy, which emphasizes the importance of allowing care decisions to cohere with patient's preferences, values, and goals. Honoring patient autonomy in decision-making has been conceptualized as a cornerstone of beneficent and trustworthy medical care,[56–58] and underpins prevailing approaches to informed consent and patient-centered practice.[59–62] DoC often problematize typical approaches to respecting patient autonomy, as patients with DoC characteristically cannot straightforwardly express their wishes, preferences or goals, and often have not previously articulated them through advance care planning due to the abrupt, acute, and often unexpected nature of brain injuries resulting in DoC.[63,64] As such, uncertainty about how to ensure goal-concordance in decision-making for patients with DoC is common and may weigh heavily on clinicians faced with challenging decisions regarding whether it is within patient's goals to continue life-sustaining and rehabilitative treatments or to focus care on comfort through palliative approaches. Compounding these challenges may be confusion regarding the ontological nature of persons incapable of ordinary self-expression due to disturbances in conscious awareness, and perspectival shifts in concepts of personhood occasioned in these settings.[65–68] These challenges are often magnified by prognostic uncertainty regarding the likelihood of functional recovery, and what degree of recovery might be considered acceptable to a given patient. In these contexts, surrogate decision-makers are commonly relied on to help guide goal-concordant decision-making; however, a surrogate decision-maker is not always available or willing to provide substituted judgement (as in the case of underrepresented or unrepresented patients), or may be uncertain of what the patient's wishes would be if they could express them.[69–71] In such circumstances, ethicists have defended mosaic approaches to decision-making ideally incorporating perspectives of diverse stakeholders in order to guide decisional outcomes in a manner most likely to approximate a patient's best interests in settings of uncertainty.[72–74] To the extent possible, clinicians should meticulously seek out ways to involve patients with liminal or reemergent agency following brain injury in medical decision-making, for example, by seeking assent or respecting dissent when reasonable, even when full-fledged consent may not be possible.[75,76] In support of these efforts, assistive technologies may be leveraged to engage emerging functional capacities to enable communication and facilitate societal reintegration.[77–81]

BENEFICENCE, NONMALEFICENCE, AND DISABILITY BIAS IN DISORDERS OF CONSCIOUSNESS REHABILITATION

The ethical principles of beneficence and nonmaleficence emphasize the importance of making medical decisions and designing rehabilitative care plans in a manner that maximizes patient well-being and minimizes potential harm. However, as patients with DoC often lack ordinary means of self-expression (eg, due to cognitive impairment, aphasia, and disruptions in wakefulness or awareness), it may be difficult for clinicians to fully understand the impact of individual decisions on a patients' well-being and subjective states. For example, if a patient is unable to clearly express when they are in pain or experience pleasure, understanding which rehabilitation approaches and environments are most likely to result in felt positive experiences for a patient, particularly in the short term, may prove challenging. In such circumstances, it is incumbent on clinicians to rely on objective data sources and surrogate input to craft and guide optimal approaches to rehabilitative management. With respect to analgesia and symptom control, a precautionary and proactive approach is necessary to optimally manage symptoms, potentially using complementary measures of perception,[82,83] recognizing that patients who are behaviorally unresponsive may nonetheless be covertly aware of their self and/or environment.[84–88] Accordingly, clinicians should not categorically assume that a patient who is behaviorally unresponsive or who lacks clear capacities of self-expression cannot hear or understand those around them; instead, ethical principles of beneficence, nonmaleficence, and respect for autonomy require that clinicians generally relate to and communicate with patients experiencing DoC under the default presumption that they can perceive what is occurring in their environment. Task-based and stimulus-based neuroimaging and electrophysiologic techniques carry further promise to clarify what patient's perceptual capacities might be when standard neurobehavioral assessment techniques fail to demonstrate signs of awareness. To operationalize these imperatives, the Minimum Competency Recommendations for Programs That Provide Rehabilitation Services for Persons With Disorders of Consciousness developed by the American Congress of Rehabilitation Medicine and the National Institute on Disability, Independent Living and Rehabilitation Research Traumatic Brain Injury Model Systems emphasize that: "*As patients progress through rehabilitation, validated assessment methods should be used to monitor progress across multiple outcome domains, including arousal, pain, mobility, and communication ability. Assessments should be repeated regularly to determine the rate of recovery and, as performance reaches ceiling on a particular instrument, transition to measures capable of capturing more complex functions. When behavioral responses are ambiguous or infrequent, Individualized Quantitative Behavioral Assessment can be considered to address case-specific questions in a standardized manner. The frequency of assessment depends on the nature of the problem, measurement variability, magnitude of effect, and speed of onset of the treatment being assessed. It may not be possible to determine the effectiveness of a medication in the context of slow and variable background recovery, especially when the medication has a gradual onset of action and must be slowly titrated… When bedside examination findings remain ambiguous, functional imaging (eg, single photon-emission computed tomography, positron emission tomography, functional MRI) and electrophysiological studies (eg, electroencephalography, evoked potentials, event-related potentials) may be considered to detect covert signs of consciousness revealed by specific patterns of brain activation".*[12] However, it should be recognized that the such techniques are not yet widely available, and the phenomenological significance of the results produced by these advanced techniques is not yet fully understood; for example, while consistent volitional modulation of brain activity in response to command is likely to indicate conscious awareness, it is unknown whether a patient who demonstrates passive cortical responses on fMRI or EEG to language truly understands the stimulus or whether this might be a reflexive, nonconscious response.[89,90] Further research into the determinants of quality of life and well-being of patients with DoC as well as caregivers through the rehabilitative care continuum are necessary to support evidence-based, beneficent systems of care that optimally promote patient autonomy and to preempt unintended burdens or harms.[91–95]

REVISITING GOALS OF CARE AND PROGNOSTIC UNCERTAINTY IN THE REHABILITATION SETTING

Neuroprognostication (ie, prediction of outcome) for patients with DoC is particularly challenging due to the complexity of the brain and the multifactorial influences on individual patient courses. Because no single factor can yield infallible outcome predictions in patients with DoC, responsible neuroprognostication requires a multimodal approach with consistent and transparent communication with surrogates as patient's clinical profile evolves; in discussions with surrogates, the limits of medical knowledge and elements of uncertainty should be explained. This is especially true in the acute phase following injury, where American Academy of Neurology (AAN), American Congress of Rehabilitation Medicine (ACRM), and National Institute on Disability, Independent Living, and Rehabilitation Research (NIDILRR) guidelines have emphasized as a level A recommendation that "[w]hen discussing prognosis with caregivers of patients with a DoC during the first 28 days post injury, clinicians must avoid statements that suggest these patients have a universally poor prognosis."[96] Minimum competency guidelines further emphasize that *"it may not be clinically or ethically appropriate to limit care early after injury, particularly when these limits are based on early prognostic signs. Most caregivers want treatment to continue as long as uncertainty remains. Unfortunately, by the time accurate prognostication is feasible, most patients are no longer in the care of specialists with the knowledge to assess and discuss prognosis with family members. The current system too often fosters premature termination of treatment based on overly pessimistic early predictions yet may also lead to continued aggressive care after treatment is futile".* In developing prognostic assessments and in discussions with surrogates, it is also vital to avoid conflating prognostic assessments regarding the likelihood of recovery or loss of particular functional capacities with subjective value judgements about expected quality of life because such judgments vary from patient to patient based on personal, cultural, philosophical, and other idiosyncratic factors.[3]

Multidisciplinary supports within postacute settings are necessary to facilitate revisiting goals of care decisions should a patient's trajectory not meet expectations or hopes that may have motivated decisions made earlier on in a patient's course. To support patient autonomy and promote beneficent care systems, rehabilitation teams should regularly reassess the alignment of care strategies with patients' values, preferences, and goals, in close collaboration with surrogate decision-makers. When deciding about transitions or discharge to less intensive or alternative care environments, effective communication between clinicians, patients and surrogates is crucial to ensure that support needs are met and expectations are reasonably met,[5,12] with adequate planning for appropriate follow-up, recognizing that patients with DoC are at high risk of suboptimal, "custodial" care, neglect, or loss to follow-up.[97–101] Potential cognitive biases that could unduly influence decision-making and outcomes should also be proactively acknowledged and mitigated, including the disability paradox, ambiguity aversion, and self-fulfilling prophecy.[8,102–106]

ETHICS AND EPISTEMOLOGY IN DISORDERS OF CONSCIOUSNESS NOSOLOGY AND DIAGNOSTIC CRITERIA

The nosology of DoC and their diagnostic criteria raise an underexplored set of ethical and philosophical issues requiring further ethical and clinical study. Given that current approaches to classifying and diagnosing DoC (eg, coma, vegetative state/unresponsive wakefulness syndrome, minimally conscious state and acute confusional state) rely heavily on behavioral criteria, questions have arisen concerning the accuracy of prevailing nomenclature in light of the essential disjunction between consciousness, which is an inherently subjective phenomenon, and volitional behavior, which is an outward motor manifestation of some but not all forms of mental life.[107–110] Given the possibility of dissociation between a patient's state of awareness and their motor and language capacities, some have argued that diagnostic terms, such as "minimally conscious state," "coma" or "unresponsive wakefulness syndrome," which rest on behavioral criteria for their clinical ascription, may misrepresent what a patient's level of consciousness might actually be.[107–110] For example, a patient who is fully aware but has severe motor impairment with only intermittently preserved abilities to respond to verbal commands may, by prevailing behavioral criteria, be considered to be in a "minimally conscious state," even if their level of consciousness (ie, subjective awareness and experience) is fully preserved.[111] Misleading diagnostic labels could thereby inappropriately skew how clinicians or family members communicate with and interact with patients. In light of these challenges, it is important to sensitize prevailing diagnostic labels and criteria to recent neuroscientific findings highlighting the possibility of cognitive-motor dissociation in a substantial portion of patients following brain injury,[112,113] and for rehabilitation clinicians to be forthcoming with surrogates about the limitations of prevailing clinical nomenclature and diagnostic techniques in reliably characterizing patients' levels of consciousness. Furthermore, efforts to revise diagnostic criteria and clinical nosology in a manner that incorporates findings of novel neurotechnologies including task-based, stimulus-based, and resting-state neuroimaging and electrophysiologic techniques through establishing composite reference standards is necessary to avoid misdiagnosis, and to optimize the fidelity of clinical communication and DoC research.[46]

SUMMARY

Awareness of the complex ethical, epistemic, and clinical challenges that arise in the course of rehabilitative management of patients with DoC can help to prepare clinicians to optimally support patients and surrogates following the acute phase of injury through the continuum of recovery, adaptation, and rehabilitation. Although the issues explored here are not exhaustive of the entire landscape of DoC ethics, they reflect salient and distinctive ethical dimensions and dilemmas that might be encountered by rehabilitation clinicians in caring for patients with DoC. Opportunities to advance empirical and theoretical study of the ethical, social, and philosophical issues in DoC rehabilitation should be recognized and strengthened,[114] along with efforts to educate clinicians on strategies to proactively identify and manage these issues in clinical practice. Capacity building efforts at local, national, and international levels are sorely needed to advance equitable and responsible approaches to identifying, supporting, and promoting recovery of consciousness in this vulnerable population.

CLINICS CARE POINTS

- Disorders of consciousness often problematize typical approaches to respecting patient autonomy, as patients characteristically cannot straightforwardly express their wishes, preferences or goals, and often have not previously articulated them through advance care planning due to the abrupt, acute, and often unexpected nature of brain injuries.

- To support patient autonomy and promote beneficent care systems, rehabilitation teams should regularly reassess the alignment of care strategies with patients' values, preferences, and goals, in close collaboration with surrogate decision-makers.

- Potential cognitive biases that could unduly influence decision-making and outcomes should also be proactively acknowledged and mitigated, including the disability paradox, ambiguity aversion, and self-fulfilling prophecy.

- With respect to analgesia and symptom control, a precautionary and proactive approach is necessary to optimally manage symptoms, potentially using complementary measures of perception, recognizing that patients who are behaviorally unresponsive may nonetheless be covertly aware of their self and/or environment.

- Efforts to revise diagnostic criteria and clinical nosology in a manner that incorporates findings of novel neurotechnologies including task-based, stimulus-based, and resting-state neuroimaging and electrophysiologic techniques through establishing composite reference standards is necessary to avoid misdiagnosis, and to optimize the fidelity of clinical communication.

- Avoid conflating prognostic assessments regarding the likelihood of recovery or loss of particular functional capacities with subjective value judgements about expected quality of life because such judgments vary from patient to patient based on personal, cultural, philosophical, and other idiosyncratic factors.

FUNDING/ACKNOWLEDGMENTS

M.J. Young is funded by NIH, United States BRAIN Initiative (F32MH123001) and American Academy of Neurology, United States (AAN) Palatucci Advocacy Leadership Award. The funders played no role in the preparation, review, approval, or decision to submit this article for publication.

REFERENCES

1. Fins J. Rights come to mind: brain injury, ethics, and the struggle for consciousness. Cambridge, UK: Cambridge University Press; 2015.
2. Young MJ, Bodien YG, Giacino JT, et al. The neuroethics of disorders of consciousness: a brief history of evolving ideas. Brain 2021;144(11):3291–310.

3. Young M.J. and Peterson A., Neuroethics across the disorders of consciousness care continuum. *Seminars in Neurology*, 2022, Thieme Medical Publishers, Inc., 375–392.

4. Fins JJ, Bernat JL. Ethical, palliative, and policy considerations in disorders of consciousness. Neurology 2018;91(10):471–5.

5. Fins JJ. Disorders of consciousness and disordered care: families, caregivers, and narratives of necessity. Arch Phys Med Rehabil 2013;94(10):1934–9.

6. Rohaut B, Eliseyev A, Claassen J. Uncovering consciousness in unresponsive ICU patients: technical, medical and ethical considerations. Crit Care 2019; 23:1–9.

7. Edlow BL, Fecchio M, Bodien YG, et al. Measuring consciousness in the intensive care unit. Neurocritical Care 2023;1–7.

8. Peterson A, Young MJ, Fins JJ. Ethics and the 2018 practice guideline on disorders of consciousness: a framework for responsible implementation. Neurology 2022;98(17):712–8.

9. Young MJ, Edlow BL. The quest for covert consciousness: bringing neuroethics to the bedside. Neurology 2021;96(19):893–6.

10. Edlow BL, Fins JJ. Assessment of covert consciousness in the intensive care unit: clinical and ethical considerations. J Head Trauma Rehabil 2018;33(6):424.

11. Lewis A, Claassen J, Illes J, et al. Ethics priorities of the curing coma campaign: an empirical survey. Neurocritical Care 2022;37(1):12–21.

12. Giacino JT, Whyte J, Nakase-Richardson R, et al. Minimum competency recommendations for programs that provide rehabilitation services for persons with disorders of consciousness: a position statement of the American Congress of Rehabilitation Medicine and the National Institute on Disability, Independent Living and Rehabilitation Research Traumatic Brain Injury Model Systems. Arch Phys Med Rehabil 2020;101(6):1072–89.

13. Malec JF. Guidelines for competency in providing service to patients who have disorders of consciousness are detailed, comprehensive, and need to be implemented. Arch Phys Med Rehabil 2020;101(11):2051–2.

14. Bayley M, Ponsford J, Bayley MT, et al. INCOG 2.0 guidelines for cognitive rehabilitation following traumatic brain injury: methods, overview, and principles. J Head Trauma Rehabil 2023;38(1):7–23.

15. Espinoza LF, Simko LC, Goldstein R, et al. Postacute care setting is associated with employment after burn injury. Arch Phys Med Rehabil 2019;100(11): 2015–21.

16. Lorenz LS, Doonan M. Value and cost savings from access to multi-disciplinary rehabilitation services after severe acquired brain injury. Front Public Health 2021;1855.

17. Lewis FD, Horn GJ. Comparison of TBI and CVA outcomes: durability of gains following post-hospital neurological rehabilitation. NeuroRehabilitation 2023;(Preprint):1–9.

18. Allen BC, Cummer E, Sarma AK. Traumatic brain injury in select low-and middle-income countries: a narrative review of the literature. J Neurotrauma 2023; 40(7–8):602.

19. Prasad GL, Anmol N, Menon GR. Outcome of traumatic brain injury in the elderly population: a tertiary center experience in a developing country. World neurosurgery 2018;111:e228–34.

20. Foster M, Tilse C. Referral to rehabilitation following traumatic brain injury: a model for understanding inequities in access. Soc Sci Med 2003;56(10):2201–10.

21. Asemota AO, George BP, Cumpsty-Fowler CJ, et al. Race and insurance disparities in discharge to rehabilitation for patients with traumatic brain injury. J Neurotrauma 2013;30(24):2057–65.
22. Odonkor CA, Esparza R, Flores LE, et al. Disparities in health care for black patients in physical medicine and rehabilitation in the United States: a narrative review. PM&R 2021;13(2):180–203.
23. Schnakers C, Liu K, Rosario E. Sociodemographic, geographic and clinical factors associated with functional outcome and discharge location in US inpatient rehabilitation settings. Brain Inj 2022;36(2):251–7.
24. Cnossen MC, Lingsma HF, Tenovuo O, et al. Rehabilitation after traumatic brain injury: a survey in 70 European neurotrauma centres participating in the CENTER-TBI study. J Rehabil Med 2017;49(5):395–401.
25. McQuistion K, Zens T, Jung HS, et al. Insurance status and race affect treatment and outcome of traumatic brain injury. J Surg Res 2016;205(2):261–71.
26. Lequerica AH, Sander AM, Pappadis MR, et al. The association between payer source and traumatic brain injury rehabilitation outcomes: a TBI Model Systems study. J Head Trauma Rehabil 2023;38(1):E10–7.
27. Summers J, Morrison E. Principles of healthcare ethics. Health care ethics. 2nd ed. Sudbury: Jones and Bartlett Publishers; 2009. p. 41–58.
28. Daniels N. Justice and justification: reflective equilibrium in theory and practice. Cambridge, UK: Cambridge University Press; 1996.
29. Abbasi M, Majdzadeh R, Zali A, et al. The evolution of public health ethics frameworks: systematic review of moral values and norms in public health policy. Med Healthc Philos 2018;21:387–402.
30. Daniels N. Just health: meeting health needs fairly. Cambridge, UK: Cambridge University Press; 2007.
31. Wright RW. Principles of justice. Notre Dame Law Rev 1999;75:1859.
32. Fins JJ, Wright MS, Kraft C, et al. Whither the "improvement standard"? Coverage for severe brain injury after Jimmo v. Sebelius. J Law Med Ethics 2016;44(1):182–93.
33. Wright MS, Varsava N, Ramirez J, et al. Severe brain injury, disability, and the law: achieving justice for a marginalized population. Fla St UL Rev 2017;45:313.
34. Ezer T, Wright MS, Fins JJ. The neglect of persons with severe brain injury in the United States: an international human rights analysis. Health and human rights 2020;22(1):265.
35. Meixner C, O'Donoghue CR. Access to care for persons with brain injury: ethical frameworks to promote health systems change. J Head Trauma Rehabil 2021;36(1):72–7.
36. Fins JJ. When no one notices: Disorders of consciousness and the chronic vegetative state. Hastings Cent Rep 2019;49(4):14–7.
37. Fins JJ. Disorders of consciousness, disability rights and triage during the COVID-19 pandemic: even the best of intentions can lead to bias. The Journal of Philosophy of Disability 2021;. https://www.pdcnet.org/jpd/content/jpd_2021_0999_8_17_4.
38. Peterson A, Aas S, Wasserman D. What justifies the allocation of health care resources to patients with disorders of consciousness? AJOB neuroscience 2021;12(2–3):127–39.
39. Young MJ, Edlow BL. Emerging consciousness at a clinical crossroads. AJOB neuroscience 2021;12(2–3):148–50.

40. Giacino JT, Bodien YG, Zuckerman D, et al. Empiricism and rights justify the allocation of health care resources to persons with disorders of consciousness. AJOB neuroscience 2021;12(2–3):169–71.

41. Edlow BL. Covert consciousness: searching for volitional brain activity in the unresponsive. Curr Biol 2018;28(23):R1345–8.

42. Edlow BL, Claassen J, Schiff ND, et al. Recovery from disorders of consciousness: mechanisms, prognosis and emerging therapies. Nat Rev Neurol 2021; 17(3):135–56.

43. Diserens K, Meyer IA, Jöhr J, et al. A focus on subtle signs and motor behavior to unveil awareness in unresponsive brain-impaired patients: the importance of being clinical. Neurology 2023;100(24):1144–50.

44. Egbebike J, Shen Q, Doyle K, et al. Cognitive-motor dissociation and time to functional recovery in patients with acute brain injury in the USA: a prospective observational cohort study. Lancet Neurol 2022;21(8):704–13.

45. Giacino JT, Katz DI, Schiff ND, et al. Practice guideline update recommendations summary: disorders of consciousness: report of the guideline development, dissemination, and implementation subcommittee of the American academy of neurology; the American congress of rehabilitation medicine; and the national institute on disability, independent living, and rehabilitation research. Arch Phys Med Rehabil 2018;99(9):1699–709.

46. Kondziella D, Bender A, Diserens K, et al. European academy of neurology guideline on the diagnosis of coma and other disorders of consciousness. Eur J Neurol 2020;27(5):741–56.

47. Comanducci A, Boly M, Claassen J, et al. Clinical and advanced neurophysiology in the prognostic and diagnostic evaluation of disorders of consciousness: review of an IFCN-endorsed expert group. Clin Neurophysiol 2020; 131(11):2736–65.

48. Young MJ, Bodien YG, Freeman HJ, et al. Toward uniform insurer coverage for functional MRI following severe brain injury. J Head Trauma Rehabil 2023;10: 1097.

49. Lewis A. International variability in the diagnosis and management of disorders of consciousness. Presse Med 2023;52(2):104162.

50. Mainali S, Aiyagari V, Alexander S, et al. Proceedings of the second curing coma campaign NIH symposium: challenging the future of research for coma and disorders of consciousness. Neurocritical Care 2022;37(1):326–50.

51. Maas AI, Menon DK, Manley GT, et al. Traumatic brain injury: progress and challenges in prevention, clinical care, and research. Lancet Neurol 2022;21(11): 1004–60.

52. Howe EG. Fourteen important concepts regarding moral distress. J Clin Ethics 2017;28(1):3–14.

53. Young M.J., Neuroethics in the era of teleneurology. Seminars in neurology, 2022, Thieme Medical Publishers, Inc..

54. Young MJ, Bodien YG, Edlow BL. Ethical considerations in clinical trials for disorders of consciousness. Brain Sci 2022;12(2):211.

55. Lewis A, Young MJ, Rohaut B, et al. Ethics along the continuum of research involving persons with disorders of consciousness. Neurocritical Care 2023;1–13.

56. Stirrat GM, Gill R. Autonomy in medical ethics after O'Neill. J Med Ethics 2005; 31(3):127–30.

57. O'neill O. Autonomy and trust in bioethics. Cambridge, UK: Cambridge University Press; 2002.

58. Sim J. Respect for autonomy: issues in neurological rehabilitation. Clin Rehabil 1998;12(1):3–10.
59. Stoljar N. Informed consent and relational conceptions of autonomy. J Med Philos 2011;36(4):375–84.
60. Archard D. Informed consent: autonomy and self-ownership. J Appl Philos 2008;25(1):19–34.
61. Ursin LØ. Personal autonomy and informed consent. Med Healthc Philos 2009; 12:17–24.
62. Beauchamp T.L., Autonomy and consent. In: Miller F., Wertheimer A., eds. *The ethics of consent: theory and practice.* Oxford University Press, 2010. Oxford, UK 2010:55-78.
63. Young MJ. Compassionate care for the unconscious and incapacitated. Am J Bioeth 2020;20(2):55–7.
64. Berger JT. Marginally represented patients and the moral authority of surrogates. Am J Bioeth 2020;20(2):44–8.
65. Bird-David N, Israeli T. A moment dead, a moment alive: how a situational personhood emerges in the vegetative state in an Israeli hospital unit. Am Anthropol 2010;112(1):54–65.
66. Kitzinger CC, Kitzinger J. his in-between: How families talk about death in relation to severe brain injury and disorders of consciousness: interdisciplinary perspectives, The Social Construction of Death, 2014. https://www.ncbi.nlm.nih.gov/books/NBK252967/.
67. Zulato E, Montali L, Bauer MW. Understanding a liminal condition: comparing emerging representations of the "vegetative state". Eur J Soc Psychol 2021; 51(6):936–50.
68. Zulato E, Montali L, Quagliarella C. "Is There anyone in there?": caregivers and professionals' mutual positioning to take care of vegetative state patients. Interculturality in Institutions: Symbols, Practices and Identities: Springer 2022;141–60.
69. Pope TM. Unbefriended and unrepresented: better medical decision making for incapacitated patients without healthcare surrogates. Ga St UL Rev 2016; 33:923.
70. Pope TM. Making medical decisions for patients without surrogates. N Engl J Med 2013;369(21):1976–8.
71. Courtwright A, Rubin E. Who should decide for the unrepresented? Bioethics 2016;30(3):173–80.
72. Fins JJ. Mosaic decisionmaking and reemergent agency after severe brain injury. Camb Q Healthc Ethics 2018;27(1):163–74.
73. Mukherjee D. Looking ahead: traumatic brain injury, ethics, and discharge planning. J Head Trauma Rehabil 2022;37(2):125–9.
74. Wright MS, Kraft C, Ulrich MR, et al. Disorders of consciousness, agency, and health care decision making: lessons from a developmental model. AJOB Neuroscience 2018;9(1):56–64.
75. Johnson-Greene D. Informed consent issues in traumatic brain injury research: current status of capacity assessment and recommendations for safeguards. J Head Trauma Rehabil 2010;25(2):145–50.
76. van Wijk RP, van Dijck JT, Timmers M, et al. Informed consent procedures in patients with an acute inability to provide informed consent: Policy and practice in the CENTER-TBI study. J Crit Care 2020;59:6–15.
77. Pignat J-M, Jöhr J, Diserens K. From disorders of consciousness to early neurorehabilitation using assistive technologies in patients with severe brain damage. Curr Opin Neurol 2015;28(6):587–94.

78. Young M.J., Lin D.J. and Hochberg L.R., Brain–Computer interfaces in neurore-covery and neurorehabilitation. *Seminars in neurology*, 2021, Thieme Medical Publishers, Inc., 206–216.
79. Young M.J., Brain-computer interfaces and the philosophy of action, J AJOB Neuroscience, 2020, Taylor & Francis, 4–6.
80. Luauté J, Morlet D, Mattout J. BCI in patients with disorders of consciousness: clinical perspectives. Annals of Physical and Rehabilitation Medicine 2015; 58(1):29–34.
81. Pan J, Xie Q, Qin P, et al. Prognosis for patients with cognitive motor dissociation identified by brain-computer interface. Brain 2020;143(4):1177–89.
82. Chatelle C, Thibaut A, Whyte J, et al. Pain issues in disorders of consciousness. Brain Inj 2014;28(9):1202–8.
83. Zasler ND, Formisano R, Aloisi M. Pain in persons with disorders of consciousness. Brain Sci 2022;12(3):300.
84. Graham M, Owen AM, Çipi K, et al. Minimizing the harm of accidental awareness under general anesthesia: New perspectives from patients misdiagnosed as being in a vegetative state. Anesth Analg 2018;126(3):1073–6.
85. Taylor N, Graham M, Delargy M, et al. Memory during the presumed vegetative state: Implications for patient quality of life. Camb Q Healthc Ethics 2020;29(4): 501–10.
86. Naci L. and Owen A.M., Uncovering consciousness and revealing the preservation of mental life in unresponsive brain-injured patients. *Seminars in neurology*, 2022, Thieme Medical Publishers, Inc., 299–308.
87. Morlet D, Mattout J, Fischer C, et al. Infraclinical detection of voluntary attention in coma and post-coma patients using electrophysiology. Clin Neurophysiol 2023;145:151–61.
88. Rohaut B. "DoC DoC", your attention please! Clin Neurophysiol 2023;145:106–7.
89. Edlow BL, Naccache L. Unmasking covert language processing in the intensive care unit with electroencephalography. Ann Neurol 2021;89(4):643.
90. Jain P, Conte MM, Voss HU, et al. Low-level language processing in brain-injured patients. Brain Communications 2023;5(2):fcad094.
91. Romaniello C, Simoni C, Farinelli M, et al. Emotional burden, quality of life, and coping styles in care givers of patients with disorders of consciousness living in Italy: preliminary data. Brain Impair 2016;17(3):254–64.
92. Tung J, Speechley KN, Gofton T, et al. Towards the assessment of quality of life in patients with disorders of consciousness. Qual Life Res 2020;29:1217–27.
93. Chinner A, Pauli R, Cruse D. The impact of prolonged disorders of consciousness on family caregivers' quality of life–A scoping review. Neuropsychol Rehabil 2022;32(7):1643–66.
94. Reynolds JM. The ableism of quality of life judgments in disorders of consciousness: Who bears epistemic responsibility? AJOB Neuroscience 2016;7(1):59–61.
95. Reynolds JM. The life worth living: disability, pain, and morality. Minneapolis, MN: U of Minnesota Press; 2022.
96. Giacino JT, Katz DI, Schiff ND, et al. Practice guideline update recommendations summary: disorders of consciousness: report of the guideline development, dissemination, and implementation subcommittee of the American academy of neurology; the American congress of rehabilitation medicine; and the national institute on disability, independent living, and rehabilitation research. Neurology 2018;91(10):450–60.

97. Hammond FM, Giacino JT, Nakase Richardson R, et al. Disorders of consciousness due to traumatic brain injury: functional status ten years post-injury. J Neurotrauma 2019;36(7):1136–46.

98. Hamilton JA, Ketchum JM, Hammond FM, et al. Comparison of veterans affairs and NIDILRR traumatic brain injury model systems participants with disorders of consciousness. Brain Inj 2023;37(4):282–92.

99. Fins J.J., Wright M.S. and Bagenstos S.R., Disorders of consciousness and disability law, 2020, Mayo Clinic Proceedings, Elsevier, Rochester, MN, 1732–1739.

100. Zhang B, O'Brien K, Woo J, et al. Specialized intensive inpatient rehabilitation is crucial and time-sensitive for functional recovery from disorders of consciousness. Front Neurol 2023;14:568.

101. Shapiro ZE, Golden AR, Antill GE, et al. Designing an americans with abilities act: consciousness, capabilities, and civil rights. BCL Rev 2022;63:1729.

102. Fischer D, Edlow BL, Giacino JT, et al. Neuroprognostication: a conceptual framework. Nat Rev Neurol 2022;18(7):419–27.

103. Peña-Guzmán DM, Reynolds JM. The harm of ableism: medical error and epistemic injustice. Kennedy Inst Ethics J 2019;29(3):205–42.

104. Wilkinson D. The self-fulfilling prophecy in intensive care. Theor Med Bioeth 2009;30:401–10.

105. De-Arteaga M, Elmer J. Self-fulfilling prophecies and machine learning in resuscitation science. Resuscitation 2022.

106. Lazaridis C. Withdrawal of life-sustaining treatments in perceived devastating brain injury: the key role of uncertainty. Neurocritical Care 2019;30:33–41.

107. de Jong BM. "Complete motor locked-in" and consequences for the concept of minimally conscious state. J Head Trauma Rehabil 2013;28(2):141–3.

108. Coleman D. The minimally conscious state: definition and diagnostic criteria. Neurology 2002;58(3):506–7.

109. Johnson LSM. The ethics of uncertainty: entangled ethical and epistemic risks in disorders of consciousness. Oxford, UK: Oxford University Press; 2022.

110. Hermann B, Sangaré A, Munoz-Musat E, et al. Importance, limits and caveats of the use of "disorders of consciousness" to theorize consciousness. Neuroscience of Consciousness 2021;2021(2):niab048.

111. Thibaut A, Bodien YG, Laureys S, et al. Minimally conscious state "plus": diagnostic criteria and relation to functional recovery. J Neurol 2020;267:1245–54.

112. Edlow BL, Chatelle C, Spencer CA, et al. Early detection of consciousness in patients with acute severe traumatic brain injury. Brain 2017;140(9):2399–414.

113. Arzi A, Rozenkrantz L, Gorodisky L, et al. Olfactory sniffing signals consciousness in unresponsive patients with brain injuries. Nature 2020;581(7809):428–33.

114. Young MJ, Bernat JL. Emerging subspecialties in neurology: Neuroethics: An Emerging Career Path in Neurology. Neurology 2022;98(12):505–8.

Disorders of Consciousness in Children: Assessment, Treatment, and Prognosis

Beth S. Slomine, PhD[a,b,c], Stacy J. Suskauer, MD[a,c,d],*

KEYWORDS

• Pediatric • Child • Coma • Vegetative state • Minimally conscious state

KEY POINTS

• Many children with acquired brain injury experience disorders of consciousness.
• Assessment tools studied in adults with disorders of consciousness (DoC) may require additional consideration and/or modification for use in young children.
• In light of limited data specific to evaluation and management of children with DoC, it is reasonable to apply clinical standards that have been developed in adults with DoC to children while considering developmental differences.

INTRODUCTION

Disorders of consciousness (DoC) including coma, vegetative state/unresponsive wakefulness syndrome (VS/UWS), and minimally conscious state (MCS) have been described in children. In fact, soon after the Aspen Neurobehavioral Conference workgroup published definition and diagnostic criteria for MCS,[1] Ashwal and Cranford[2] presented a case series describing the clinical and neuroimaging data for five children diagnosed with DoC following acquired brain injury and associated with neurodevelopmental disorders. Since that time, there has been a growing body of literature focusing on diagnosis, prognosis, and treatment in pediatric DoC. In this review, the authors provide an overview of the state-of-the-art literature in each of these areas.

[a] Kennedy Krieger Institute, 707 North Broadway, Balitmore, MD 21205, USA; [b] Department of Psychiatry and Behavioral Health, Johns Hopkins University School of Medicine, 600 North Wolfe Street, Baltimore, MD 21205, USA; [c] Department of Physical Medicine & Rehabilitation, Johns Hopkins University School of Medicine, 600 North Wolfe Street, Baltimore, MD 21205, USA; [d] Departments of Pediatrics, Johns Hopkins University School of Medicine, 600 North Wolfe Street, Baltimore, MD 21205, USA
* Corresponding author. 707 North Broadway, Balitmore, MD 21205.
E-mail address: suskauer@kennedykrieger.org

Phys Med Rehabil Clin N Am 35 (2024) 223–234
https://doi.org/10.1016/j.pmr.2023.06.012
1047-9651/24/© 2023 Elsevier Inc. All rights reserved.

DISCUSSION
Diagnosis

In adults, there are relatively recent guidelines developed for evaluation and management of DoC. The practice guideline recommendations developed by the American Academy of Neurology (AAN) and the American Congress of Rehabilitation Medicine (ACRM) provide 18 recommendations, only 3 of which focus on children.[3] According to the AAN/ACRM practice guidelines recommendations, neurobehavioral assessment is recommended to diagnose prolonged DoC (DoC lasting ≥28 days). Clinicians should use standardized neurobehavioral assessment measures that have adequate psychometric properties to diagnosis states of DoC. In addition, serial standardized neurobehavioral assessments should be used, and clinicians should attempt to increase arousal and treat confounding conditions before assessment. Further when there is ambiguity regarding evidence of awareness, multimodal assessment (eg, electroencephalography [EEG], fMRI) may be considered, and if there is evidence of consciousness on these functional and electrophysiological measures, frequent neurobehavioral reevaluation may be conducted to identify emerging signs of DoC.[3] Given the paucity of literature exploring tools and methods for diagnosing state of DoC in children with prolonged DoC, it is reasonable to apply the recommendations developed for adults.

The European Academy of Neurology (EAN) Scientific Panel on Coma and Chronic Disorders of Consciousness generated a guideline on the diagnosis of coma and other DoC focused exclusively on adults.[4] Although the guideline was not based on pediatric literature, such as the AAN/ACRM guideline, it is reasonable that these recommendations may also be applied to children. Like the AAN/ACRM guideline, the EAN guideline focused on the importance of thorough and repeated neurobehavioral assessment. Specific recommendations were provided related to stimuli used and measurement tools to include in a neurobehavioral assessment. A summary of the strong recommendations is provided below.

Strong recommendations included passively opening eyes of patients who do not display spontaneous eye opening, use of a mirror to diagnose visual pursuit, and the use of the Coma Recovery Scale Revised (CRS-R) to classify level of consciousness for patients in the subacute state (or later), including in the intensive care setting once sedation is stopped and when patients are in rehabilitation and long-term care facilities. Owing to ease of use and improved detection of signs of consciousness over the Glasgow Coma Scale, the Full Outline of Unresponsiveness score should be used in the intensive care setting. In addition, serial assessment was also recommended and the guideline states that classification of state of DoC should never be made based on an isolated assessment. The EAN guideline also included a strong recommendation for the use of EEG-based techniques to detect preserved consciousness. Overall, this guideline highlighted that patients should receive multimodal assessment and be given the highest level of consciousness identified by any of these three approaches (neurobehavioral assessment, EEG, and neuroimaging).[4]

Neurobehavioral assessment tools and qualitative assessment of behavioral features have been used to delineate state of DoC in children. There is a growing literature demonstrating the efficacy of several tools and methods that have also been used to diagnose VS/UWS and MCS, including MCS+ and MCS− in children. In children, several measures have been used to diagnosis DoC. Measures reported in the pediatric literature including the CRS-R,[5] Coma Near Coma Scale (CNCS),[6] Post-Acute Level of Consciousness Scale (PALOC-s),[7] Western Neurosensory Stimulation Profile (WNSSP).[8] Despite the use of standardized neurobehavioral assessment measures, reports of reliability and validity is lacking in these measures. See **Table 1** for more details about these measures.

Although the CRS-R is the gold standard tool for adults,[9] the use of the CRS-R has only been reported recently in pediatric DoC. Three studies recently came out of the Alarm Clock Clinic, described as a model hospital for children with severe brain injury, in Warsaw, Poland.[10–12] These three studies examined multimodal assessment in children ages 6 to 18 years. In all three, the CRS-R was used to delineate state of DoC based on five administrations over a 2-week period. The performance on the administration indicating the highest level of consciousness was used to determine state of DoC.

More recently, Frigerio and colleagues examined the CRS-R in children with DoC.[13] In this prospective observational study, children were assessed with both the CRS-R and the Rappaport CNCS for clinical purposes. The investigators found moderate agreement between the two scales; however, the investigators noted that the CRS-R has high motor demands and may be particularly challenging in children emerging from MCS who have significant motor impairment. These investigators recommend using multiple neurobehavioral scales to assess the full spectrum of behavior in children emerging from DoC.

The CNCS has also been described in the pediatric literature. In addition to the study described above, it was used by Pham and colleagues combined with behavioral observations to determine state of DoC.[14] More recently, the CNCS was used in combination with the Levels of Cognitive Function Assessment Scale (LOCFAS) to diagnosis state of DoC in children.[15] In that study, the investigators using both measures more accurately characterized states of DoC.

The PALOC-s[7] was recently revised.[16] The PALOC-s has been used to examine the levels of consciousness in children and young adults. When the measure was initially developed, it included eight levels of consciousness. The various levels mapped on to coma (level 1), VS (levels 2–4), MCS (levels 5–7), and consciousness (level 8). The recent revision, PALOC-sr, includes a table where these levels of consciousness are mapped onto the currently accepted DoC terminology, including MCS+, MCS−, and confusional state. The investigators recommend its use for patients from 2 years of age and older but combined with other standardized neurobehavioral assessment measures.

Diagnosing states of DoC is particularly challenging in young children given the limited range of expected developmental skills that are required for diagnosing DoC, especially language skills. Recently, a pediatric version of the CRS-R was developed (Coma Recovery Scale for Pediatrics, CRS-P).[17] The CRS-P was developed by modifying the CRS-R assessment and scoring. For example, toys were added to the stimuli, language was simplified, and some items were based on observation of spontaneous behavior rather than requiring the child to respond to commands. The measures were examined in a group of typically developing children ages 6 months to 4 years. Inter-rater reliability was strong. With modifications of stimuli, administration, and scoring, children as young as 12 months of age were able to demonstrate signs consistent with emergence from MCS (eg, functional object use). In contrast, the other marker of emergence from a Minimally Conscious State (eMCS), functional communication, was not observed in any child under 2 years of age and not observed consistently, even with the CRS-P modifications, until age 3 years.

A qualitative assessment of neurobehavioral features has also been used to categorize states of DoC in the youngest patients. In the same period that the CRS-P was being developed, another study examined behavioral features of DoC in young children with acquired brain injury who were admitted to an inpatient neurorehabilitation facility.[18] In that study, medical records were reviewed to identify behavioral features outlined in the

Table 1
Neurobehavioral assessment tools used to assess children with disorders of consciousness

Tool	Description	Developed for Children	Developed to Assess DoC Only	Designed to Diagnose Recognized States of DoC	Estimated Administration Time (Minutes)
CALS[24]	20 items to assess cognitive recovery after brain injury in children admitted to an inpatient rehabilitation setting, two items relevant to DoC are rated based on administration of another measure, typically CNCS and/or CRS-R or informal observation	Y	N	N	30
CNCS[6]	11 items assessing responses to visual, auditory, and tactile stimulation. Items are rated based on observed responses such as eye opening, postural and motor movements, yawning, and some degree of arousability on stimulation	N	Y	N	10
CRS-P*,[17]	Modifications of the CRS-R (below) to include pediatric appropriate stimuli, administration, and scoring guidelines	Y	Y	Y	15–25
CRS-R[5]	23 items that comprise six subscales addressing auditory, visual, motor, oromotor, communication, and arousal functions. CRS-R subscales are composed of hierarchically arranged items associated with brain stem, subcortical, and cortical processes.	N	Y	Y	15–25
LOCFAS[15]	10 levels of recovery after brain injury, rated based on observation. Levels I–III described as corresponding with DoC	N	N	N	10
PALOC-sr[16]	Levels of consciousness from 1 to 8 based on observations during administration of a structured examination of the patient such as the WNSSP	Y	Y	N	NA
WNSSP[8]	32 items making up six subscales including auditory comprehension, visual comprehension, visual tracking, object manipulation, arousal/attention, and tactile/olfactory	N	Y	N	45

Abbreviations: CALS, cognitive and linguistic scale; CNCS, coma near coma scale; CRS-P, coma recovery scale for pediatrics; CRS-R, coma recovery scale, revised; LOCFAS, levels of cognitive functioning assessment scale; PALOC-sr, post-acute level of consciousness scale revised; WNSSP, western neuro sensory stimulation profile.

*not validated in patients with DoC.

Aspen Neurobehavioral Conference workgroup.[1] Common features of MCS were contingent affective responding, visual fixation or tracking, automatic motor behavior, and contingent communicative intent. No children in MCS showed command following or intelligible verbalization. In addition, although all of the children diagnosed as emerged from MCS showed functional object use, only a subset of children considered emerged from MCS showed higher level language skills including command following, intelligible verbalizations, and functional communication.

Taken together, several standardized neurobehavioral assessment measures have been used with children to diagnose states of DoC, although assessment of reliability and validity is lacking. Especially in the youngest children, who have not yet developed necessary language skills to demonstrate signs of eMCS, clinicians need to rely more heavily on visual and motor responses. When visual and motor impairment is present, multimodal assessment may be beneficial.

Multimodal Assessment

Data regarding the use of multimodal assessment tools (ie, specialized functional imaging, electrophysiologic studies) in children with DoC after acquired brain injury (ABI) are very limited though recently beginning to grow. Wijnen and colleagues studied visual evoked potentials (VEPs) in children and young adults with DoC.[19] It is important to note that despite behavioral improvements in visual function over the course of recovery, no change in VEPs was identified in association with improved cognitive function, suggesting that VEPs are not meaningful for this purpose. Ishaque and colleagues described preserved resting-state functional MRI (rsfMRI) networks in a cohort of 11 children with a history of anoxic brain injury from drowning and associated spastic quadriplegia felt to masking true cognitive function.[20] A case report of an 11-year-old boy demonstrates potential benefit of rsfMRI for identifying both the existence of intact functional networks which may suggest better potential for recovery as well as the possibility of simultaneously identifying potentially treatable coexisting conditions, in this case concern for high likelihood of seizures despite no epileptiform activity on EEG.[21]

Evidence from two different research groups supports the potential for use of EEG for evaluating cognitive function in pediatric patients presenting in DoC and throughout the stages of cognitive recovery after ABI. Passive EEG assessment provides an advantage of no active demands on the child (other than tolerating the EEG equipment/positioning). Zieleniewska and colleagues demonstrated that features of EEG recordings from sleep (eg, power of sleep spindles, spectral entropy) differ in children with differing clinical states within DoC.[11] Duszyk and colleagues[10] and Kim and colleagues[22,23] have both reported on the use of auditory oddball paradigms and observed differential responses (based on EEG) to different tones; further, Kim and colleagues demonstrated an effect of cognitive state, across the spectrum of recovery, on magnitude of EEG responses.

Both of these research groups have also demonstrated the use of EEG-based techniques to identify "covert" command following in children with DoC and no evidence of command following on neurobehavioral evaluation. Dovgialo and colleagues studied patients treated at the aforementioned "Alarm Clock Clinic" and used personalized stimuli as the basis for EEG paradigms designed to evaluate command following and reported that 2/7 children in UWS and 3/9 children in MCS− showed command following based on EEG.[12] More recently, using an expanded battery of EEG paradigms in addition to motor imagery and spatial navigation fMRI paradigms, Kim and colleagues reported the identification of cognitive-motor dissociation in two adolescents (ages 15 and 18 years old) based on physiologic evidence; one presented clinically in MCS− and the other in VS/UWS.[22,23]

Prognosis

According to the AAN/ACRM guideline, the natural history of pediatric DoC is not well-defined, and clinicians should counsel families of children in DoC that there are no evaluations that can improve prognosis. Although the literature is scant, there is emerging evidence that specific factors can be used to help prognosticate when children experience prolonged DoC. Factors that are emerging to be important include initial state of DoC on entrance into rehabilitation and etiology.

Several studies suggest that early signs of responsiveness are associated with subsequent emergence from MCS. Most of these studies have focused on children with TBI; however, there is some evidence in children with a range of etiologies. Pham and colleagues found that in a group of children in DoC after TBI, initial CNCS score was associated with emergence from MCS.[14] In addition, higher admission score on the responsiveness item of the Cognitive and Linguistic Scale (CALS)[24] was also associated with emergence from MCS. The CALS responsiveness item is a rating based on behavioral observation of the consistency of responsiveness throughout a 30-minute neurobehavioral assessment. More recently, when examined very long-term outcome in survivors of pediatric DoC following TBI, 68% of those who were admitted to inpatient neurorehabilitation in VS emerged from MCS, whereas all of those in MCS at admission emerged from MCS.[25] Similarly, in a cohort of the youngest children admitted to one inpatient neurorehabilitation facility after ABI, none of the patients admitted in VS emerged from MCS, whereas a third of those in MCS emerged before discharge.[26] In a mixed sample PALOC-s scores at admission and discharge to a specialized neurorehabilitation program predicted long-term disability.[27]

There is also evidence to suggest etiology of DoC is associated with outcome with better outcome noted after traumatic brain injuries relative to anoxic brain injuries. The larger studies that compared children with traumatic and anoxic brain injuries, however, are several decades old. In 1993, in a cohort of 60 children who were "unconscious" for 90 days and admitted to an inpatient rehabilitation unit, none of the 13 children with anoxic injury regained cognitive or motor skills, although three were described as socially responsive. In contrast, of the 36 children with TBI, 27 regained consciousness and displayed functional cognitive skills.[28] Kriel and colleagues compared outcomes in 127 children and adolescents who were reported to be in a "persistent vegetative state" for at least 30 days following either traumatic or hypoxic brain injury.[29] At 3-month post-injury 34% of the traumatic brain injury (TBI) group and 13% of the hypoxic group regained consciousness, and by 19-month post-injury 84% of traumatic group and 55% the hypoxic group regained consciousness. Of note, the definition of regaining consciousness is similar to what we think of as MCS today. Specifically, in that study, regaining consciousness was defined as at least one recognizable and reproducible behavior, including turning eyes and head to sound. More recently, in a study of 10 to 12 year follow-up of children and young adults admitted to inpatient rehabilitation in DoC, of the 23 surviving patients with follow-up data, 18/20 of those with TBI emerged from MCS, whereas of the three with other etiologies, one emerged, one remained in MCS, and one remained in VS. In addition, of those who died, most (7/11, 64%) had etiologies other than traumatic.[30]

Treatment

The AAN/ACRM guideline states that there are no established therapies for children with a prolonged DoC.[3] In adults, guideline recommendations for treatment include systematically facilitating prevention, early identification, and treatment of medical complications common in the first few months; treating suspected pain; and prescribing amantadine for patients with traumatic etiology of injury within 4 to 16 weeks post-injury.[3] Similar to considerations regarding assessment, in the absence of pediatric-specific evidence, these recommendations should be considered in the care of children with DoC.

Inpatient rehabilitation programs for children with DoC[31,32] facilitate repeated neurobehavioral assessment, caregiver education, and the systematic treatment approach to prevention and treatment highlighted by the Guideline.[3] Comprehensive treatment for children with DoC encompasses environmental modifications to optimize arousal and responsiveness, therapy-based interventions, and pharmacologic management. Emerging data suggest that other types of brain stimulation also merit additional evaluation.

Environmental modifications are used to facilitate return of normal circadian rhythm to facilitate daytime arousal and nighttime sleep to aid with optimal assessment and engagement in therapeutic activities during the day as well as to improve ease of care in the home setting.[31] Environmental recommendations often include upright positioning and use of light to stimulate daytime arousal along with a bedtime routine and good sleep hygiene to facilitate nighttime sleep.[32] Therapy sessions may need to incorporate a daytime rest/nap time; for very young children, more than one naptime may be needed.

Structured preference assessments are designed to identify stimuli which are arousing and/or calming and can be used to facilitate optimal engagement in therapeutic activities. Amari and colleagues published a caregiver interview called the Preference Assessment for Youth with Disorders of Consciousness which is an adaptation of the Reinforcer Assessment for Individuals with Severe Disabilities.[33] In this work, the investigators demonstrated the utility of a standardized evaluation methodology for identifying highly idiosyncratic stimuli that elicit often subtle behavioral signs of responsiveness and how identified preferred items are used in varying ways as part of a treatment program. Music has been identified as a particularly important stimulus for consideration in treatment of children with DoC; music is both salient and familiar to children, and there is evidence that music activates and fosters interactions between regions of the brain involved in cognition and affective processing.[34]

Therapy (eg, physical, occupational, speech) interventions for children with DoC include improving arousal and awareness and laying the foundation for additional recovery of function through rebuilding fundamental motor skills such as head control and treating and/or preventing complications such as joint contracture.[31,32] Given that well-fitted wheelchairs and other positioning devices intentionally restrict active movement, Yeh and colleagues highlighted the importance of therapy activities out of the wheelchair (eg, positioned with therapist support on a mat table or using body weight support devices).[32] Some children seem to respond best to more challenging activities, and providing support for standing and/or gait may elicit motor responses.[32]

Pharmacologic intervention in children with DoC comprises most of the literature related to treatment in this population; however, all of the pediatric-specific clinical trials are limited by small sample sizes.[35] Consistent with amantadine having the most data to support use in adults with DoC[3,36] amantadine has been the focus of much of the limited literature on pharmacologic intervention for children with DoC (and acquired brain injury more broadly). One hospital system reported on the use of neurostimulant medications in children with TBI severe enough to require admission to the intensive care unit; amantadine was the most frequently prescribed neurostimulant.[37] Only 1.4% of greater than 30,000 children in this broad group of children with TBI (eg, not DoC-specific) received amantadine, with a significant increase in prescription over the study years (from 2005 to 2014). Neurostimulant prescription was more common in older children and those with markers of more severe injury (injury sustained in motor vehicle collision, ICP monitoring, craniotomy/craniectomy, mechanical ventilation).[37]

Recently, McLaughlin and colleagues published retrospectively collected data on amantadine use in children with TBI across eight different inpatient rehabilitation units in the United States.[38] In this cohort, 21% of all children with TBI, and 45% of children with TBI admitted to rehabilitation in a DoC, received amantadine during the inpatient admission. The children who received amantadine were older (mean 11.6 vs 3.0 years) and had longer rehabilitation lengths of stay (mean 47 vs 31 days) than children who did not receive amantadine. Importantly, data demonstrated the use of amantadine in children as young as 1 year of age and at a wide range of weight-based dosing, including higher than that previously reported in the literature.[38] Particularly in light of a previous, small pharmacokinetic study suggesting that younger/smaller children may benefit from higher doses of amantadine,[39] the multisite data presented by McLaughlin and colleagues[38] set the stage for exploration of evaluating tolerability and efficacy of higher doses of amantadine in this population.

Levodopa/carbidopa has been described as a pharmacologic therapy for adults with DoC in case reports/case series.[40] More recently, Yeh and colleagues reported that retrospective review of clinical data from a pediatric DoC inpatient rehabilitation program yielded anecdotally higher positive response rate to levodopa/carbidopa and methylphenidate compared with other neurostimulant medications, including amantadine; however, adverse effects were also noted more frequently with these two agents compared with others.[32] Fridman and colleagues demonstrated, using PET in a small group of adults with DoC, that use of levodopa/carbidopa to restore dopamine is necessary to elicit benefit from medications that inhibit dopamine reuptake, such as amantadine and methylphenidate.[41]

The use of zolpidem has been somewhat sporadically reported in children with DoC.[32,35,42] There remain no published cases of significant behavioral recovery associated with use in a child with DoC, in contrast to the adult literature.[43] Given the safety and ease of trialing zolpidem as well as the known low rate of adult responders (suggesting that there may be pediatric responders identified as more children with DoC are exposed to zolpidem), a brief trial of zolpidem remains a reasonable option to consider for a child with DoC who is not showing rapid gains in arousal and responsiveness. Anecdotally, some caregivers of pediatric patients prefer not to proceed with a trial of zolpidem for their child due to the short window of improved function and reported habituation with ongoing administration.[44]

Noninvasive brain stimulation is emerging as an intervention for DoC with applicability for children.[42] In adults, a meta-analysis showed favorable response in adults with DoC, with increasing CRS-R scores in response to transcranial direct current stimulation (tDCS).[45] Potential benefit of tDCS has been established in other pediatric brain injury populations (ie, children with cerebral palsy).[46] Although a protocol for the study of safety and tolerability of tDCS in children with DoC has been published[47]; thus far, there is no pediatric-specific evidence for this intervention in children with DoC.

SUMMARY

As is evident from this review, much of current evaluation and care of children with DoC is based on adult practices. Although the literature surrounding assessment of children with DoC is growing, more research is needed to optimize evaluation particularly of very young children and to translate laboratory-based use of neurophysiological assessments into clinical practice. The standardization of assessment techniques will improve precision in prognostication for children with DoC and thus set the stage for improving homogeneity and/or subgroup evaluation in treatment trials to ultimately optimize outcome after pediatric DoC.

CLINICS CARE POINTS

- A number of neurobehavioral measures have been used to diagnose states of disorders of consciousness (DoC) in children; however, studies exploring the psychometric properties of these measures in children with DoC are limited.
- Early signs of responsiveness and traumatic (vs hypoxic) brain injury are variables associated with greater likelihood of emergence from minimally conscious state after pediatric DoC.
- Recent advancements in description of fMRI and EEG approaches to evaluating cognitive function in children with DoC may herald the beginning of development of clinical measures to complement neurobehavioral assessment in this population
- Growing data from clinical use of amantadine in children can be used to increase confidence in use with young children and at higher doses than were previously reported.

DISCLOSURE

Dr B. Slomine receives royalties from an edited book from Cambridge University Press. Dr S. Suskauer discloses participating in the scientific advisory board for Myomo and receiving related stock options.

REFERENCES

1. Giacino JT, Ashwal S, Childs N, et al. The minimally conscious state: Definition and diagnostic criteria. Neurology 2002;58(3). https://doi.org/10.1212/WNL.58.3.349.
2. Ashwal S, Cranford R. The minimally conscious state in children. Semin Pediatr Neurol 2002;9(1). https://doi.org/10.1053/spen.2002.30334.
3. Giacino JT, Katz DI, Schiff ND, et al. Practice guideline update recommendations summary: Disorders of consciousness. Neurology 2018;91(10). https://doi.org/10.1016/j.apmr.2018.07.001.
4. Kondziella D, Bender A, Diserens K, et al. European Academy of Neurology guideline on the diagnosis of coma and other disorders of consciousness. Eur J Neurol 2020;27(5). https://doi.org/10.1111/ene.14151.
5. Giacino JT, Kalmar K, Whyte J. The JFK Coma Recovery Scale-Revised: Measurement characteristics and diagnostic utility. Arch Phys Med Rehabil 2004;85(12). https://doi.org/10.1016/j.apmr.2004.02.033.
6. Rappaport M, Dougherty AM, Kelting DL. Evaluation of coma and vegetative states. Arch Phys Med Rehabil 1992;73(7):628–34.
7. Eilander HJ, van de Wiel M, Wijers M, et al. The reliability and validity of the PALOC-s: A Post-Acute Level of Consciousness scale for assessment of young patients with prolonged disturbed consciousness after brain injury. Neuropsychol Rehabil 2009;19(1). https://doi.org/10.1080/09602010701694822.
8. Ansell BJ, Keenan JE. The Western Neuro Sensory Stimulation Profile: A tool for assessing slow-to-recover head-injured patients. Arch Phys Med Rehabil 1989;70(2).
9. Ronald TS, Mark S, John W, et al. Assessment Scales for Disorders of Consciousness: Evidence-Based Recommendations for Clinical Practice and Research. Arch Phys Med Rehabil 2010;91(12).

10. Duszyk A, Dovgialo M, Pietrzak M, et al. Event-related potentials in the odd-ball paradigm and behavioral scales for the assessment of children and adolescents with disorders of consciousness: A proof of concept study. Clin Neuropsychol 2019;33(2). https://doi.org/10.1080/13854046.2018.1555282.

11. Zieleniewska M, Duszyk A, Rózański P, et al. Parametric Description of EEG Profiles for Assessment of Sleep Architecture in Disorders of Consciousness. Int J Neural Syst 2019;29(3). https://doi.org/10.1142/S0129065718500491.

12. Dovgialo M, Chabuda A, Duszyk A, et al. Assessment of Statistically Significant Command-Following in Pediatric Patients with Disorders of Consciousness, Based on Visual, Auditory and Tactile Event-Related Potentials. Int J Neural Syst 2019;29(3). https://doi.org/10.1142/S012906571850048X.

13. Frigerio S, Molteni E, Colombo K, et al. Neuropsychological assessment through Coma Recovery Scale-Revised and Coma/Near Coma Scale in a sample of pediatric patients with disorder of consciousness. J Neurol 2022. https://doi.org/10.1007/s00415-022-11456-6.

14. Pham K, Kramer ME, Slomine BS, et al. Emergence to the conscious state during inpatient rehabilitation after traumatic brain injury in children and young adults: A case series. J Head Trauma Rehabil 2014;29(5). https://doi.org/10.1097/HTR.0000000000000022.

15. Molteni E, Colombo K, Pastore V, et al. Joint neuropsychological assessment through coma/near coma and level of cognitive functioning assessment scales reduces negative findings in pediatric disorders of consciousness. Brain Sci 2020;10(3). https://doi.org/10.3390/brainsci10030162.

16. Eilander HJ, van Erp WS, Driessen DMF, et al. Post-Acute Level of Consciousness scale revised (PALOC-sr): adaptation of a scale for classifying the level of consciousness in patients with a prolonged disorder of consciousness. Brain Impairment; 2022. https://doi.org/10.1017/BrImp.2022.7.

17. Slomine BS, Suskauer SJ, Nicholson R, et al. Preliminary validation of the coma recovery scale for pediatrics in typically developing young children. Brain Inj 2019;33(13–14):1640–5.

18. Alvarez G, Suskauer SJ, Slomine B. Clinical Features of Disorders of Consciousness in Young Children. Arch Phys Med Rehabil 2019;100(4):687–94.

19. Wijnen VJM, Eilander HJ, de Gelder B, et al. Visual processing during recovery from vegetative state to consciousness: Comparing behavioral indices to brain responses. Neurophysiol Clin 2014;44(5). https://doi.org/10.1016/j.neucli.2014.08.008.

20. Ishaque M, Manning JH, Woolsey MD, et al. Functional integrity in children with anoxic brain injury from drowning. Hum Brain Mapp 2017;38(10). https://doi.org/10.1002/hbm.23745.

21. Boerwinkle VL, Torrisi SJ, Foldes ST, et al. Resting-state fMRI in disorders of consciousness to facilitate early therapeutic intervention. Neurol Clin Pract 2019;9(4): e33–5.

22. Kim N, Watson W, Caliendo E, et al. Objective Neurophysiologic Markers of Cognition after Pediatric Brain Injury. Neurol Clin Pract 2022;12(5):352–64.

23. Kim N, O'Sullivan J, Olafson E, et al. Cognitive-Motor Dissociation Following Pediatric Brain Injury: What About the Children? Neurol Clin Pract 2022;12(3). https://doi.org/10.1212/CPJ.0000000000001169.

24. Slomine BS, Grasmick PH, Suskauer SJ, et al. Psychometric properties of the cognitive and linguistic scale: A follow-up study. Rehabil Psychol 2016;61(3):328–35.

25. Rodgin S, Suskauer SJ, Chen J, et al. Very Long-Term Outcomes in Children Admitted in a Disorder of Consciousness After Severe Traumatic Brain Injury. Arch Phys Med Rehabil 2021;102(8). https://doi.org/10.1016/j.apmr.2021.01.084.
26. Alvarez G, Suskauer SJ, Slomine B. Clinical Features of Disorders of Consciousness in Young Children. Arch Phys Med Rehabil 2019;100(4):687–94.
27. Eilander HJ, van Heugten CM, Wijnen VJM, et al. Course of recovery and prediction of outcome in young patients in a prolonged vegetative or minimally conscious state after severe brain injury: An exploratory study. J Pediatr Rehabil Med 2013;6(2). https://doi.org/10.3233/PRM-130241.
28. Kriel RL, Krach LE, Jones-Saete C. Outcome of children with prolonged unconsciousness and vegetative states. Pediatr Neurol 1993;9(5). https://doi.org/10.1016/0887-8994(93)90104-K.
29. Heindl UT, Laub MC. Outcome of persistent vegetative state following hypoxic or traumatic brain injury in children and adolescents. Neuropediatrics 1996;27(2). https://doi.org/10.1055/s-2007-973756.
30. Eilander HJ, Wijnen VJM, Schouten EJ, et al. Ten-to-twelve years after specialized neurorehabilitation of young patients with severe disorders of consciousness: A follow-up study. Brain Inj 2016;30(11). https://doi.org/10.3109/02699052.2016.1170881.
31. Eilander HJ, Wijnen VJM, Scheirs JGM, et al. Children and young adults in a prolonged unconscious state due to severe brain injury: Outcome after an early intensive neurorehabilitation programme. Brain Inj 2005;19(6). https://doi.org/10.1080/02699050400025299.
32. Yeh N, Slomine BS, Paasch V, et al. Rehabilitation in Children with Disorder of Consciousness. Curr Phys Med Rehabil Rep 2019;7(2):94–103.
33. Amari A, Suskauer SJ, Paasch V, et al. Conducting preference assessments for youth with disorders of consciousness during rehabilitation. Rehabil Psychol 2017;62(3). https://doi.org/10.1037/rep0000152.
34. Pool J, Magee WL. Music in the Treatment of Children and Youth with Prolonged Disorders of Consciousness. Front Psychol 2016;7. https://doi.org/10.3389/fpsyg.2016.00202.
35. Suskauer SJ, Trovato MK. Update on Pharmaceutical Intervention for Disorders of Consciousness and Agitation After Traumatic Brain Injury in Children. PM and R 2013;5(2). https://doi.org/10.1016/j.pmrj.2012.08.021.
36. Giacino JT, Whyte J, Bagiella E, et al. Placebo-Controlled Trial of Amantadine for Severe Traumatic Brain Injury. N Engl J Med 2012;366(9). https://doi.org/10.1056/nejmoa1102609.
37. Morrison A, Houtrow A, Zullo J, et al. Neurostimulant Prescribing Patterns in Children Admitted to the Intensive Care Unit after Traumatic Brain Injury. J Neurotrauma 2019;36(2). https://doi.org/10.1089/neu.2017.5575.
38. McLaughlin MJ, Caliendo E, Lowder R, et al. Prescribing Patterns of Amantadine during Pediatric Inpatient Rehabilitation after Traumatic Brain Injury: A Multicentered Retrospective Review from the Pediatric Brain Injury Consortium. J Head Trauma Rehabil 2022;37(4). https://doi.org/10.1097/HTR.0000000000000709.
39. Vargus-Adams JN, McMahon MA, Michaud LJ, et al. Pharmacokinetics of Amantadine in Children With Impaired Consciousness due to Acquired Brain Injury: Preliminary Findings Using a Sparse-sampling Technique. PM and R 2010;2(1). https://doi.org/10.1016/j.pmrj.2009.10.010.
40. Barra ME, Edlow BL, Brophy GM. Pharmacologic Therapies to Promote Recovery of Consciousness. Semin Neurol 2022;42(3):335–47. https://doi.org/10.1055/s-0042-1755271.

41. Fridman EA, Osborne JR, Mozley PD, et al. Presynaptic dopamine deficit in minimally conscious state patients following traumatic brain injury. Brain 2019;142(7). https://doi.org/10.1093/brain/awz118.

42. Irzan H, Pozzi M, Chikhladze N, et al. Emerging Treatments for Disorders of Consciousness in Paediatric Age. Brain Sci 2022;12(2). https://doi.org/10.3390/brainsci12020198.

43. Schnakers C, Monti MM. Disorders of consciousness after severe brain injury: Therapeutic options. Curr Opin Neurol 2017;30(6). https://doi.org/10.1097/WCO.0000000000000495.

44. Whyte J, Rajan R, Rosenbaum A, et al. Zolpidem and restoration of consciousness. Am J Phys Med Rehabil 2014;93(2). https://doi.org/10.1097/PHM.0000000000000069.

45. Feng Y, Zhang J, Zhou Y, et al. Noninvasive brain stimulation for patients with a disorder of consciousness: a systematic review and meta-analysis. Rev Neurosci 2020;31(8). https://doi.org/10.1515/revneuro-2020-0033.

46. Saleem GT, Crasta JE, Slomine BS, et al. Transcranial Direct Current Stimulation in Pediatric Motor Disorders: A Systematic Review and Meta-analysis. Arch Phys Med Rehabil 2019;100(4):724–38.

47. Saleem GT, Ewen JB, Crasta JE, et al. Single-arm, open-label, dose escalation phase i study to evaluate the safety and feasibility of transcranial direct current stimulation with electroencephalography biomarkers in paediatric disorders of consciousness: A study protocol. BMJ Open 2019;9(8). https://doi.org/10.1136/bmjopen-2019-029967.

Moving?

Make sure your subscription moves with you!

To notify us of your new address, find your **Clinics Account Number** (located on your mailing label above your name), and contact customer service at:

Email: journalscustomerservice-usa@elsevier.com

800-654-2452 (subscribers in the U.S. & Canada)
314-447-8871 (subscribers outside of the U.S. & Canada)

Fax number: 314-447-8029

Elsevier Health Sciences Division
Subscription Customer Service
3251 Riverport Lane
Maryland Heights, MO 63043

*To ensure uninterrupted delivery of your subscription, please notify us at least 4 weeks in advance of move.

Printed and bound by CPI Group (UK) Ltd, Croydon, CR0 4YY

03/10/2024

01040474-0010